The Emergency Room Nurse
A Complete Guide to Emergency Care

SEVENTH EDITION

Patricia Ann Bemis

Contributing Authors
Katherine Scholl, RN SANE-A CMI-3 CHS-3 DABFN FACFE
Virginia J. Duffy, PhD APRN-BC
Linda O. Lathan, RN MSN CCRN FNP-C
Cynthia D. Conklin, RN MSN
Pamela D. Miles, RN EMT-P
Albert Scott Praetorius, EMT-P
Katie Morales, RN-C BSN
Kim Bunker, RN BSN GCM
I Jeanne Heltzel, RN MSN ANP FNP ACNP CDE CEN
Amy J. Dietz, RN MSN NP-C
Debra E. King, RN CEN
Cynthia Price, RN CPAN
Perry Overton, RN BSN CCRN
Karen Ezell, BS RRT RPSGT
Jodi Bodenhamer, RN CDES

Published by Patricia Ann Bemis

Notice—the author of this work has made every effort to ensure that the therapy and drug doses are accurate and in accordance with the standards accepted at the time of the publication. The related information at the end of each chapter is intended as a planning tool for Emergency Room staff to anticipate medical care and is not intended for medical provider use when prescribing care. Readers are advised to check the product information provided by the manufacturer of each product or drug. The author accepts no liability for the acts of the reader or for injury or damage to persons or property.

ISBN: 978-0-9795950-2-8

Seventh Revised Edition

First edition published as the
Clinical Practice Guide of Emergency Care
Library of Congress #0-9678112-0-1

Photography by L. Warren Bemis, BPA

CONTENTS

"IT IS TRULY THE ER BIBLE."
Laura Gasparis Vonfrolio, RN PhD

"A STRAIGHTFORWARD REALISTIC TEAM APPROACH"
Thomas Knight, MD Emergency Medicine Physician

"A MUST FOR FIELD AND HOSPITAL PARAMEDICS"
Brian Reiselbara, NREMT BS BA, International speaker and EMS Educator

INTRODUCTION

This book is a ready reference for all ER nurses covering complaints seen in the ER in an easy to read format. During an emergency, it may be necessary to perform the steps simultaneously or out of sequence. No problem, this guide will give you a ready reference to the facts and show you how to adapt. When the ER turns into a zoo, you will have a plan and the ability to be flexible.

For example, if you are assigned a patient with abdominal pain, this book will point out the diseases associated with abdominal pain. It will even show different abdominal pain locations and review the disease processes found in that area. Only information related to abdominal pain is in the chapter making the review quick and easy. Another example is seizures; this book will quickly show you different types of seizures, the care necessary, and how to tell the difference between syncope and seizures. All the information you need regarding seizures will be at your fingertips.

All nursing actions are in an easy to read format from admission to discharge. They are the organized part of the ER chaos leading to professional practice defendable in court and improved patient care.

> The Certification of Nursing (CEN) is scenario-based, making this complaint-based book an excellent CEN review.

This book was originally published in 1999 under the title *Clinical Practice Guide of Emergency Care: The Ultimate Core Curriculum,* Library of Congress Catalog number 00-090370, ISBN 0-9678112-0-1. The AACN Certification Corp approved it for 26 nursing contact hours, category A. Hospitals in the U.S. and abroad used the book for emergency nurse internship programs and seminars to review for the CEN. Over the past twenty years, the book has been revised, updated, and often renamed. This edition is the seventh publication.

Some information is repeated throughout the book as it pertains to many different types of patients. The goal is to make the information readily available in each chapter with no need to refer to other areas in the book.

I hope you enjoy the book and find it helpful.

Patricia Ann Bemis

Retired RN CEN CCRN

ABOUT THE AUTHOR

Patricia Ann Bemis is a retired registered nurse certified in emergency nursing, critical care, and entrepreneurship. Bemis has written several books, including Self-Employed RN: Choices, Business Aspects, and Marketing Strategies; and Nurse Entrepreneurs, Tales of Nurses in Business. She also developed home-study courses on DVDs for RN self-employment, emergency nursing, forensic nursing and for the business side of legal nurse consulting. She traveled throughout the country, teaching on-site classes for hospitals to prepare nurses to sit for the emergency nursing certification exam.

Bemis was the writer and online instructor for the University of Florida's Forensic Nursing Science Certificate Program. She taught marketing for the legal nurse consulting course for the University of Central Florida and worked in the arena of legal nurse consulting as an expert witness on healthcare employment.

Bemis currently lives in the Ozark mountain region of Arkansas with her Chihuahua, Carlos, and works passionately keeping her books updated.

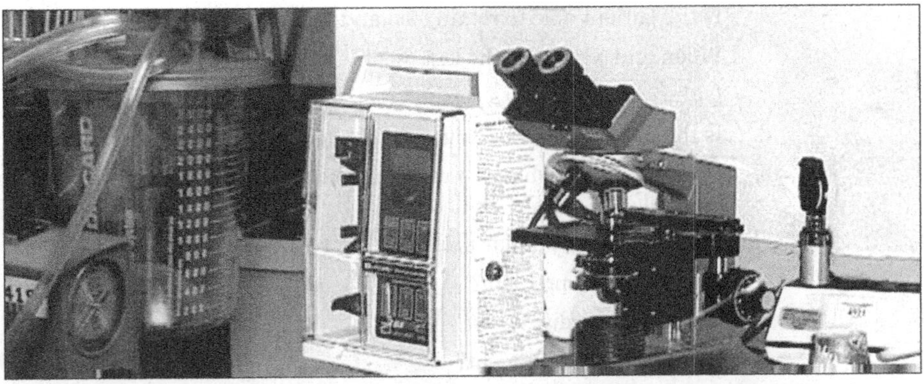

01 ABDOMINAL PAIN AND ABDOMINAL EMERGENCY

For details on triage see Chapter 34, Triage in a Nutshell.

PATIENT'S STORY – INTERVIEW QUESTIONS

Epigastric pain and indigestion are considered heart ischemia until proven otherwise in males and females over 30 years and for patients with a cardiac history. Consider using chapter #10 Chest Pain as the nature of the emergency.

1. Have you had a recent injury?
2. When did the symptoms begin?
3. Where is the pain located?
   a. Does it radiate or spread elsewhere?
   b. Are any other symptoms associated with the chief complaint; e.g., nausea; vomiting (specify when the last retained fluids were taken); diarrhea; constipation; change of stool color; and back, flank, or groin pain?
   c. What is the intensity of the pain?
   d. The pain scale commonly referred to in emergency medicine textbooks is 0 to 10.
   e. Zero to 2 being no pain ranging towards 10 as unbearable pain.
   f. The same scale must be used throughout treatment.
   g. Does anything in particular make the pain better or worse?
4. Does the patient know why the pain is present?
   a. Has the patient suffered any recent abdominal trauma?
   b. For abdominal pain associated with vomiting or diarrhea. Is ingestion of contaminated food a possibility?
5. How do the symptoms affect normal function?

a. Is the patient able to retain food and fluids?

b. When and what was the last meal?

c. Is the patient able to sleep and rest?

d. Is the patient experiencing excessive flatus?

e. Does the patient have to remain in any particular position to attain pain relief?

6. Has the patient had similar problems before?1

   a. When was the problem?

   b. What was the diagnosis?

   c. What was the treatment?

7. Was any treatment started before coming to the hospital and did it help, e.g., diet, medications?

8. Has the patient had any abdominal surgery in the past?

   a. When was the surgery?

   b. What was the surgery?

9. Does the patient have any pertinent past history?

10. Does the patient take any routine medications?

    a. What is the name, dosage, route, and frequency of each medication?

    b. When was the last dose?

11. Does the patient take any complementary or alternative therapies, herbal products, over-the-counter medications, supplements, or natural therapies?

    a. What is the name, dosage, route, and frequency of each therapy?

    b. When was the last dose or therapy?

12. Does the patient have allergies to drugs or foods?

    a. What is the name of the allergen?

    b. What was the reaction?

13. If the patient is female and between the ages of 10 to 50 years, when was the first day of her last menstrual period?

> Large majorities of females with lower abdominal pain have gynecological problems. These problems put the patient at risk for damage to the reproductive system and cause anxiety regarding sexuality.

14. Questions for females with suspected gynecology problems:

    a. Are menses normal?

    b. Is the patient sexually active and if so, is intercourse painful?

    c. Does the patient use birth control and if so, what kind?

d. Is a vaginal discharge, swelling, itching, redness, or pain present?

e. If vaginal bleeding is present, what is the estimated blood loss, e.g., how many pads are saturated in an hour/day?

f. What is the pregnancy history?

> The estimated blood loss from vaginal bleeding can be determined by the number of pads or tampons being used in a day or in an hour. One pad or tampon holds approximately 30 ml of blood. Symptoms may include positive orthostatic vital signs and subjective findings of lightheadedness, nausea, and sweating.

NURSING DOMAIN

The nursing domain, nursing diagnosis and plan of care can only be determined after an in-depth interview and consideration of the patient's story.

Domain 12. Comfort Class 1. Physical comfort.
Domain 3. Elimination and Exchange Class 1. Urinary function Class 2. Gastrointestinal function
Domain 2. Nutrition Class 5. Hydration

ANTICIPATED MEDICAL CARE

Review of the Anticipated Medical Care of Abdominal Emergencies	
Exam	Full body
Urine tests	Urine dip test or urinalysis; pregnancy test for women of reproductive age unless they have had a hysterectomy
Blood tests	CBC with differential, electrolytes, BUN, creatinine, glucose, ESR, liver function tests, lactic acid, lipase (more sensitive and specific than amylase), PT, PTT (WBC >20,000 suggests sepsis and may require rapid surgery), stool analysis and culture, pregnancy test in women of reproductive age
Radiographic studies	Abdominal bedside ultrasound, pelvic ultrasound, spiral CT (no oral contrast needed), abdominal CT (oral contrast needed), x-rays of the chest and abdomen, intravenous pyelogram (CT has replaced the use of IVP in detection of ureteral stones), CT angiography
Other tests	Pelvic exam, orthostatic vital signs, stool analysis and culture
Diet	NPO
IV	Intravenous access with large bore cannula, normal saline or Ringer's solution for fluid resuscitation

Review of the Anticipated Medical Care of Abdominal Emergencies	
Medications	Anti-inflammatory, antipyretic, antiemetic, narcotic analgesic
Management issues	The level of consciousness is the most important consideration when determining the need for a gastric tube. An unconscious patient is at high risk for aspiration.
Disposition	Hospital admission may be required if surgery is indicated or the patient is unstable.
Worst-case scenario	The worst-case scenario is an unsuspected abdominal aortic aneurysm rupture resulting in sudden circulatory collapse from loss of volume. Anticipate STAT arrangements for surgery by a vascular surgeon, type and cross for 20 units, blood replacement, and consents for both surgery and anesthesia. An older adult male with a history of diabetes, hypertension, and smoking is the most common patient type for an aneurysm.

If the patient is ambulatory and not bleeding vaginally, collect a clean-catch urine specimen before asking the patient to undress.

INITIAL CARE PLAN

Alcohol-based hand sanitizers are the preferred method for cleaning your hands in most clinical situations. Wash your hands with soap and water whenever they are visibly dirty, before eating, and after using the restroom.

1. Ask the patient to undress, remove jewelry that might interfere with the examination, and put on an exam gown. Assist as needed.

Pain control in patients with abdominal pain is a controversial subject. The traditional teaching was that giving pain medications before diagnosis was an unsafe practice and to avoid analgesics, especially narcotics, until a diagnosis was made. The newer teaching is that analgesia before diagnosis is a safe practice. Recent studies reveal that morphine sulfate effectively relieves pain in patients suffering from acute abdominal pain without altering the ability of medical providers to evaluate and treat patients. Antiemetic and nonsteroidal anti-inflammatory medications are given promptly in both schools of thought.

2. Obtain initial vital signs including pulse oximetry or test capillary refill. Consider obtaining a rectal temperature. Perform an orthostatic blood pressure and pulse rate. Positive results are a decrease in blood pressure >20 mmHg or increase in pulse > 20 beats/min.
3. Place on oxygen if saturation < 94% or capillary refill more than 2 to 3 seconds. Severe COPD patients may be unable to maintain saturation >88% to 92%.

4. Perform a focused physical exam.
   a. Auscultate the lungs.
   b. Perform a focused abdominal physical assessment. The sequence of steps in an abdominal examination is STOP and direct undivided attention to the abdomen, LOOK, LISTEN, and FEEL.
      i. LOOK: Inspect the abdomen for injury and scars of past surgeries. Ask the patient to name the surgery associated with the scars and when the surgery was done. Inspect for the following signs:
      Gray-Turner's sign, bruising of the flank, a sign of retroperitoneal bleeding.
      Cullen's sign, periumbilical bruising, a sign of intraperitoneal bleeding.
      ii. LOOK: Inspect for distention and ascites.
      iii. LISTEN: Auscultate abdominal bowel sounds.
      iv. FEEL: Percuss the abdomen.
      v. FEEL: Palpate the abdomen for tenderness. Evaluate for the following signs:
         1. Costovertebral tenderness: pain upon striking the patient with the heel of a closed fist firmly over both the costovertebral angles, a sign of renal disease.
         2. Murphy's sign: severe pain and inspiratory arrest on palpation of the right upper quadrant, a sign of cholecystitis.
         3. Obturator sign: flexion and internal rotation of the thigh at the hip causes hypogastric pain, a sign of pelvic abscess and/or appendicitis.
         4. Psoas sign: (iliopsoas test), extension and elevation of the right leg causes pain, a sign of appendicitis.
         5. Rebound tenderness: increased pain upon quick release of pressure during palpation of the abdomen, a sign of peritoneal irritation.
         6. Rovsing's Sign: palpation of the lower left quadrant results in increased pain in the lower right quadrant, a sign of appendicitis.
5. If the orthostatic test is positive, establish intravenous access with a large bore intravenous cannula. Administer a 200 ml fluid bolus of isotonic solution such as normal saline or Ringer's solution.
6. If the patient has vaginal bleeding, collect a catheterized urine specimen.

An indwelling urinary catheter is necessary to evaluate hourly urine output in the patient with shock, to obtain an obstetrical abdominal pelvic ultrasound, and for the patient with activity intolerance. The goal in treating all forms of shock is restoration of oxygenation and tissue perfusion.

7. Instruct the patient not to eat or drink and teach the patient and family the rationale for the NPO status.
8. Elevate the siderails and place the stretcher in the lowest position.
9. Inform the patient, family, and caregivers of the usual plan of care. Include time involved for each aspect of the stay and the expected overall time in the ER.
10. Provide the patient with a device to reach someone for assistance and explain how to use it. Ask the patient to call for help before getting off the stretcher.

ONGOING CARE PLAN

Inform the medical provider of adverse changes noted during ongoing evaluation. Document that the medical provider was notified of the adverse change. Document if orders were or were not received.

1. Monitor vital signs. Report negative changes to the medical provider.
2. Monitoring of hourly urine output is the most efficient method to assess for impending shock. If the patient is in shock, hourly urine output measurement is essential.

Normal urinary output in a child is 1 to 2 ml/kg per hour and normal adult urinary output is > 30 ml/hr.

3. Monitor change in bowel sounds, abdominal tenderness, and distention every hour. Determine if the symptoms are progressing towards a more severe problem that would warrant a change of treatment, e.g., from medical management to surgical intervention. Report negative changes to the medical provider.
4. Monitor therapy closely for the patient's therapeutic response.
   a. The usual time for a medication effectiveness check is 20 to 30 minutes after giving the drug.
   b. If therapy is not effective, ask the medical provider for a repeat dose or an alternative.
5. Monitor closely for the development of adverse reactions to therapy.
   a. Perform interventions to relieve the adverse reaction.
   b. Ask the medical provider for a remedy.
6. If not NPO, provide the patient with food at mealtimes and fluids during the stay.

7. Keep the patient, family, and caregivers well informed of the plan of care and the anticipated remaining time before disposition.
8. Monitor the patient's laboratory and radiographic results and notify the medical provider of critical abnormalities. Remedy abnormalities as ordered. In mesenteric ischemia, all tests may be normal including abdominal CT. There is usually a history of circulatory problems.
9. Notify the medical provider when all diagnostic results are available for review. Ask for establishment of a diagnosis and disposition.

DISCHARGE INSTRUCTIONS

1. Provide the patient with the name of the nurse and doctor in the emergency room.
2. Inform the patient of their diagnosis or why a definitive diagnosis couldn't be made. Explain what caused the problem if known.
3. Give the patient instructions on how to advance their fluid and food intake.
4. Instruct patients with irritable bowel syndrome to avoid food containing sorbitol because it can cause a gas bubble to form in the intestine and increase motility. Sorbitol is a sugar substitute and used in many diet drinks and foods. Sorbitol is made naturally in the body, yet it is poorly digested.
5. Instruct the female with a vaginal discharge to:
   a. cleanse the perineum from front to back with soap and water;
   b. wear cotton underwear;
   c. do NOT use vaginal douches;
   d. void before and after sexual intercourse;
   e. use barrier protection.
6. Instruct females with abnormal vaginal bleeding to:
   a. abstain from sexual intercourse;
   b. immediately report severe or persistent bleeding, abdominal pain on one side, fever, vomiting, or passage of tissue;
   c. return to the emergency room if there are any severe symptoms or delay in seeing the referral doctor.
7. Instruct patients with STD (sexually transmitted diseases) to:
   a. abstain from sexual intercourse;
   b. anticipate contact from the Health Department if a STD is diagnosed on culture or blood test;
   c. suggest follow up in 2 to 3 days for HIV and hepatitis testing;
   d. suggest follow up with repeat STD tests 2 weeks after completing any medication therapy.

8. Teach the patient how to take the medication as prescribed and how to manage the common side effects. Instruct the patient not to drive or perform any dangerous tasks while taking narcotic pain medications.
9. Recommend a medical provider for follow-up care. Provide the name, address, and phone number with a recommendation of when to schedule the care.
10. Instruct the patient to call the follow-up medical provider immediately or return to the emergency room if the pain or problem persists for over eight hours, worsens in any way, or any unusual symptoms develop. Encourage the patient NOT to IGNORE WORSENING OR PERSISTENT SYMPTOMS.
11. Ask for verbal confirmation or demonstration of understanding and reinforce teaching as needed.

COMMONLY ORDERED MEDICATIONS

DILAUDID

Dilaudid (hydromorphone)	
Indications	Moderate to severe pain
Dose	Typical dose 1 to 5 mg IV. Titrate to response. No maximum dose.
Onset	IV onset rapid, peak 15 to 30 minutes, duration 3 to 4 hours
Side effects	Drowsiness, dizziness, confusion, sedation, increased intracranial pressure, nausea, vomiting, urinary retention, respiratory depression
Monitor	CNS changes, respiratory effectiveness, allergic rash
Note	Dilaudid 5 mg equivalent to Morphine 10 mg IM. Dilute to 4 or 5 ml with NS or sterile water for injection and administer slowly over at least 2 to 3 min. Antidote is naloxone.

TORADOL

Toradol (ketorolac tromethamine)	
Indications	Severe acute pain that requires analgesia at the opioid level
Dose	60 mg IM, decrease to 30 mg IM in a patient >65 years of age, less than 110 pounds, or with renal impairment 30 mg IV, decrease to 15 mg IV in a patient >65 years of age, less than 110 pounds, or with renal impairment
Onset	IV onset 1 to 3 minutes, IM onset 10 minutes, peak 50 minutes, duration 4 to 6 hours
Side effects	Nephrotoxicity, dysuria, hematuria, oliguria, azotemia, blood dyscrasias

PEPCID

Pepcid (famotidine)	
Indications	Symptoms of duodenal or gastric ulcers
Adult dose	20 mg IV every 12 hours
Onset	IV onset immediate, peak 1 to 3 hours, duration 6 to 12 hours
Compatibility	Y-site compatible with dopamine, dobutamine, epinephrine, nitroglycerin, potassium chloride, sodium nitroprusside, theophylline, thiamine
Side effects	Seizure, bronchospasm

PHENERGAN

Phenergan (promethazine)	
Indications	Nausea, vomiting
Dose	12.5 to 25 mg IV every 4 to 6 hours When used intravenously, promethazine injection should be given in concentration no greater than 25 mg/ml at a rate not to exceed 25 mg/min. Preferably inject through a medication port in IV tubing that is known to be functioning satisfactorily. 25 mg IM every 6 hours
Pediatric dose	More than 2 years 0.25 to 0.5 mg/kg IM or IV every 4 to 6 hours
Onset	IV onset 3 to 5 min., duration 4 to 6 hours IM onset 20 min., duration 4 to 6 hours
Side effects	Drowsiness, sedation, hypotension, palpitations, tachycardia
Monitor	Vital signs, sedation level, respiratory effectiveness
Note	IV use can cause chemical induced phlebitis. Risk is reduced by using midline IVs, dilution with 10 cc NS, and administering slowing over 3 to 4 min.

ZOFRAN (ONDANSETRON)

Zofran (ondansetron)	
Indications	Nausea, vomiting
Dose	4 mg IV
Onset	IV onset rapid, peak 15 to 30 minutes, duration 4 to 8 hours
Side effects	Headache, drowsiness, constipation, diarrhea, extrapyramidal reactions

RELATED CONDITIONS AND INFORMATION

ABDOMINAL PAIN LOCATIONS RELATED TO POSSIBLE DIAGNOSES

RIGHT UPPER QUADRANT	LEFT UPPER QUADRANT
Duodenal ulcer Gallbladder disease Gallstones Liver disease, hepatitis Biliary colic Pancreatitis Kidney stones, right side Myocardial ischemia Pneumonia, right lung	Diverticulitis Gastric ulcers and gastritis Kidney stones, left Myocardial ischemia Pneumonia, left lung Pulmonary embolus Pericarditis Splenic rupture
RIGHT LOWER QUADRANT Appendicitis Crohn's disease Diverticulosis Ectopic pregnancy Fecal perforation Hernia Intestinal obstruction Ovarian cyst or salpingitis, right Ureteral stone, right	**LEFT LOWER QUADRANT** Early appendicitis Colon perforation Ectopic pregnancy Hernia Ovarian cyst or salpingitis, left Sigmoid perforation Sigmoid diverticulitis Ulcerative colitis Ureteral stone, left

ABORTION

Review of Abortions	
Definition	An abortion is a spontaneous or induced termination of pregnancy < 20-week-old fetus. Threatened abortion is characterized by mild to moderate uterine bleeding, uterine cramping, and a closed cervical os, and no expulsion of products of conception. Occurs in up to 15-20% of pregnancies and is the most common complication of pregnancy.
Symptoms	Symptoms may include vaginal bleeding, abdominal pain, and amenorrhea. First trimester vaginal bleeding is seen in about 25% of pregnancies and about 50% of these women will ultimately miscarry.
Tests	Tests may include serum pregnancy level, obstetrical ultrasound, pelvic examination, hemogram, type, Rh factor, and screen.

Review of Abortions	
Management	Management includes observation for hemodynamic changes and blood loss and may include fluid resuscitation with normal saline. Dilatation and curettage may be done in the emergency room for incomplete and inevitable abortions, and patients discharged home after 2 to 3 hours when stable.
Disposition	Incomplete abortions or those with uncontrolled bleeding may require surgical suction curettage or stable patients with pregnancies greater than 8 weeks gestational age by ultrasound may be managed by traditional vacuum evacuation. If RhoGAM has been ordered by the medical provider, answer any questions the patient may have, obtain consent, and administer this product to the patient prior to release from the ER.
Discharge instruction	Instructions include no douches, no intercourse, rest in bed, and notify the follow-up medical provider for increased abdominal pain, bleeding, fever, chills, or passage of tissue.

ALCOHOLIC CIRRHOSIS

Review of Alcoholic Cirrhosis	
Definition	Cirrhosis is a chronic liver disease characterized by abnormal changes in the architecture of the liver tissue, gradual loss of functioning liver cells, and increased resistance to flow of blood through the liver (portal hypertension). When disease is severe, it causes ammonia toxicity.
Causes	Causes of cirrhosis include nutritional deficiency, poisons including alcohol (20% of chronic alcoholics develop cirrhosis), and viral (B, C, D) or bacterial infections.
Symptoms	Symptoms may include anorexia, nausea, vomiting, diarrhea, fatigue, jaundice, and gastrointestinal bleeding.
Signs	A protuberant abdomen is secondary to portal hypertension. A firm and lumpy area in the right upper quadrant from scarring and nodules. Bulging flanks and a flattened, protruding umbilicus is often associated with the ascites of alcoholic cirrhosis. Spider telangiectasis, hepatosplenomegaly, ascites, esophageal varices, and hepatic encephalopathy are associated with cirrhosis.
Laboratory findings	Laboratory findings may include anemia, prolonged PT, hyponatremia, hypokalemic alkalosis, glucose disturbances, hypoalbuminemia, and elevated AST.

Review of Alcoholic Cirrhosis	
Management	Management may include: Fluid resuscitation with normal saline Treatment of symptoms such as vomiting, diarrhea, or gastrointestinal bleeding Administration of multivitamins, thiamine, folic acid Correction of potassium, magnesium, and phosphate deficiencies Transfusion of packed red blood cells and fresh frozen plasma to reverse coagulopathy. Monitoring for hypoglycemia
Disposition	Admission to the hospital may be required for abstinence, the first step and an absolute requirement for treatment success, continued daily support and work-up for liver transplantation in chronic, irreversible, and progressive liver disease.

ASCITES

Review of Ascites	
Definition	Ascites is an accumulation of fluid in the abdominal cavity.
Causes	Causes of ascites include interference with the venous return associated with cardiac disease and obstruction of the flow in the vena cava or portal vein. Cirrhosis is the underlying cause in at least 80% of patients.
Symptoms	Symptoms may include a protuberant abdomen secondary to portal hypertension. Bulging flanks and a flattened protruding umbilicus is often associated with the ascites of alcoholic cirrhosis. The accumulated fluid in the abdomen causes a shifting dullness as the patient changes position.
Management	A paracentesis is often necessary.
Disposition	Hospital admission may be required for severe ascites impeding respiratory effort.

ASPIRIN, NON-STEROIDAL ANTI-INFLAMMATORY, AND STEROIDAL MEDICATIONS

Aspirin, many other nonsteroidal anti-inflammatory medications and steroidal medications ingested may cause gastric irritation which may lead to ulcer formation and resultant perforation.

ANEURYSMS

Review of Aneurysms

Review of Aneurysms	
Definition	An aneurysm is a localized weakness of the arterial wall. Aneurysms can occur anywhere along the aorta. Eighty percent occur along the abdominal aorta. Abdominal aortic aneurysms (AAA) are attributed to atherosclerosis, smoking, diabetes, and hereditary influence. They are most common between the ages of 50 to 70 years. Aneurysms may develop in the left ventricle of the heart, cerebral arteries, and in any other central or peripheral artery.
Types of dissection	Type I is a dissection of the descending aorta to and beyond the arch. Type II is a dissection of the ascending aorta alone. Type III is a dissection from beyond the left subclavian artery.
Types of aortic aneurysms	A dissecting aneurysm is one in which the blood has made its way between the layers of the aortic walls and separated them. Commonly a result of necrosis of the medial portion of the aorta. A fusiform aneurysm is one in which all the walls of the aorta dilate equally creating a tubular effect. A saccular aneurysm is one that produces a saclike protrusion through a weak area on one side of the wall. A pseudoaneurysm is an outpouching of a blood vessel, involving a defect in the two innermost layers (tunica intima and media) with continuity of the outermost layer (adventitia) or all three layers are damaged and the bleeding is contained by a blood clot or surrounding structures.
Causes of dissection	The aneurysm in the arterial wall enlarges over the years and the weakened wall begins to stretch under the pressure of the circulating blood. A dissecting aneurysm results from a tear in the artery's inner layer. The dissecting artery can rupture causing hemorrhage, exsanguination, and death.
Symptoms	Symptoms of abdominal aneurysms may include abdominal distention, a pulsatile mass, and low back pain. Symptoms of thoracic aneurysms may include hoarseness, dysphagia, and mid-scapular back pain. Early signs of a rupture may include pallor, dyspnea, tachycardia, hypertension, and absence of pulses unilaterally. Late signs may include profound shock, syncope, and unilateral absence of major pulses.
Tests	The most common diagnostic test is a bedside portable ultrasound or a CT.

Review of Aneurysms	
Management	Medical management may include: immediate arrangement for STAT surgery; administering high flow oxygen; establishing intravenous access with two large bore intravenous cannulas; intravenous fluids of normal saline or Ringer's solution at a high flow rate; placement of a urinary catheter; surgical consents. If hypertension is present, the blood pressure may be lowered with drugs such as Nipride. The main objective of anti-hypertensive drugs is to maintain the systolic blood pressure at 100 to 120 mm Hg systolic for the first 24 to 48 hours. Hypovolemic shock is combated with fluid resuscitation, blood replacement, and surgery to repair the aorta. The goal in treating all forms of shock is restoration of oxygenation and tissue perfusion.

ANTACIDS

Antacids that contain magnesium have a laxative effect.

APPENDICITIS

Review of Appendicitis	
Description	Appendicitis is an inflammation of the vermiform appendix. All people are susceptible, but it is most common between the ages of 10 and 30 years and very rare before the second year and after the fiftieth year.
Signs and symptoms	Signs and symptoms may include a dull right lower quadrant pain with rebound at McBurney's point (just inside the iliac crest), Rovsing's sign, slightly elevated temperature, moderate elevated WBC (rarely greater than 20,000 cells/mm3), anorexia, tachycardia, nausea, and vomiting. Appendicitis should be suspected in any child over two years who has symptoms of persistent abdominal pain. Appendix rupture in younger children (over 2 years) is more apt to be misdiagnosed as gastroenteritis because they are less able to describe the character and location of the pain. They become more restless or assume a fetal position as the pain increases. Young children are more prone to infection, but do not have a higher incidence of perforation.

Review of Appendicitis	
Management	The main goal is diagnosis and hospital admission for surgical removal before rupture. Consents are needed for both surgery and anesthesia. Appendectomy is the most common reason for surgery in children. Laparoscopic surgery is preferred. A prophylactic broad-spectrum antibiotic may be administered preoperatively. Surgery is urgent and delay can lead to complications of perforation, peritonitis, or abscess formation. If the appendix ruptures, the patient may have momentary relief followed by an increase of involuntary guarding and fever.

BACK PAIN

Back Pain Location	Visceral disease
T10 to 12	Peptic ulcers and tumors of the stomach, duodenum, or pancreas
Low back pain	Ulcerative colitis, diverticulitis, PID, cancer of the ovary, uterus, or prostate
Costovertebral angle	Renal disease
Thoracic-lumbar	Aortic dissecting aneurysm
Note	Back pain referred from visceral disease reveals no stiffness and movement of the back does not increase the pain

BARTHOLIN'S GLAND

The Bartholin's gland is a small gland that secretes fluid into a duct on the labia. If the duct becomes obstructed, the gland can become infected. The labia become swollen and tender. Management may include incision, drainage, drain placement, and antibiotics.

BLOOD LOSS

	Class I	Class II	Class III	Class IV
Blood loss	Up to 750 cc	750 to 1500 cc	1500 to 2000 cc	> 2000
HR	< 100	> 100	> 120	> 140
BP	Normal	Normal	Decreased	Decreased
RR	14 to 20	20 to 30	30 to 35	> 35
Cap refill	Normal	Slight delay	From 2 to 3 seconds	No filling
Skin	Pink and cool	Pale and cold	Pale, cold, moist	Mottled
Urine	> 30 cc/hr	20 to 30 cc/hr	5 to 15 cc/hr	< 5 cc/hr
Behavior	Slight anxiety	Mild anxiety	Anxious, confused	Lethargic, confused

	Class I	Class II	Class III	Class IV
Fluid	Crystalloid	Crystalloid	Crystalloid and blood	Crystalloid and blood

BOTULISM

There are three main kinds of botulism: foodborne botulism, infant botulism, and wound botulism.

Foodborne botulism is a foodborne illness caused by eating foods that contain the botulinum toxin. Symptoms include dry mouth, difficulty swallowing, slurred speech, muscle weakness, vomiting and diarrhea, and progress to paralysis and death.

Infant botulism is caused by ingested spores of the botulinum bacteria which grow in the intestines of the infant and release toxin. Symptoms include dry mouth, difficulty swallowing, slurred speech, muscle weakness, vomiting and diarrhea, and progress to paralysis and death. This is the rarest form of botulism and affects about 100 infants a year. It is rarely diagnosed in countries other than the U.S. Fifty percent of the cases are in California. Infants less than 12 months are susceptible.

Wound botulism is caused by toxin produced from a wound infected with Clostridium *botulinum*. Symptoms progress to paralysis and death.

Intensive care nursing and a ventilator are needed for all forms of botulism for several weeks. If diagnosed early, patients can be treated with an antitoxin if it is available. Supply is extremely limited.

All forms of botulism can be fatal and are considered medical emergencies.

BOWEL OBSTRUCTION

Review of Bowel Obstruction	
Causes	The most common cause of bowel obstruction is adhesions from previous abdominal surgeries and can occur at varying ages in both males and females. When obstruction occurs, fluid accumulates above the obstruction causing distention with increased peristalsis that causes more secretions to be released and worsens the distention. Hyperactive high-pitched bowel sounds are present in both large and small bowel obstruction. The abdomen is not tender unless the bowel is ischemic.
Large bowel obstruction	Large bowel obstructions generally cause colicky cramping pain, abdominal distention, and constipation. Radiographic studies show large dilated, fluid-filled loops of bowel. Carcinoma is the primary cause in an adult. The next most common cause is diverticulitis.
Small bowel obstructions	Small bowel obstructions generally cause copious vomiting with minimal abdominal distention. The patient may be able to pass feces. Pain is often around the umbilicus.

Review of Bowel Obstruction	
Management	Management may include decompression by nasogastric tube connected to low intermittent suction, intravenous fluids, and antiemetic medications. If the problem does not resolve, surgery may be necessary. Life threatening complications include peritonitis, strangulation of the bowel, and perforation. The definitive treatment for life threatening abdominal obstruction is surgery.
Mortality Rate	Untreated severe obstruction with shock has a 70% mortality rate. The goal in treating all forms of shock is restoration of oxygenation and tissue perfusion.

CROHN'S DISEASE

Crohn's disease is a chronic disorder that causes inflammation of the intestinal tract. It can involve the tract from mouth to anus; but commonly affects the small intestine and/or colon. A related disease, ulcerative colitis, is so similar it is hard to differentiate. Both illnesses are marked by an abnormal response by the body's immune system. The main symptoms are loose, watery, and frequent bowel movements, crampy abdominal pain, fever and at times, rectal bleeding. The goal of treatment is to suppress the inflammatory response. Treatment includes hydration, pain medication, and antiemetics. Treatment may include steroids and antibiotics.

CLOSTRIDIUM DIFFICILE

Enterocolitis is caused by *Clostridium difficile*, a species of bacteria that produces a toxin. It is found in the soil and in the intestinal tract. The bacterium has been associated with antibiotic treatment and may occur four to nine days after the start of antibiotic therapy. The infection causes diarrhea and fever. Diagnosis is made by detection of the cytotoxin in the stool. Management may include replacement of fluid and a change of current antibiotic treatment.

CLOSTRIDIUM PERFRINGENS

Clostridium perfringens is a bacterium that causes an infectious process approximately eight to fourteen hours after ingestion of contaminated meat, poultry, or legumes. The infection causes diarrhea and cramping abdominal pain lasting less than twenty-four hours. Management includes fluid replacement.

CHOLECYSTITIS

Review of Cholecystitis	
Definition	Cholecystitis is an acute inflammation of a distended gallbladder usually caused by an impacted stone in the cystic duct.
Symptoms	Symptoms may include sudden or gradual onset of right upper quadrant or gastric pain, nausea, vomiting, anorexia, and fever. Jaundice is a sign of common bile duct obstruction.
Tests	Test findings may include a CBC, LFT, amylase, lipase, urinalysis, and ultrasound scan or a nuclear medicine HIDA (hepatobiliary iminodiacetic acid) scan of the abdomen.

Review of Cholecystitis	
Management	Management may include bowel rest, nasogastric suction, intravenous fluids with electrolytes, analgesia with opioids, and antibiotics. Symptoms resolve in 75% of patients. Surgery is definitive and is performed as soon as feasible. Gallstones usually cause chronic cholecystitis. Surgery is indicated if the patient has symptoms.

CHOLELITHIASIS

Cholelithiasis	
Definition	Cholelithiasis is stones in the gallbladder consisting of cholesterol or pigments such as calcium salts and bilirubin. In the United States, over 80% of the stones are cholesterol.
Symptoms	Symptoms occur when the stones cause inflammation or obstruction. The pain may be colicky in the right upper quadrant or epigastric area. It occurs thirty to ninety minutes after a fatty meal and lasts for several hours associated with nausea and vomiting. Murphy's sign is when palpation of the right upper quadrant and liver causes increased pain during inspiration and is usually a sign of cholecystitis.
Tests	Ultrasound is the best diagnostic test. Laboratory findings may include a mild elevation of the bilirubin.
Management	Management may include bowel rest, nasogastric suction, intravenous fluids with electrolytes, antiemetics, analgesia, and antibiotics for the acute inflammation. Elective laparoscopic surgery resolves the problem.

DIVERTICULITIS

Review of Diverticulitis	
Definition	Diverticulitis is an inflammation or infection of herniations or saclike protrusions of the mucosal wall at points of nutrient artery penetration. It commonly occurs in the sigmoid colon.
Causes	Cause of diverticulitis has been attributed to a low-fiber diet and intraluminal pressure.
Acute symptoms of diverticulitis	Symptoms may include left lower quadrant pain relieved by defecation, fever, colon tenderness, bloody stools, and leukocytosis.
Tests	Tests may include CT of the abdomen with oral contrast.
Management	Management may include NPO status, intravenous normal saline for fluid resuscitation, antibiotics, and hospital admission for surgical resection.

DYSFUNCTIONAL VAGINAL BLEEDING

Review of Dysfunctional Vaginal Bleeding

Review of Dysfunctional Vaginal Bleeding	
Description	Dysfunctional vaginal bleeding is vaginal bleeding not associated with a normal menses and can occur in both pregnant and non-pregnant females. Vaginal bleeding in a post-menopausal female is a sign of benign or malignant tumor.
Estimated blood loss	Blood loss can be estimated by counting the number of pads or tampons saturated in a day or an hour. A saturated peri pad or tampon holds approximately 30 ml of blood. Approximately 600 ml is 15% of circulating volume and can cause significant orthostatic hypotension.
Causes	Causes include infections, unusual exercise, injury, ovarian problems, breakthrough bleeding while on contraceptives, and endometriosis.
Management	Management is symptomatic. Some cases of bleeding will resolve without treatment and some require outpatient treatment with a course of hormones.

ECTOPIC PREGNANCY

Review of Ectopic Pregnancy	
Definition	A pregnancy is considered ectopic when the fertilized ovum implants itself outside the uterus. Common locations may include fallopian tube (93 to 97% occur in the tube), ovary, and abdominal cavity. The ovum may rupture the tube as it grows. The most common time frame for rupture is at 12 weeks gestation.
Symptoms	Symptoms may include amenorrhea, intermittent left or right lower quadrant pain, and vaginal bleeding. If the ectopic pregnancy is leaking or ruptured, Kehr's sign may be present as the blood irritates the diaphragm causing referred pain to the shoulder.
Tests	The most accurate diagnostic tests include a transvaginal ultrasound. Tests may include serum pregnancy, CBC, type and screen, and abdominal ultrasound (indwelling urinary catheter may be required in some facilities for abdominal ultrasound).
Management	Management may include intravenous access and pelvic examination. If the tube is not ruptured, Methotrexate may be given to terminate the pregnancy in conjunction with obstetrical consult and close followup. Admission and immediate surgery may be indicated if the tube has ruptured, the patient is in shock, or non-surgical methods are not available. Consents are needed for both surgery and anesthesia.

EPIDIDYMITIS

Review of Epididymitis	
Definition	Epididymitis is an inflammation of the epididymis that constitutes the first part of the excretory duct of each testis.
Causes	The major cause of epididymitis in heterosexual men is *Chlamydia trachomatis.*
Symptoms	Symptoms may include unilateral scrotal pain, fever, epididymal tenderness, and swelling.
Tests	Tests may include CBC, urinalysis and culture, urethral swab culture, and scrotal ultrasound to rule out testicular torsion.
Management	Medical management is prescription of antibiotics, bedrest, scrotal support, ice packs, and analgesics and/or anti-inflammatories.

ERYTHROMYCIN

Erythromycin can cause drug induced inflammatory colitis with bloody stools.

ESOPHAGEAL VARICES

Esophageal varices are dilated tortuous veins in the submucosal lining of the lower esophagus. The varices may extend throughout the esophagus and into the stomach. The cause is commonly portal hypertension resulting from obstruction of the portal venous circulation or cirrhosis from excessive alcohol ingestion.

GASTROENTERITIS

Review of Gastroenteritis	
Definition	Gastroenteritis is an inflammation of the stomach caused by a virus, bacteria, parasite, or chemical agent.
Symptoms	Symptoms may include nausea, vomiting, diarrhea, abdominal cramps, hyperactive bowel sounds, and occasionally fever. Persistent vomiting for 6 to 8 hours is the usual course for viral gastritis.
Management	Management may include symptomatic relief with antiemetics, analgesia, fluid replacement, and treatment of the underlying cause.

GYNECOLOGY PROBLEMS

Gynecology problems commonly seen in the ER include ovarian cysts, Bartholin's cyst, dysfunctional vaginal bleeding, and sexually transmitted diseases such as pelvic inflammatory disease (PID), genital herpes, and gonorrhea. Primary syphilis saw resurgence in the 1990s.

HEMORRHOIDS

Hemorrhoids are dilated, tortuous veins on the exterior or interior of the anorectum. Symptoms include pain. Management depends on the severity. Minor hemorrhoids are treated with anal hygiene and ointments. Major varicosities are surgically removed. A strangulated external hemorrhoid is a varicosity entrapped by the anal sphincter with no blood supply. The vein must be reduced from its entrapment and blood flow restored to avoid death of the tissue.

HEPATITIS

Review of Acute Hepatitis	
Definition	Acute hepatitis is an infection of the liver caused by a hepatotropic virus (A, B, C, D, E) and other viruses.
Symptoms	Symptoms may include nausea, vomiting, diarrhea, malaise, low-grade fever, dark urine, clay-colored stools, jaundice, and a tender liver.
Cause	A: Fecal to oral transmission B: Percutaneous (needle stick), sexual, perinatal transmission C: Percutaneous transmission (Intravenous drug use accounts for over 50% of the reported cases.) D: Intravenous transmission (IV drug users and transfusions) Endemic among HBV (hepatitis B virus) carriers in the Mediterranean bases and areas of South America. E: Waterborne transmission (epidemic in India, Africa, and Mexico)
Management	Management may include symptomatic treatment, fluid resuscitation with normal saline, and hospital admission or outpatient follow-up care.
Outcome	A: Recovery within 6 to 12 months with occasional relapses B: Recovery in > 90% of the cases C: Incubation period 7 to 8 weeks, course clinically mild, > 50% likelihood of chronicity, leading to cirrhosis in 20% of the cases D: Progresses to chronic hepatitis E: May need a liver transplant

HERNIA

A hernia is a protrusion of an organ or part of an organ through the wall of the cavity that normally contains it. The more common hernias are umbilical, femoral, and inguinal. The intestine becomes trapped outside the abdominal cavity through a natural opening that has failed to close normally, deteriorated with age, injury, or been weakened by surgical procedures. The intestine can be felt in the sac and bowel sounds heard if the bowel contents are still flowing. If the intestine is strangulated, blood flow is stopped, and bowel contents cannot flow through the strangulated intestine. The herniated intestine must be immediately returned to the abdominal cavity by pushing it through the opening (reducing) or by surgically replacing it inside the cavity. If the bowel is infarcted, the infarcted (dead) areas are removed at surgery. Consents must be obtained for both surgery and anesthesia.

JEJUNUM AND ILEUM

The jejunum and the ileum are not common sites of ulcers.

KEHR'S SIGN

Kehr's sign is pain referred from the epigastrium to the right shoulder, a phenomenon associated with biliary colic or acute cholecystitis. A ruptured spleen can also cause Kehr's sign when the diaphragm is irritated by blood in the peritoneal cavity.

KIDNEY STONES

Review of Kidney Stones	
Definition	Kidney stones are stones anywhere in the urinary tract.
Symptoms	Symptoms may include severe pain (constant, migrating, or colicky) and hematuria.
Tests	Tests may include CBC, urinalysis, KUB x-ray, and dual energy CT to assess for kidney stones or soft tissue urate crystals.
Management	Management may include large amounts of intravenous fluids (regardless of the location of the stone) and control of pain and nausea. All urine must be strained. Any obtained stones should be sent for analysis. Demerol is the narcotic agent of choice; morphine is thought to causes spasms in the ureter that intensifies the pain.
Treatment	Treatment is determined by the location of the stone, the degree of obstruction, and the presence of infection or impaired kidney function. Surgical removal of the stone by cystoscopy might be necessary for an obstructing stone that does not migrate. Lithotripsy is often an alternative to surgery. Consents for surgery and anesthesia must be obtained. Kidney stones are common in 1% of the population and recurrent 50% to 80% of the time.

OVARIAN CANCER

Review of Ovarian Cancer	
Definition	Cancer of the ovaries
Symptoms	Called the silent killer. Most women experience abdominal pressure bloating or discomfort, nausea, indigestion or gas, feeling full even after a light meal, urinary frequency, constipation or diarrhea, abnormal vaginal bleeding, unexplained fatigue or shortness of breath, pain during intercourse, or unexplained weight loss or gain.
Tests	Pelvic examination, pelvic ultrasound, CA125 is elevated in 80% of the cases.
Management	Admission for complete evaluation and intervention.

PROLAPSE

A prolapse is a falling or dropping down of an organ or internal part, commonly the uterus or rectum. Medical management may involve putting the organ back into its normal cavity to protect the mucous membrane and recommend the use of a pessary. Surgical correction may be needed for chronic prolapse.

PROSTATITIS

Review of Prostatitis	
Definition	Prostatitis is an inflammation of the prostate gland.
Causes	Prostatitis is usually caused by gram-negative urinary pathogens.
Tests	Diagnosis is by urine culture.
Management	Management may include intravenous antibiotics, oral antibiotics, and referral to a medical provider for follow-up.

PAIN SEVERITY

The severity of the pain is not related to the seriousness of the problem.

Review of Pain Associated with the Abdomen	
Dull pain	Dull pain is commonly associated with inflammation and low-grade infection.
Intermittent pain	Intermittent pain is commonly associated with gastroenteritis and small bowel obstruction.
Severe pain	Severe pain controlled by medication is commonly associated with pancreatitis, peritonitis, small bowel obstruction, renal colic, and biliary colic. Severe pain not controlled by medications is commonly associated with infarction or rupture.

PANCREATITIS

Review of Pancreatitis	
Definition	Pancreatitis is an inflamed condition of the pancreas that can be acute or chronic.
Cause	In the United States, the most common cause of pancreatitis is alcohol intake. The second most common is cholelithiasis. A perforated duodenal ulcer that erodes through the pancreatic wall and into the pancreas can progress to pancreatitis. Heredity is not a causal factor.

Review of Pancreatitis	
Symptoms	Symptoms may include sudden, intense, steady, boring pain in the epigastrium radiating to the back, often increasing in the supine position. Associated symptoms may include nausea, vomiting, low-grade fever, tachycardia, hypotension, basilar crackles, abdominal tenderness, rigidity, and diminished bowel sounds. A palpable upper abdominal mass is often present. Cullen's sign (blue discoloration about the umbilicus due to hemoperitoneum) and Turner's sign (discoloration of the flanks due to tissue catabolism of hemoglobin) are often present in acute hemorrhagic pancreatitis, a form of pancreatitis that causes hemorrhage into the pancreatic tissue.
Diagnostic findings	The amylase and lipase are elevated. In acute pancreatitis, amylase is often elevated more than three times normal within a few hours of onset and remains elevated for three days. After twenty-four hours, serum lipase levels rise and remain elevated for ten days. In chronic pancreatitis, levels are often normal. CT confirms the diagnosis. Ultrasound often does not visualize the pancreas because of overlying gas but may detect gallstones.
Management	Management may include analgesics and intravenous fluids. Demerol is used for pain associated with pancreatitis because traditionally it is believed that it does not cause spasms of the sphincter of Oddi like other narcotics. No studies are readily available to substantiate that tradition. Antibiotics are rarely used except when infection has been established.
Complications	Acute respiratory distress syndrome may result from acute pancreatitis or the associated sepsis and hypovolemia. The pancreatic exudates are thought to destroy the surfactant. Hypokalemia and hyperglycemia are common complications of pancreatitis. Approximately 90% of the cases subside after three to seven days.
Discharge Instructions	Home instructions include a low-fat, no-alcohol, and no-caffeine diet. Limiting fat intake and avoiding alcohol helps prevent stimulation of the pancreas. No caffeine prevents stimulation of gastric acid that activates the pancreas.

PELVIC INFLAMMATORY DISEASE

Pelvic inflammatory disease (PID)	
Definition	PID is an acute or chronic infection of the fallopian tubes and surrounding tissue.
Symptoms	Symptoms may include moderate to severe pain in the lower abdomen. Fever, abnormal vaginal discharge, and vaginal bleeding may be present.

Pelvic inflammatory disease (PID)	
Risk Factors	PID risk factors include an intrauterine device for birth control, recent abortion, and multiple sex partners.
Tests	Tests may include cervical culture for *Gonorrhea*, *Chlamydia*, and *Gardnerella*.
Management	Management includes pain control, antibiotics, and teaching.

PERFORATED GASTRIC ULCERS

Perforated gastric ulcers often cause abdominal pain radiating to the neck. Gastric ulcers comprise only 20% of the total ulcer perforations. The referred pain is caused by irritation of the diaphragm and phrenic nerves. Other symptoms may include absent bowel sounds, hypotension, tachycardia, anxiety, and respiratory difficulty.

PERITONITIS

Peritonitis is an inflammation of the peritoneal and visceral surfaces of the abdominal cavity. It is usually caused by leakage of gastric or intestinal content after a perforation of the stomach or intestine. The pain of peritonitis is caused by the peritoneum's primary response to injury, edema, and bowel hypermotility.

ROTAVIRUS VACCINE

The RotaTeq® vaccine is an oral vaccine administered in three doses, at 2, 4, and 6 months of age.

The Rotarix® vaccine is an oral vaccine administered to infants at 2 and 4 months of age.

The vaccinated babies are much less likely to have diarrhea. The rotavirus vaccines may be given at the same time as other childhood vaccines.

ROVSING'S SIGN

Rovsing's sign is an increase in right lower quadrant pain initiated by palpation of the left lower quadrant. It is suggestive of acute appendicitis.

STAPHYLOCOCCUS AUREUS

Staphylococcus aureus is a bacterium that causes an infectious process associated with diarrhea. The bacterium most commonly appears in confections, meat, and milk. Onset of symptoms is one to six hours post ingestion. Duration of the process is often ten hours or more. Management includes treatment of symptoms and fluid replacement.

SALMONELLA

Salmonella causes an inflammatory process with nausea, watery diarrhea, and fever. The bacterium most commonly appears in poultry, eggs, and meat. Onset of symptoms is six to forty-eight hours post ingestion.

SHIGELLA

Shigella infection develops from human fecal contamination and causes a watery bloody diarrhea with mucus and fever. Onset is one to seven days post ingestion. Diagnosis is made from a finding of fecal leukocytes in the stool and stool cultures. The fever lasts three to four days. The diarrhea lasts for one to two weeks. Management includes treatment of symptoms, fluid replacement, and antibiotics.

SPICY FOOD

Spicy food, alcohol, and tobacco are sometimes linked to esophageal carcinoma.

SEXUALLY TRANSMITTED INFECTIONS

GENITAL HERPES

Review of Genital herpes	
Definition and cause	Genital herpes is caused by a virus that lives in the nerve cells that supply feeling to the skin and reactivates itself to cause painful blisters for one to three days followed by slow healing with scabs on the genital and rectal areas. The problem recurs at random intervals and is sometimes related to stress. Infection of a sexual partner may occur at any time but is more likely when sores are present. Condoms may help decrease the spread of the infection but are not 100% effective. There is no cure.
Management	Management in the ER may include pelvic examination, cervical culture, and diagnosis.
Treatment	Outpatient instruction includes keeping the area clean with soap and water three to four times a day to reduce the risk of a secondary bacterial infection. A prescription antiviral cream such as acyclovir may help.

GONORRHEA

Review of Gonorrhea	
Definition	Gonorrhea is a specific, contagious, inflammation of the genital mucous membrane of either sex.
Cause	The cause of gonorrhea is unprotected sex with a partner infected with the bacteria *Neisseria gonorrhea.*
Locations	Infection can be located on the pharynx, vagina, penis, anal canal, and secondarily in the eyes.
Symptoms	Symptoms begin one week after infection. Males may present with a mucopurulent discharge and dysuria. Females may have mild symptoms such as vaginal discharge, lower abdominal discomfort, and abnormal menses. The mild symptoms in females are often overlooked.

Review of Gonorrhea	
Management	Some gonococcal strains may be resistant to penicillins, tetracyclines, spectinomycin, and fluoroquinolones. Resistance to ciprofloxacin and ofloxacin exceeds 40% in some Asian countries. CDC guidelines recommend treatment may include a dual therapy with a cephalosporin plus either azithromycin or doxycycline. The patient should be instructed to abstain from sex until the treatment is completed. Untreated gonorrhea can lead to systemic involvement.
Prevention	Prevention and control of sexual transmitted disease require: • education of those at risk; • detection of infected individuals; • effective diagnosis and treatment; • evaluation, treatment, and counseling of sex partners of persons who have an STD; • changing the sexual behaviors that place people at risk.
Tests	Diagnosis is by cervical culture.
Note	Gonorrhea is the second most frequently reported communicable disease in the United States, an estimated 820,000 new cases each year. Most states have laws that allow minors of any age to consent to birth control counseling and the treatment of sexually transmitted disease such as gonorrhea.

SYPHILIS

Syphilis is a sexually transmitted disease that has seen a recent resurgence. It is confirmed by a blood test and treated with antibiotics.

TESTICULAR TORSION

Review of Testicular Torsion	
Definition	Testicular torsion is a twisting of the testicle within the scrotum often causing an obstruction of the blood supply to the testicle.
Symptoms	Symptoms of testicular torsion may include unilateral scrotal pain, tenderness, and swelling.
Tests	Tests may include ultrasound.
Management	Management may include EMERGENT surgical repair to restore blood supply to the testicle.

PEDIATRIC CONSIDERATIONS RELATED TO ABDOMINAL PAIN

Pediatric Considerations
Appendicitis is the most common major surgical disease in school age children and most frequently occurs between the ages of 10 and 12 years of age.
Celiac disease is a congenital autoimmune disorder characterized by an inability to tolerate and absorb gluten resulting in damage to the lining of the small intestine. It becomes apparent when gluten foods are introduced into the diet of children between the ages of 6 and 18 months. Symptoms include diarrhea, steatorrhea, signs of malnutrition and failure to thrive.
Hirschsprung's disease is a congenital disorder and is defined by the absence of parasympathetic ganglion cells in a segment of the large intestine. This results in a dilation of the colon and obstruction.
Intussusception is a telescoping of the intestines into itself. It is seen from 6 months to three years of age and most commonly seen in males and children with cystic fibrosis. This may be fatal if treatment is delayed more than 24 hours. Children with suspected intussusception may present with grunting, sweating, screaming, and drawing their knees to their chest; parents may report red currant jelly like stools.
Rotavirus Vaccine vaccinated babes are much less likely to have diarrhea. Rotarix® is a live, monovalent, human attenuated vaccine given in 2 doses (one course) at 2 and 4 months of age. RotaTeq® is a live, pentavalent, human–bovine reassortant vaccine given in 3 doses (one course) at 2, 4 and 6 months of age.
Volvulus is torsion of the intestine 180° around itself. This results in vascular compromise to the intestines, ischemia and necrosis. The child may present with distended abdomen, bilious vomiting, and severe abdominal pain and absent bowel sounds. Parents may report bloody stool.
Pyloric stenosis (bowel obstruction) occurs in infants and is commonly seen at age 2 to 10 weeks. The incidence in the U.S. is 2 to 4 per 1000 live births. 30% of the infants are first-born males.

PAIN IN CHILDREN

To avoid a procedure, children may not admit to pain.

SEXUALLY TRANSMITTED DISEASES IN CHILDREN UNDER 12 YEARS OF AGE

Children with suspected STDs should be considered in abuse cases and reported according to area statutes.

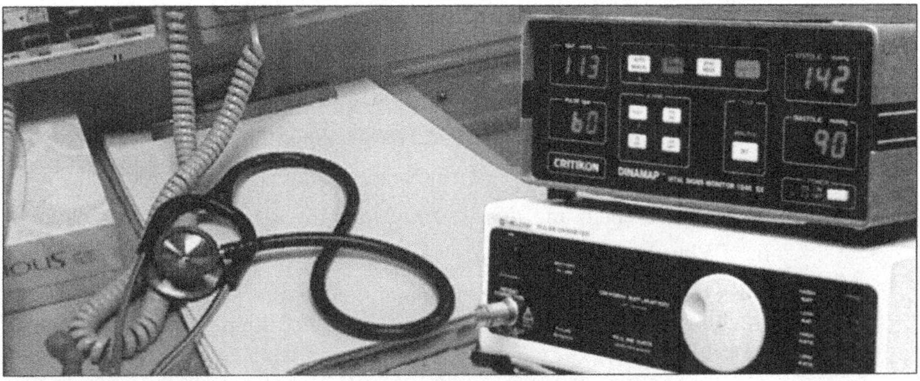

02 ALLERGIC REACTIONS AND STINGS

For details on triage see Chapter 34, Triage in a Nutshell.

PATIENT'S STORY – INTERVIEW QUESTIONS

1. Have you had a recent injury?
   a. When did the symptoms begin?
   b. If the symptoms are no longer active, how long did they last?
   c. If the symptoms were intermittent, how long did each episode last and how frequent were they?
2. Where is the sting or allergic reaction?

> Localized redness, swelling, and tenderness are a normal reaction to a sting.

   a. What is the appearance of the area?
   b. Are any other symptoms associated with the chief complaint, e.g., nausea, vomiting, difficulty swallowing, hoarseness, shortness of breath, swelling the lips or tongue, lightheadedness?
3. Is the cause known?
   a. Did the patient ingest or encounter a known allergen, e.g., eating shellfish, peanuts, or MSG?
   b. Has the patient recently ingested or been exposed to a new medication or potential allergen?
   c. Was the patient stung or bitten by an insect, spider, or marine animal?
4. How do the symptoms affect normal function?
   a. Is any itching or pain present?
   b. Is the patient able to rest or sleep?
5. Has the patient ever had similar reactions in the past?

   a. What was the diagnosis?
   b. What was the treatment?
   c. Has any treatment been initiated, and has it helped?
6. What is the pertinent medical and surgical history?
7. Does the patient take any routine medications?
   a. What is the name, dosage, route, and frequency of each medication?
   b. When was the last dose?
8. Does the patient take any complementary or alternative therapies, herbal products, over-the-counter medications or supplements, or natural therapies?
   a. What is the name, dosage, route and frequency of each therapy?
   b. When was the last dose or therapy?
9. Does the patient have allergies to drugs or foods?
   a. What is the name of the allergen?
   b. What was the reaction?
10. When was the patient's last tetanus immunization?
11. If the patient is female and between the ages of 10 to 50 years, when was the first day of her last menstrual period?

NURSING DOMAIN

The nursing domain, nursing diagnosis and plan of care can only be determined after an in-depth interview and consideration of the patient's story.

Domain 12. Comfort. Class 1. Physical comfort.
Domain 11. Safety/Protection Class 5. Defensive processes.

ANTICIPATED MEDICAL CARE

Review of the Anticipated Medical Care of Allergic Reactions and Stings	
Medical provider exam	Systemic reactions require a full body exam. Local reactions require examination of the involved area.
Tests	A pregnancy test may be ordered for women of reproductive age unless they have had a hysterectomy
Diet	NPO
Fluids	Normal saline or Ringer's solution
Medications	Epinephrine, Benadryl, Zantac, steroids
Disposition	Hospital admission may be required if the symptoms do not resolve.

Review of the Anticipated Medical Care of Allergic Reactions and Stings	
Worst case scenario	The worst-case scenario is sudden anaphylaxis with a compromised airway and hypotension. Management may include providing supplemental oxygen and administering epinephrine IV or SC, Benadryl IV or IM, and steroids IV or PO. Epinephrine can cause cardiac ischemia in an elderly patient. Cardiac and blood pressure monitoring are essential. Endotracheal intubation with rapid sequence anesthesia induction or tracheotomy may be necessary to restore the patent's airway.

INITIAL CARE PLAN

Alcohol-based hand sanitizers are the preferred method for cleaning your hands in most clinical situations. Wash your hands with soap and water whenever they are visibly dirty, before eating, and after using the restroom.

Breathing difficulty (oxygen saturation < 94 or capillary refill < 2 seconds), hoarseness, swelling of the tongue or lips, or lightheadedness (hypotension) can be signs of developing anaphylaxis. Stay with the patient and summon help. Place the patient in high Fowler's position to optimize breathing efforts. Establish intravenous access. Perform ongoing evaluations by continuous heart monitor, automatic blood pressure cuff every 15 minutes (or perform manually), and pulse oximetry. Obtain an order for an antihistamine or epinephrine and administer. Carefully look at the mg/ml dose of the epinephrine to avoid giving the incorrect amount. Use epinephrine 0.3 to 0.5 mg (1:10,000 for IV route and 1:1,000 for IM route). Pediatric dose is epinephrine 0.01 mg/kg SC or IV.

1. Ask the patient to undress, take off jewelry that might interfere with the exam, and put on an exam gown. Assist as needed.
2. Perform a focused physical examination.
   a. Inspect the skin for rash, hives, or edema.
   b. Auscultate the lungs.
   c. Evaluate the level of consciousness based on the mnemonic **AVPU** or **ACDU** level of consciousness score.
   AVPU: **A**lert, **V**erbal, **P**ain, **U**nresponsive.
   ACDU: **A**lert, **C**onfused, **D**rowsy, **U**nresponsive.
3. Instruct the patient not to eat or drink. Teach the rationale for the NPO status.
4. If appropriate, circle the identified injury site.
5. Start therapy for local reaction at injury site.
6. Administer medications covered by hospital protocol, e.g., tetanus toxoid.

ALL patients who have received ANY type of bite should receive a tetanus toxoid booster if their last booster was over ten years ago. The purpose for the toxoid is to update their immunization status, not to prevent tetanus.

7. Instruct the patient to call for assistance immediately if breathing difficulty, hoarseness, swelling of the tongue or lips, or lightheadedness develops.
8. Provide the patient with a device to reach someone for assistance and explain how to use it. Ask the patient to call for help before getting off the stretcher.
9. Elevate the bedside rails and place the stretcher in the lowest position.
10. Inform the patient, family, and caregivers of the usual plan of care. Include time involved for each aspect of the stay and the expected overall time in the ER.

ONGOING CARE PLAN

Inform the medical provider of adverse changes noted during ongoing evaluation. Document that the medical provider was notified of the adverse change. Document if orders were or were not received.

1. Monitor vital signs and effectiveness of breathing. Frequency of monitoring is every 15 minutes for patients with allergic reactions until stability is determined.
2.
3. Monitor the patient's physical status.
4. Auscultate the lungs
5. Inspect the skin for rash, hives, or edema.
6. Evaluate the level of consciousness based on the mnemonic **AVPU** or **ACDU** level of consciousness score.
   AVPU: **A**lert, **V**erbal, **P**ain, **U**nresponsive.
   ACDU: **A**lert, **C**onfused, **D**rowsy, **U**nresponsive.
7. Provide fluids to liquefy secretions. Antihistamines cause dryness of the mucous membranes and thicken secretions.
8. Monitor therapy closely for the patient's therapeutic response.
   a. The usual time for a medication effectiveness check is 20 to 30 minutes after giving the drug.
   b. If the therapy is not effective, ask the medical provider for a repeat dose or an alternative.
9. Monitor closely for the development of adverse reactions to therapy.
   a. Perform interventions to relieve the adverse reaction.
   b. Ask the medical provider for a remedy.
10. If appropriate, provide the patient with food at mealtimes.

11. Keep the patient, family, and caregivers well informed of the plan of care and the remaining time anticipated before disposition.
12. Monitor the patient's laboratory and radiographic results and notify the medical provider of critical abnormalities. Remedy abnormalities as ordered.
13. Notify the medical provider when all symptoms have abated, and patient has been observed for one hour. Ask for disposition.

DISCHARGE INSTRUCTIONS

1. Provide the patient with the name of the nurse and doctor in the emergency room.
2. Inform the patient of their diagnosis or why a definitive diagnosis couldn't be made. Explain what caused the problem if known.
3. Instruct the patient with an allergic response to insect bites to wear protective clothing when working or playing outdoors to reduce the risk of bites. Check the protective clothing before each use to reduce the risk of infestations.
4. Instruct the patient who suffered an insect-related allergic reaction to wear a medical alert indicating the allergy, to carry an anaphylaxis kit, and to avoid perfumed sprays and brightly colored clothing that attract insects.
5. The patient may have serum sickness from several days to several weeks post administration of antiserum (human or animal serum containing antibodies that are specific to one or more antigens). Symptoms may include fever, enlarged lymph nodes and spleen, skin rash, and painful joints. If symptoms occur, medical treatment is needed.
6. Instruct the patient to treat a rash with cool baths and to avoid scratching. Calamine lotion and Benadryl can be helpful. Use as directed.
7. Instruct the patient of the need to continue medication(s) as prescribed by the medical provider due to possible toxin remaining in their system for up to 24 hours post injury and recurring symptoms.
8. Antihistamines cause drowsiness. Do not use antihistamines when driving, operating dangerous machinery, when drinking alcohol, or when pregnant.
9. Teach the patient how to take the medication as prescribed. Teach the common side effects or adverse effects common to the medications and what to do if any of these occur.
10. Recommend a medical provider for follow-up care. Provide the name, address, and phone number with a recommendation of when to schedule the care.
11. Instruct the patient to watch for worsening symptoms like severe swelling or wheezing. Return to the emergency room if any of these symptoms arise. Otherwise, follow-up with the medical provider as recommended. DO NOT IGNORE WORSENING SYMPTOMS.

12. Ask for verbal confirmation or demonstration of understanding and reinforce teaching as needed.

COMMONLY ORDERED MEDICATIONS

EPINEPHRINE IN SEVERE ALLERGIC REACTIONS

Epinephrine	
Indications	Severe allergic reactions, bronchospasm, anaphylaxis
Dose	The route of the epinephrine administration depends on the severity of the symptoms. 0.2 to 0.5 mg SC or IM every 10 to 15 min. not to exceed 5 mg
Pediatric dose	0.01 mg/kg SC or IM every 15 min. times 2 doses, then every 4 hours up to a maximum of 0.5 mg
Onset	SC onset 5 to 15 min., IM onset variable, duration 1 to 4 hours
Side effects	Tremors, anxiety, tachyarrhythmias, nausea, vomiting, dyspnea, use with caution in the elderly
Monitor	Heart, blood pressure, pulse oximetry
Note	Large doses of epinephrine cause vasoconstriction and small doses cause vasodilation. May be ordered IM rather than SC because the IM route is absorbed more efficiently if edema is present.

BENADRYL

Benadryl (diphenhydramine) H1 Blocker	
Indications	Allergy symptoms
Dose	50 to 80 mg IV for anaphylaxis 10 to 50 mg IV or IM every 4 to 6 hours 25 to 50 mg PO every 4 to 6 hours, maximum 400 mg/day
Pediatric dose	For a child more than 12 kilograms, 5 mg/kg/day IV or IM, every 6 hours, maximum 300 mg/day
Onset	IV onset immediate, IM onset 30 minutes, PO onset 15 to 60 minutes, duration 4 to 8 hours for IV, IM, and PO
Side effects	Dizziness, drowsiness, urinary retention
Monitor	Respiratory status

SOLU-MEDROL

Solu-Medrol (methylprednisolone sodium succinate)	
Indications	Severe inflammation, shock, contact dermatitis, pruritus
Dose	100 to 250 mg IV
Pediatric dose	117 mcg to 1.66 mg/kg IV in 3 to 4 divided doses
Onset	IV onset rapid, IM onset unknown, duration 1 to 4 weeks

Solu-Medrol (methylprednisolone sodium succinate)	
Side effects	Circulatory collapse, thrombophlebitis, embolism, thrombocytopenia
Monitor	Hypokalemia and hyperglycemia may be an adverse effect of long-term therapy.

ZANTAC

Zantac (ranitidine) H2 Blocker	
Indications	Severe inflammation, shock, contact dermatitis, pruritus
Dose	50 mg IV, 150mg PO
Pediatric dose	4 to 5 mg/kg/d PO divided q8 to 12 h; not to exceed 300 mg/d, 1.5 mg/kg/d IV divided q12 h
Onset	IV onset rapid, PO slower onset
Side effects	Anemia, depression, sinus bradycardia, AV block
Monitor	Cardiac status

RELATED CONDITIONS AND INFORMATION

ALLERGY

An allergy is an acquired hypersensitivity to a substance (allergen) that does not normally cause a problem. It is a disorder of the immune system resulting in an antibody-antigen reaction. An allergic reaction may start the second time a person is exposed to the offending agent or may occur after years of exposure. The allergic response can start within a few seconds from exposure to the allergen and be severe. Allergic conditions include eczema, allergic rhinitis, hay fever, bronchial asthma, urticaria (hives), and anaphylaxis. Symptoms may include nasal congestion, tearing, sneezing, wheezing, coughing, itching, and rash. Management includes antihistamines, steroids, and instruction to avoid the offending agent. The cause may remain unidentified in up to two-thirds of the cases. Food appears to be the most causative agent. Shellfish and peanuts are the most frequent offenders.

ALLERGIC DRUG REACTIONS

Drug reactions commonly begin with a macular eruption on the head and proximal extremities that spreads in a symmetrical (the same on opposite sides) pattern. Onset of exanthematous type reactions is usually one week after the start of the offending drug and can be as long as 14 days after the drug is discontinued. The morphology of the rash offers no clue of the causal drug.

ANAPHYLACTIC SHOCK

Anaphylaxis is generally thought to occur in less than 1% of the population and death rarely occurs. Anaphylactic shock induces an antibody-antigen reaction that stimulates the release of vasoactive mediators. Symptoms may include laryngeal edema, bronchoconstriction, and hypotension. Management of anaphylaxis includes oxygen, epinephrine 0.3 to 0.5 mg (0.3 to 0.5 ml of 1:1000) IV or SC every 10 to 15 minutes. The goal in treating all forms of shock is restoration of oxygenation and tissue perfusion.

BLACK WIDOW SPIDER BITES

The black widow is found throughout the Continental United States and Canada, but most common in Arizona and other western states. These spiders are nocturnal and prefer dark crevices. The spider is approximately a half inch long and only the female spiders bite humans and only when disturbed. There are two common species:

The southern black widow has the shiny, black, globular abdomen with the distinctive red hourglass on the underside

The northern black widow has a row of red spots down the middle of the upper surface of its abdomen and 2 crosswise bars on the undersurface. The markings can also be yellow or white, and the spider itself may be brown or have red legs.

A black widow spider's bite is neurotoxic and causes a pinprick sensation followed several hours later by abdominal pain, a board like abdomen, severe extremity cramping, muscular rigidity, nausea, vomiting, and pruritus. In adults, the symptoms abate after several hours and typically disappear in several days. In children and the elderly, the bite can cause death. Pain can be severe and is dependent on the amount of venom injected. Management may include narcotic medications for pain and 10% calcium gluconate IV over 20 minutes for cramping. One vial antivenin Latrodectus in 50 ml NS over 15 minutes is given for severe continued pain. All patients given antivenin Latrodectus should be tested for horse serum sensitivity.

BROWN RECLUSE SPIDER BITES

A brown recluse spider's range is the south-central United States. There are 13 species of recluse spiders in the United States. Their bite often causes no immediate pain. Several hours after the bite a bluish ring, local edema, erythema, and pain develop. If pain is severe, medical management may include steroids and débridement. Brown recluse spider bites can produce large disfiguring wounds that require skin grafting to close.

CATFISH BARBS PUNCTURES

Catfish barbs inject venom. The venom is heat labile and produces severe pain. Immersing the body part in very warm water minimizes the discomfort and neutralizes the toxins. Intravenous pain and antiemetic medications are often necessary. Because benzodiazepines make the effector neurons less excitable to the transmission of stimuli to the brain, they are helpful with the anxiety and fear.

CORAL

Coral causes lacerations and abrasions that are complicated by the presence of foreign bodies, envenomation from tiny nematocysts, and inoculation with microorganisms. Management consists of aggressive hydrogen peroxide cleansing, débridement, and applications of chloramphenicol ointment. The wounds often heal leaving an unsightly scar and may result in a granuloma formation.

DORSAL FINS AND TAILS PUNCTURES

The dorsal fins of bullhead sharks, dogfish, ratfish, catfish, and the tail of the stingray are venomous. The venom is heat labile and produces pain. Treat the pain by immersing the injured body part in hot water. Irrigate with saltwater to remove fragments.

FIRE ANTS BITES

Fire ants are from the southern United States and tropical America. They build large mounds and are capable of inflicting a painful sting. Fire ants bite multiple times causing localized pain, erythema, and wheals that expand into vesicles and eventually a pustule. Fire ant bites are a common cause of anaphylaxis.

HALDOL AND COMPAZINE ADVERSE REACTIONS

Dystonia is a reaction to medications that causes muscle spasm or contractions that typically involve the tongue, neck, and jaw. Medications that cause dystonia include Haldol and Compazine. Management includes Cogentin (benztropine mesylate) and Benadryl.

HIVES

Urticaria (hives) involves the superficial dermis and presents as circumscribed wheals with raised spreading borders and blanched centers. Angioedema involves the deeper layers of the skin and subcutaneous tissue. Management includes antihistamines and instruction to avoid the offending agent.

HONEYBEES

Honeybees are widely domesticated as a source of honey and beeswax. Their stings leave a puncture wound that often has the stinger protruding. Do not grasp and pull the stinger out as this contracts the venom sacs and releases more poison. Remove the stinger by scraping off with a dull object. The local reaction is sharp pain, a wheal, erythema, and itching. Management includes washing with an antiseptic or soap and water, applying ice, and elevating the body part. Oral antihistamines and steroids may be needed.

HORNET STINGS

Hornets characteristically build large papery nests. Their stings leave a painful puncture wound. The reaction is sharp local pain, a wheal, erythema, and itching. The wheal expands to a large vesicle, purulence develops, and the area reddens followed by crusting. Management includes washing with an antiseptic or soap and water, applying ice, and elevating the body part. Oral antihistamines and steroids may be needed.

JELLYFISH STINGS

Jellyfish are free-swimming, gelatinous, tentacled, invertebrate marine animals. Their tentacles contain thousands of venom containing nematocysts that fire with changes in osmotic pressure. A sting can occur from handling a dead jellyfish. The sting causes a linear, erythematous, and painful eruption. Management is debatable. Soaking the wound in dilute acetic acid (vinegar) or sodium hydroxide is the most accepted management. The part should not be immersed in freshwater until the tentacles are removed. Use of antihistamines and topical steroids may be warranted. Jellyfish stings are usually mild.

PORTUGUESE MAN-OF-WAR STINGS

A Portuguese man-of-war is a complex invertebrate animal of warm seas, having a bluish bladder-like float with a broad sail-like crest from which hang numerous long stinging tentacles. The tentacles embed themselves in the skin. Welts or streaks appear causing intense pain. The therapy is debatable. Soaking the wound in dilute acetic acid (vinegar) or sodium hydroxide is the most accepted. The injured body part should not be immersed in freshwater until the tentacles are removed. Use of antihistamines and topical steroids may be warranted.

SCORPIONS

A scorpion is any of various arachnids of warm dry regions with a segmented body and an erectile tail tipped with a venomous sting. Scorpions are not dangerous in most parts of the United States. A dangerous species, Centruroides (Bark Scorpion), lives in Arizona, New Mexico, Southern California, and Texas. The tail of the scorpion contains a telson where venom is produced and stored. A stinger injects potent venom with at least 5 neurotoxins. Immediate local reaction occurs with pain and swelling. Systemic reactions range from mild symptoms to anaphylaxis. Local reactions resolve in a few hours. Systemic reactions may continue for several days. Its sting is very painful, though the wound may not swell much at first. It is generally not life-threatening to healthy adults. Adults may experience mild twitching of the facial muscles, cramps, nausea and anxiety. Infants are especially at risk of respiratory failure. Treat severe reactions with goat serum scorpion antivenin and diazepam. Combat shock and dehydration with fluid replacement.

SEA SNAKES BITES

Sea snakes are any of the various venomous tropical snakes that are adapted to living in the sea, especially in the Pacific and Indian oceans, which bear live offspring. Sea snakes are venomous fish that inject a short-chain polypeptide poison. They have short fangs that inject neurotoxin capable of causing marked malaise, ascending paralysis, and death. An antivenin is available, but the key to survival is application of an immobilization dressing to delay the spread of venom until it is less potent.

SEAWEED AND ALGAE

Seaweed and algae can cause dermatitis. The lesions occur in the swimsuit distribution. Vigorous washing and cool compresses help the discomfort.

SPINY SEA URCHINS PUNCTURES

Spiny sea urchins are any of various echinoderms having a soft body enclosed in a round, symmetrical, calcareous shell covered with long spines. They can produce dirty puncture wounds and deliver a mild toxin. Possible sequela is a painful irritation. Management consists of hot water irrigation and spine removal.

STINGRAYS STINGS

A stingray is any of various rays having a whiplike tail armed with one or more venomous spines capable of inflicting severe injury. They carry a short-chain polypeptide poison and inject the venom by means of a dorsal spine. Envenomation is associated with local erythema, ecchymosis, and severe pain. The venom is heat labile. Immersing the injured part in hot water minimizes the discomfort.

TICKS

Ticks are any of numerous small bloodsucking parasitic arachnids many of which transmit febrile diseases. Ticks pierce the skin and borrow their heads in the tissue.

Rocky Mountain spotted fever is caused by the rickettsia parasite that is maintained in nature by a cycle that involves an insect vector and an animal reservoir. Host factors associated with death are male, chronic alcohol abuse, advanced age, and African American race.

Lyme disease is the most common tick-borne disease in North America and Europe. It is named after the town of Old Lyme, Connecticut. The cause of Lyme disease is a bacterial infection with a spirochete. The disease may include a rash and flu-like symptoms followed by musculoskeletal, arthritic, neurologic, psychiatric, or cardiac problems. Treatment is by doxycycline or amoxicillin therapy. There is controversy regarding the prevalence of the disease, diagnosis, and treatment of later stages among public health agencies.

Squeezing the body of the infected tick during removal may inject more viruses into the victim. Local lore describes various ways to kill the tick and the virus with ether, gasoline, or a hot match before removal. Symptoms start three to twelve days after being bitten by an infected tick. Management with antibiotics is effective when given early with the onset of the rash. In mild or moderate cases, symptoms abate within 2 weeks without therapy. Mortality in severe cases is about 7% and usually occurs during the second week of illness.

SWIMMER'S ITCH

Swimmer's itch is cercarial dermatitis. The larva, found in fresh water in the Midwest and eastern United States, attaches itself inside the epidermis and then dies. A local reaction with maculopapular pruritic eruption appears and lasts about a week. Antipruritics provide relief.

YELLOW JACKETS STINGS

Yellow jacket stings leave a painful puncture wound, do not leave a stinger, and can sting repeatedly. The reaction is sharp local pain, a wheal, erythema, and itching. Management includes washing with antiseptic or soap and water, applying ice, and elevating the body part. Oral antihistamines and steroids may be needed.

PEDIATRIC CONSIDERATIONS

Food sensitivities in the pediatric population
Ninety-five percent of children's food allergies are due to cow's milk protein, egg whites, wheat proteins, soybeans, shellfish, fish, peanuts, and tree nuts (like walnuts). Other common allergens include corn, peanut butter, citrus fruits, chocolate, and food additives.
Children under the age of three are most likely to have food sensitivities, because their immune systems cannot yet tolerate a wide range of new substances. Children with a family history of food allergies should not be given peanuts or peanut products until the age of three for this reason. Also, eggs should not be given to a high-risk child until the age of 18 months.

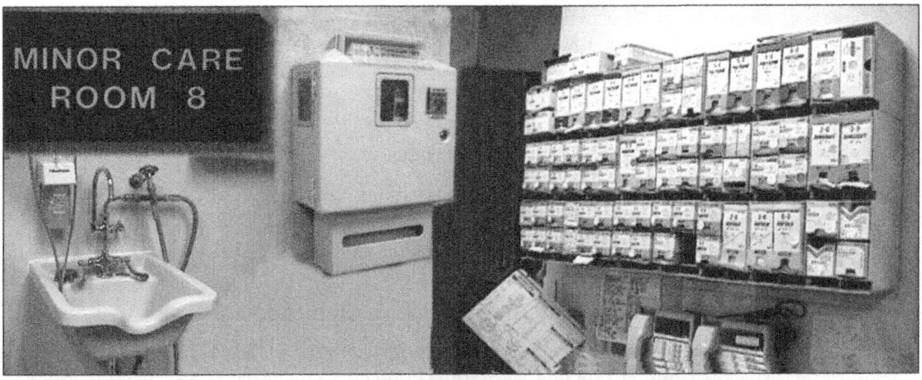

03 ANIMAL ATTACK AND SNAKEBITE

For details on triage see Chapter 34, Triage in a Nutshell.

PATIENT'S STORY – INTERVIEW QUESTIONS

1. When did the attack take place?
2. What kind of reptile or animal was involved?
3. Where are the injuries?
    a. What is the appearance of the injured area?
    b. Are any other symptoms associated with the chief complaint, e.g., nausea, vomiting, headache, sweating, respiratory distress, or irregular heartbeat?
4. Did anything cause the attack, e.g., playing, provoking, or feeding?
5. How do the injuries affect normal function?
    a. Is cardiovascular function compromised?
    b. Is neurovascular function normal distal to the injury?
    c. Does the patient have normal use of the injured area?
6. Were animal control authorities notified?

Animal control authorities should be notified on ALL animal bites even if rabies is not suspected.

7. Was any treatment initiated and has it helped?
8. Does the patient have any pertinent past history?
9. Does the patient take any routine medications?
    a. What is the name, dosage, route, and frequency of each medication?
    b. When was the last dose?

10. Does the patient take any complementary or alternative therapies, herbal products, over-the-counter medications or supplements, or natural therapies?
    a. What is the name, dosage, route, and frequency of each therapy?
    b. When was the last dose or therapy?
11. Does the patient have allergies to drugs or foods?
    a. What is the name of the allergen?
    b. What was the reaction?
12. When was the patient's last tetanus immunization?
13. If the patient is female and between the ages of 10 to 50 years, when was the first day of her last menstrual period?

NURSING DOMAIN

The nursing domain, nursing diagnosis and plan of care can only be determined after an in-depth interview and consideration of the patient's story.

Domain 12. Comfort. Class 1. Physical comfort.
Domain 11. Safety/Protection Class 1. Infection.

ANTICIPATED MEDICAL CARE

Review of the Anticipated Medical Care of Animal Attacks and Snakebites	
Medical provider exam	Full body exam if multiple injury sites are present or the patient has systemic involvement.
Urine tests	Urine pregnancy test for women of reproductive age unless they have had a hysterectomy
Blood	CBC, PT, aPTT, electrolytes, glucose, renal function studies for snakebites (BUN, creatinine), fibrogen, fibrin split products, type and cross 4 units PRBC; No specific labs for animal bites
ECG	ECG for snakebite.
X-ray	X-ray injured area if bone involvement is suspected.
Diet	NPO
IV	Normal saline or Ringer's solution
Medications	Tetanus toxoid, rabies immunization, prophylactic antibiotics IV or IM Antivenin for snakebite
Other	Cleansing, irrigation of the wound, approximation of wound edges (The need for sutures depends on severity and contamination. A contaminated wound is often packed or left open.)

Review of the Anticipated Medical Care of Animal Attacks and Snakebites	
Disposition	Hospitalization may be required for snakebite or severe injuries.
Worst-case scenario	The worst-case scenario is sudden anaphylaxis to antivenin. Treatment includes oxygen, Epinephrine 0.2 to 0.5 mg IV or SC, and Benadryl 50 to 80 mg IV or IM.

INITIAL CARE PLAN

> Alcohol-based hand sanitizers are the preferred method for cleaning your hands in most clinical situations. Wash your hands with soap and water whenever they are visibly dirty, before eating, and after using the restroom.

1. Ask the patient to undress and take off jewelry that may interfere with the exam.
2. Put on an exam gown.
3. Assist as needed.

SNAKEBITE INITIAL ASSESSMENTS AND INTERVENTIONS

Snakebite Interventions	
1.	EMERGENT — NOTIFY THE PHYSICIAN IMMEDIATELY
2.	KEEP THE BITTEN AREA STILL
3.	Elevate to the level of the heart. May elevate above the level of the heart if needed to control pain.
4.	NO ICE
5.	NO TOURNIQUET (A constricting band may be ordered if within 30 minutes of the bite. Do not constrict arterial flow.)
6.	NO FOOD OR DRINK
7.	Establish intravenous access with normal saline and draw blood for CBC, ProTime, levels of fibrinogen, fibrin splint products, electrolytes, glucose, BUN and creatinine. Type and cross for 4 unites of PRBC. Pregnancy test for all women of reproductive age with no history of a hysterectomy. Obtain ECG. Obtain urinalysis.
8.	Perform a cursory body surface inspection for unnoticed bites. Auscultate the lungs. If the bite occurred on an extremity, mark the bite site. Measure, mark, and document the extremity circumference above and below the bite; also mark the leading edge of the swelling. Monitor these measurements for any changes. Monitor pulses distal to the bite.
9.	Observe the patient carefully for evidence of sequential venom effects. Measure the edema caused by the bite by marking the skin at the leading edge with a pen every 15 to 30 minutes as well as the circumferential measurements.

Snakebite Interventions
10. Give antivenin for evidence of coagulopathy, systemic venom effects, or progression of the local tissue injury. Give within the golden hour if possible. Antivenin is less effective if given more than 8 hours after the snakebite.
11. Give tetanus prophylaxis. Treat pain with narcotic analgesia if the patient is stable.
12. Repeat CBC, PT, aPTT to monitor progression.
13. Note: Envenomation cannot be assumed. The patient must be closely monitored for symptoms and treated accordingly.

ANIMAL ATTACKS INITIAL ASSESSMENTS AND INTERVENTIONS

Animal attack interventions
Obtain a wound culture if drainage is purulent.
Cleanse the area with antiseptic solution and cover the area with a sterile dressing.
Protect, rest, ice, compress, and elevate the injured body part.
Administer tetanus toxoid if the last tetanus booster was more than 5 years ago. Consider the need for rabies prophylaxis. Consider the need for prophylactic antibiotics in high-risk patients.
Order x-rays of areas with suspected bony damage.
Notify animal control authorities.

GENERAL INTERVENTIONS

1. Instruct the patient not to eat or drink. Explain the rationale for the NPO status.
2. Elevate the side rails and leave the stretcher in the lowest position.
3. Inform the patient, family, and caregivers of the usual plan of care. Include time involved for each aspect of the stay and the expected overall time in the ER.
4. Provide the patient with a device to reach someone for assistance and explain how to use it. Ask the patient to call for help before getting off the stretcher.

ONGOING CARE PLAN

Inform the medical provider of adverse changes noted during ongoing evaluation. Document that the medical provider was notified of the adverse change. Document if orders were or were not received.

1. Monitor swelling and redness at the site, circulation of the extremity or digit, changes in level of consciousness, and vital signs.
2. Monitor therapy closely for the patient's therapeutic response.

   a. The usual time for a medication effectiveness check is 20 to 30 minutes after giving the drug.
   b. If therapy is not effective, ask the medical provider for a repeat dose or an alternative.
3. Monitor closely for the development of adverse reactions to therapy.
   a. Perform interventions to relieve the adverse reaction.
   b. Ask the medical provider for a remedy.
4. If not NPO, provide the patient with food at mealtimes and fluids during the stay.
5. Keep the patient, family, and caregivers well informed of the plan of care and the remaining time anticipated before disposition.
6. Monitor the patient's radiographic and laboratory results. Notify the medical provider of critical abnormalities. Remedy abnormalities as ordered.
7. Notify the medical provider when all diagnostic results are available for review. Ask for establishment of a diagnosis and disposition.

DISCHARGE INSTRUCTIONS

1. Provide the patient with the name of the nurse and doctor in the emergency room.
2. Inform the patient of their diagnosis or why a definitive diagnosis couldn't be made. Explain what caused the problem if known.
3. Teach the patient how to take the medication as prescribed and how to manage the common side effects. Instruct the patient not to drive or perform any dangerous tasks while taking narcotic pain medications.
4. Instruct the patient with damaged skin that:
   a. The injured area should be kept clean and dry.
   b. The dressing applied in the ER should be removed in one to two days and the wound left open to the air. Some lacerations of the face and scalp are not covered with a dressing in the ER. Wounds may be covered with a dry sterile dressing if needed to protect the area.
   c. Elevation of the area when possible reduces the risk of swelling.
   d. Lacerations should be kept clean with a mild soap, rinsed with water, dried thoroughly, and an antibiotic over-the-counter ointment applied two times a day for the first three days.
   e. Follow-up is recommended for suture removal.
5. Some lacerations contaminated with dirt or bacteria are not sutured. These are considered dirty wounds and further care is necessary at home.
   a. Soak the area in warm water and prescribed solution for twenty minutes three times a day for the first three days.

b. Keep the wound covered with a dry sterile dressing between soaks. If the wound is dry and clean after three days of soaks, stop the soaking, and keep it clean, dry, and covered.

c. Not all dirty wounds need antibiotics. If antibiotics are prescribed, take them until the pills are gone. Do not stop when the wound looks better.

> Signs of infection are redness, swelling, red streaks, and pus. Notify the follow-up medical provider if any of these symptoms develop.

6. Teach the mnemonic **PRICE.** When the injured area is not managed properly, the patient pays the PRICE of increased pain and disability.

   Protect the injured area and keep out of harm's way; do not leave an injured foot in the way of a passerby. Cover skin that is not intact with a sterile dressing when in a dirty environment.
   Rest the area. Do not use the injured extremity. Use crutches or a wheelchair to rest an injured lower extremity.
   Ice the area. Cool the region of injury to decrease the potential for swelling.
   Compress the area with light pressure from a compression bandage or ice pack to reduce the risk of swelling.
   Elevate the injured area above the level of the heart.

7. Recommend a medical provider for follow-up care. Provide the name, address, and phone number with a recommendation of when to schedule the care.

8. Instruct the patient to watch for worsening symptoms, e.g., redness, swelling, pus, fever, and red streaks near the wound. Encourage the patient NOT to IGNORE WORSENING SYMPTOMS. Call the follow-up medical provider if any of these signs develop.

9. Ask for verbal confirmation or demonstration of understanding and reinforce teaching as needed.

COMMONLY ORDERED MEDICATIONS

HUMAN RABIES IMMUNE GLOBULIN

Human Rabies Immune Globulin (HRIG)	
Indications	A bite from a rabies infected animal
Dose	20U/kg ½ SC and ½ IM passive immunization is given on the day of exposure. Give half the dose subcutaneous at the site of the bite and the other half IM into the gluteal region. Five days of Human Diploid Cell Vaccine (HDCV) 1 ml doses IM are given for active immunization on days 0, 3, 7, 14, and 28 after exposure.

SNAKE ENVENOMATION GRADES AND ANTIVENIN DOSAGE

Snake Envenomation Grades	FabAV Antivenin

Snake Envenomation Grades	FabAV Antivenin
Grade 0 (minimal) envenomation: No local changes, no systemic symptoms, no laboratory changes	None
Grade I (minimal) envenomation: Snakebite suspected. There may be fang marks present. Changes confined to area of bite with minimal edema and erythema immediately beyond that area. Pain is localized to the wound. No signs of systemic symptoms present and no laboratory changes.	None
Grade II (moderate) envenomation: Manifestations extend beyond the immediate bite area with systemic symptoms, such as nausea, vomiting, and a mild elevation in temperature may be present.	4 to 6 vials
Grade III (severe) envenomation: Manifestations extend beyond the bite area with serious systemic symptoms and very significant laboratory changes or hemorrhage.	5 to 10 vials
Grade IV (severe) envenomation: Severe compromise occurring within 15 minutes of the bite.	10 to 20 plus vials

TETANUS AND DIPHTHERIA TOXOID, ADSORBED FOR ADULTS

Tetanus and Diphtheria Toxoid Adsorbed for Adults	
Indications	Immunization against tetanus and diphtheria
Dose	0.5 ml IM for adults and children 7 years and older
Side effects	Erythema, induration, tenderness, fever, chills, myalgias, headache
Note	The goal is to keep tetanus immunization current not specifically to prevent tetanus infection from the current wound. Persons in the United States have a right not to be immunized. Children can receive a religious exception and be in public school without the recommended immunizations.

RELATED CONDITIONS AND INFORMATION

ANIMAL AND HUMAN BITES

Both animals and humans inflict bites. Human bites have the highest incidence of infection of all bite injuries. The bite injury usually involves a contusion, avulsion, laceration, or puncture wound. Teeth cause extensive crushing and tearing injuries. Dog bites account for 85% of the reported animal bite cases. All bites are considered contaminated. Severe complications such as infection, rabies, tetanus, and loss of the body part can occur. Human and animal bites to the hands are at high risk for infection. Hepatitis B can be transmitted through human salvia. Human bites are explored, copiously irrigated, débrided, and initially left open. Prophylactic antibiotics are commonly given. Animal bites are cleansed and débrided. Wound closure is dependent on site, size, and contamination.

ANESTHESIA

Anesthesia for closure of bite injuries is usually by local infiltration or regional block. Sedation or conscious sedation may be used.

ANESTHESIA DURATION

Local Anesthesia Duration	
Lidocaine (Xylocaine)	Lasts for 30 to 60 minutes
Lidocaine with epinephrine	Lasts 60 to 90 minutes
Marcaine 0.5% (bupivacaine)	Lasts for 3 to 6 hours Marcaine can be used as a regional block to avoid injection directly into the wound. It is used for the face to avoid distortion of the wound that impairs edge matching.

AVULSION

An avulsion is a tear that causes full-thickness skin loss and is impossible to approximate.

CONTUSION

A contusion is an altered area of skin integrity caused by blunt trauma. Large wounds on an extremity can develop into compartmental syndrome commonly occurring within 12 to 72 hours after the injury.

FACIAL LACERATIONS

Facial lacerations require special care. Keep the tissue moist with a saline moistened dressing while waiting for suturing to minimize devitalization of the tissue. Prevention of devitalized tissue is essential for optimal skin layer matching. All lacerations cause scarring; the goal is to minimize the scar. Do not use Betadine or peroxide because it can be caustic to tissue. Facial sutures should be removed in 3 to 5 days to further minimize scarring.

GILA MONSTER (BEADED LIZARD)

This lizard is native to the United States southwest desert area. Envenomation is dependent upon how long the lizard bites and chews on the victim. Symptoms are similar to those experienced with rattlesnake bites including weakness, dizziness, and shock.

LACERATIONS

Lacerations are open cuts caused by blunt force trauma. They can be superficial, through the epidermis and dermis, or can involve the deep muscle layers.

LIZARD BITES

Lizard bites are usually from the iguana, a large tropical American lizard with spiny projections along the back. The bite is generally nontoxic but medical treatment should be sought due to risk of salmonellosis infection especially with high-risk populations, e.g. pregnant individuals, children under 5 years old, and immunocompromised individuals.

POISON CONTROL CENTER

A poison control center is an emergency telephone service. They have information about animal bites and specific treatments. They have the most accurate and up-to-date information. A call to the Poison Control Center is the standard of emergency care for snakebite. The phone number is 1-800-222-1222. Call the Antivenom Index at (602) 626-6016 in Tucson, Arizona for help with treatment of exotic snakebites.

PUNCTURE WOUNDS

Puncture wounds inflicted by animals are considered contaminated wounds. They are often opened, irrigated, and left open to facilitate drainage.

RABIES

Rabies is rare in the United States. Eighty-five percent of the cases occur in wildlife and 3% occur in domestic dogs and cats. Rabies is found in dogs, cats, cattle, horses, goats, sheep, llamas, pigs, raccoons, skunks, bats, and foxes. Rabies has not been found in rodents, such as mice, rats, chipmunks, hamsters, gerbils, and squirrels. Authorities should be notified of ALL animal bites. The virus is passed by infected salvia. The mean incubation time is 1to 2 months. The range of incubation is 10 days to > 1 year. A good source of information related to possible need for rabies prophylaxis is the state veterinarian school.

SNAKEBITES

Pit vipers are any of the various venomous snakes of the family Crotalidae, such as copperhead, rattlesnake, and water moccasins. A small sensory pit below each eye characterizes them. Snakebite symptoms may include burning at the site, local swelling, gangrene of the skin, fever, nausea, vomiting, circulatory collapse, bleeding, muscle cramping, pupillary constriction, delirium, and convulsions.

Key Points:

- Anaphylaxis can occur whenever antivenin is administered.
- The smaller the patient, the larger the relative initial dose that may be required.
- Pregnancy is not a contraindication to antivenin therapy.
- Administration of the antivenin at or around the site of the bite is not recommended.
- The need for subsequent doses is based on the patient's clinical response.
- Patients with severe envenomation should be treated with a dilute form of antivenin and epinephrine even without a history or signs of allergy.
- All victims of bites by the eastern coral snake should be given antivenin.

SNAKEBITES STATISTICS

Of the approximately 7000 snakebites per year, most in the Southeast and Gulf States, less than 0.2% (1 out of 500) is fatal. Factors affecting the severity of the snakebite symptoms are the patient's age, size and health, the amount of venom injected, the location of the bite, the amount of exercise after the snakebite, and the size of the snake. About one-half of the venomous snakebites are dry (the snake did not inject venom).

SUTURE REMOVAL

Review of Suture Removal Times	
Face	3 to 5 days

Review of Suture Removal Times	
Scalp, trunk, hands, and feet	7 to 10 days
Arms and legs	10 to 14 days
Over joints	14 days

TETANUS PRONE WOUNDS

Tetanus prone wounds are greater than six hours old, are wounds with avulsed crushed devitalized tissue and wounds contaminated with dirt, feces, or salvia.

WOUND AGE

Wound age is a critical factor in deciding whether a wound should undergo primary closure. A wound more than six hours old is considered high risk for infection.

TYPES OF WOUNDS

Types of Wounds	
Open	Abrasion: a superficial wound in which the topmost layers of the skin are scraped off Avulsion: a forcible separation or detachment of skin Gunshot wound: caused by a projectile driving into or through the body Incision: caused by a sharp-edged object Laceration: rough, irregular wounds caused by blunt force trauma Puncture: caused by an object puncturing the skin Penetrating wound: caused by an object entering the body
Closed	Contusion (bruise): caused by blunt force trauma that damages tissue under the skin Crush injury: caused by an extreme amount of force applied over a long period of time. Hematoma: caused by damage to a blood vessel that causes blood to collect under the skin

WOUND MANAGEMENT

Review of Wound Management
Control bleeding with pressure
Ask that local anesthesia be initiated. Clean the wound. Scrub if necessary. If contaminated, irrigate for five to 30 minutes with normal saline. Soak puncture wounds for 15 to 30 minutes.
Set up for débridement of devitalized tissue and approximation of wound edges with sutures, staples, or Steri-Strips by assembling and arranging instruments, light, sutures, and a kick bucket.

Review of Wound Management
After the wound is débrided and approximated, apply a thin layer of antibiotic ointment and dress with a dry sterile dressing. DO NOT USE PLASTIC BAND-AIDS. Plastic coverings macerate the skin and prevent healing. Facial lacerations are covered with ointment and normally no dressing is applied.
Instruct the patient in proper home wound care. Recommend the time and place for suture or staple removal.

WOUND CLOSURES

Review of Wound Closures	
Tape closures (Steri-Strips)	Used for superficial wounds under minimal tension. An anesthetic is not necessary, and a lower rate of infection is associated with tape closures than with no closure. No follow-up visit is required for tape removal.
Sutures	Sutures approximate wound edges, decrease infections, promote wound healing, and minimize scarring. A local anesthetic is required. A follow-up visit is required for suture removal.
Staples	Staples approximate the wound edges, have a low rate of infection, but do not approximate the wound edges close enough to minimize scarring. A follow-up visit is required to remove the staples.
Tissue Adhesive (Dermabond®)	Dermabond® is a cyanoacrylate tissue adhesive that forms a strong bond across apposed wound edges providing a flexible water-resistant protective coating and eliminates the need for suture removal. Tissue adhesive should not be used on jagged wounds, animal bites, severely contaminated wounds, ulcers, puncture wounds, mucous membranes (including mucocutaneous junctions) or areas of high moisture content, such as the groin or axillae. The adhesive may be used for sutures of 5-0 or smaller to selected wounds on the face, torso, and extremities.

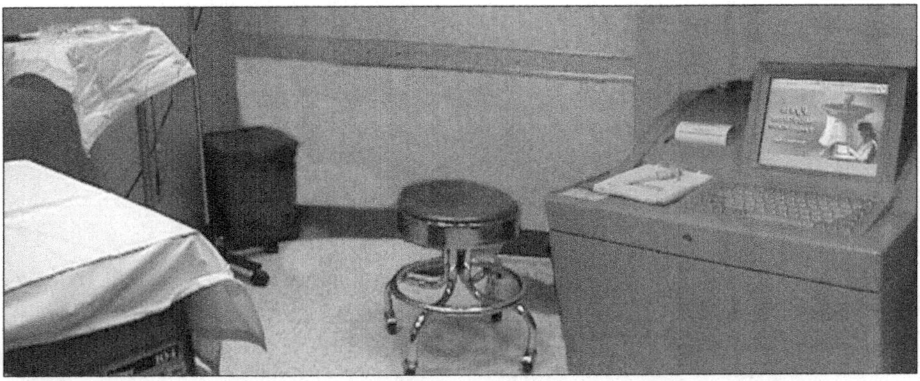

04 Battery, Sexual Assault, Abuse, and Intimate Partner Violence

For details on triage see Chapter 34, Triage in a Nutshell.

Patient's Story – Interview Questions

Patients with complaints of chest pain, shortness of breath, loss of consciousness or altered consciousness, severe abdominal pain, active bleeding, or an obvious deformity to an extremity require immediate medical attention prior to evidence collection considerations.

1. Where is the alleged perpetrator?
2. Does the patient know the alleged perpetrator?
3. How many alleged perpetrators were involved in the assault?
4. When did the alleged battery take place?
5. Are any physical injuries present?
    a. Where are the injuries, e.g., bites, stab wounds, abrasions, bruises?
    b. Is bleeding present?
    c. Was a weapon used?
    d. Did the patient lose consciousness?
    e. What body orifices were penetrated?
    f. Were any foreign objects used?
    g. What sexual acts were performed?
6. Is the patient able to function normally since the assault?
    a. Is neurovascular function normal distal to all injuries?
    b. Is the patient able to use the injured areas normally?

   c. Has the patient showered, bathed, ingested anything, defecated, smoked, urinated, or douched since the event?
   d. Has the patient had consensual sex within the past 72 hours?
7. Is unlawful activity suspected?
   a. Was law enforcement at the scene?
   b. Where did the event occur?
   c. What agency?
   d. Does this event require mandatory reporting in your state, e.g., did it involve a child, elderly, or disabled person?

> Medical personnel are legally obligated to report suspected unlawful acts. Battery is a crime when a person actually and intentionally touches or strikes another person against the will of the other or intentionally causes bodily harm to another. Assault is an intentional unlawful threat by word or act to do violence to the person of another, coupled with an apparent ability to do so, and doing some act that creates a well-founded fear in such other person that violence is imminent.

1. Does the patient have any pertinent past history?
2. Does the patient or law enforcement agent report use or suspected use/ingestion/inhalation of mind-altering drugs including alcohol?
3. Does the patient take any routine medications?
   a. What is the name, dosage, route, and frequency of each medication?
   b. When was the last dose?
4. Does the patient take any complementary or alternative therapies, herbal products, over-the-counter medications or supplements, or natural therapies?
   a. What is the name, dosage, route, and frequency of each therapy?
   b. When was the last dose or therapy?
5. Does the patient have allergies to drugs or foods?
   a. What is the name of the allergen?
   b. What was the reaction?
6. When was the patient's last tetanus immunization?
7. If the patient is female and between the ages of 10 to 50 years, when was the first day of her last menstrual period?

NURSING DOMAIN

The nursing domain, nursing diagnosis and plan of care can only be determined after an in-depth interview and consideration of the patient's story.

> Domain 12. Comfort.
> Class 1. Physical comfort.

Domain 8. Sexuality Class 2. Sexual function
Domain 11. Safety/Protection Class 2. Physical Injury Class 3. Violence
Domain 8. Sexuality Class 1. Sexuality
Domain 9: Coping/Stress tolerance Class 1. Post-trauma response

ANTICIPATED MEDICAL CARE

Review of the Anticipated Medical Care of Battery, Sexual Assault, and Survivors of Violence	
Exam	Full body
Urine test	Pregnancy test for women of reproductive age unless they have had a hysterectomy and possible toxicology
Blood tests	Syphilis serology, pregnancy test, Gonococcus and Chlamydia culture. Other labs as indicated by injuries and possible ETOH
ECG	None
X-ray	X-ray of suspected bony damage
Other	Cervical smears for wet prep and cultures (A separate set of slides may be collected and included with the evidence.)
Diet	NPO before the examination
IV	None
Medications	Prophylactic PO, IM or IV antibiotics, PO pills to reduce the risk of pregnancy
Other	Wound treatment, collection of legal evidence
Disposition	Home or to a safe environment. Preferably with a supportive family member, friend, or caregiver.
Worst-case scenario	The worst-case scenario is when the perpetrator comes to the ER to finish the attack and in the process kills anyone who represents an obstruction. CALL 911.

INITIAL CARE PLAN

Alcohol-based hand sanitizers are the preferred method for cleaning your hands in most clinical situations. Wash your hands with soap and water whenever they are visibly dirty, before eating, and after using the restroom.

1. The first priority is to establish the stability of the patient and determine whether any life-threatening injuries are present by performing a full body exam.

2. If no serious injuries are present, the next priority is to place the survivor of violence in a safe environment. A secure private waiting area is more appropriate than an exam room.
3. Instruct the patient, their support persons, and other emergency staff that the patient should not urinate or defecate (if possible), change clothes, rinse the mouth, smoke, or wash any body part or wound until after the exam. Evidence is lost when the area of penetration is washed, rinsed, or wiped.
4. Ask the patient not to eat or drink until the examination is completed.
5. Inform the patient that clothes worn during the rape are collected as evidence and determine what the patient will wear home.
6. Notify the appropriate law enforcement and support agencies.

> Many states have a rape crisis center and a Sexual Assault Response Teams (SART) that consist of non-medical provider medical providers, law enforcement, prosecuting attorney, and victim advocate services. The team is on call and responds to hospitals when a sexual assault victim arrives.

7. In compliance with each state's laws, either the team or the nurse and medical provider collect the evidence.
   a. The nurse should not collect evidence until the support agency personnel has described the methods to the patient and outlined the patient's options.
   b. The American College of Emergency Medical providers, in the association document titled *Evaluation and Management of the Sexually Assaulted or Sexually Abused Patient*, stated that sexual assault nurse examiners (SANE) programs are an excellent option for acute and chronic sexual assault evaluations, because they standardize the sexual assault evaluation and collection of evidence.
8. Decline to discuss the case with staff members.
9. Let the patient know you will be available to testify about the collection of the evidence and that your job is to collect the evidence in a manner to make it acceptable in court.
   a. Obtain the patient's permission to conduct the examination. Explain that the evidence collection process is detailed and time consuming.
   b. Written consent from the law enforcement agency may be needed if the hospital charges the cost of evidence collection to the agency. Many states reimburse the cost of the exam to the hospital and no charge is made to the survivor.
   c. Be sure all releases and consents are signed prior to the beginning of the examination.
10. For the sexual battery patient, anticipate collecting evidence for a law enforcement agency.

a. An official sexual assault kit approved by the state's law enforcement agencies is needed to collect evidence.

b. Kits are not standardized and may be different from state to state.

c. To maintain the validity of the evidence, an opened kit cannot leave the vision of the nurse until the kit is properly sealed and a law enforcement officer officially receives the evidence. A list of all transfers of the evidence is logged on the hospital record and on the evidence itself. This is part of the chain of evidence.

d. The nurse commonly collects most of the evidence. A sexual assault nurse examiner (SANE) or the medical provider usually collects the evidence requiring a speculum exam. The kit contains detailed instructions. Read the instructions carefully.

e. Blood specimens may be needed. The medical provider may need blood test results for treatment. The law enforcement agent may request separate urine and blood specimens be collected for toxicology studies at their designated crime lab if drug use is considered a factor in the incident.

> If the blood needed for hospital testing is drawn early in the patient's stay, the results will be available for the medical provider to prescribe treatment and not delay the patient's disposition when the legal exam is completed.

f. Order a pregnancy test. A negative pregnancy test is needed before medications can be ordered.

g. Order a test for syphilis, gonorrhea, Chlamydia, and a wet prep for trichomoniasis, and possible sperm identification.

h. Have a Wood's lamp available. Body fluids including semen are visible under the light from a Wood's lamp and glows fluorescent orange or blue green.

11. Inform the patient, family, and caregivers of the usual plan of care and the expected overall time in the ER.

12. Provide the patient with a device to reach someone for assistance and explain how to use it.

> If the law enforcement agent requests photographs, allow him/her to take the photographs with their own equipment and to retain the photographs in their custody to maintain the chain of evidence. ALL PHOTOGRAPHS SHOULD REMAIN IN THE POSSESSION OF THE LAW ENFORCEMENT AGENT.

13. The following table shows examples of evidence collection for the male and female sexual assault survivor. Actual evidence collection varies from state to state.

Generic Example of Legal Evidence Collection for Male and Female Survivors of Sexual Assault

Generic Example of Legal Evidence Collection for Male and Female Survivors of Sexual Assault	
Evidence	Method of Collection
Clothing	Place each piece of collected clothing in a separate paper bag. Underwear may be collected even if the victim has changed clothing and showered/bathed since the incident due to possible drainage of secretions. Other clothes are not usually collected if they were not worn at the time of the sexual battery.
Fingernail Scraping	Collect, if indicated. Hold each hand over a piece of paper and use a wooden stick to scrap under the nail.
Genitalia	Examine with the Wood's lamp. Collect dried material and matted hair that glows.
Oral Cavity	Swab the oral cavity if penetration occurred within the past 6 hours regardless of ingestion of liquids/food since the incident.
Penis	Collect dried secretions using two swabs, one from the urethral meatus and one from the glans and shaft. Examine the penis for injury.
Pubic Hair	Trim pubic hair with dried secretions and place the specimen in an evidence envelope. Comb pubic hair. The comb, the collected debris, and any combed-out hair are placed in an evidence envelope.
Rectum	Collect dried secretions using two sets of swabs and dry mounted slides.
Skin	Scan the body with a Wood's lamp and collect dried and moist secretions using cotton-tipped swabs. When dried secretions are collected using a moistened swab, a control sample should be taken from the same area where there are no secretions.
Vagina	Deferred to the medical provider or trained forensic examiner e.g. SANE, SAFE, FNE. Anticipate three separate sets of swabs and possibly slides from the vaginal pool, one wet-prep and two dry-mounts. Drying of swabs and slides before placing in evidence envelops preserves the DNA markers.
Bite, Lick, or Kiss Marks	Utilize a Woods Lamp to identify secretions which may be present on all parts of the body and should be collected into evidence. Use distilled water to collect dry secretions from these sites. Swab from the periphery toward the center of the area with a cotton swab. Be sure to collect a control swab from an unaffected area. Take a final, additional dry swab to remove any residue from the area, label each with information concerning the types of specimen and the site where it was collected, and also place in an evidence envelope. If distilled water is not available, use normal saline.

Ideally, a shower and clean clothing will be available for the patient after the exam is completed.

DATE RAPE DRUG INFORMATION

Date Rape Drug Information	
GHB (Gamma-Hydroxybutyrate) G, Liquid G, Georgia Home Boy, Easy Lay, Grievous Bodily Harm, soap, salty water	Tablet, white powder or clear liquid. Effects are weight related and potentiated when combined with alcohol. Effects may be noticed within 15 minutes of ingestion. May cause headaches, shaking, spasms, seizures, drowsiness, and nausea, irregular heartbeat, vomiting, altered LOC, loss of consciousness, coma and death. May be detected in urine up to 12 hours after ingestion.
Rohypnol (flunitrazepam) Roofies, roaches, Roche, forget pill, trip and fall	White tablet. Effects are weight related and potentiated when combined with alcohol. Effects may be noticed within 30 minutes of ingestion and last as long as 12 hours. May cause memory impairment, amnesia, drowsiness, visual disturbances, dizziness, impaired motor skills and judgment, slurred speech, confusion, gastrointestinal disturbances, urinary retention, loss of consciousness, coma, and death. May be detected in urine up to 48 hours after ingestion.
Ecstasy MDMA (3,4-methylenedioxymethamphetamine) X, XTC, Adam, Clarity, Lover's Speed	Homemade colored tablets. May cause increased energy, nausea, hallucinations, chills, sweating, shaking, blurred vision, rapid heartbeat, high blood pressure, muscle cramping, heat stroke, severe dehydration, possible changes in brain functioning, memory problems, serious depression. Memory difficulties may last as long as 3 weeks after ingestion. May be detected in serum, urine, hair, and sweat up to 7 days after ingestion.
Alcohol (ethanol or ethyl alcohol)	Liquid. Effects related to weight of the person, amount consumed, and other drugs ingested. May cause feelings of relaxation, lowered inhibitions, increased sociability, dizziness, kills pain, nausea, slurred speech, slower reflexes, sleepiness, bad judgment, dehydration and a hangover the next day. Alcohol may cause a loss of motor control, black-outs, temporary coma, brain and liver damage, and death. May be detected in urine and serum up to 24 hours after ingestion.

Date Rape Drug Information	
Ketamine (ketamine hydrochloride) Special K, K, kit kat, cat Valium	Snorted, swallowed, smoked, injected. Symptom onset dependent on route of consumption but may begin as soon as 5 minutes and last up to 24 hours. Effects may include lack of coordination, confusion, seizures, high blood pressure, depression, numbness in legs, death due to respiratory collapse, kidney damage, difficulty moving, coma, and death. May be detected up to 14 days after ingestion.

ONGOING CARE PLAN

Inform the medical provider of adverse changes noted during ongoing evaluation. Document that the medical provider was notified of the adverse change. Document if orders were or were not received.

1. Monitor vital signs.
2. Monitor the patient's emotional state and effectiveness of coping mechanisms.
3. Keep the patient, family, and caregivers well informed of the plan of care and the remaining time anticipated before disposition.
4. Monitor the patient's pregnancy results. Results are needed to determine what antibiotics and medications to use.

Pregnancy prevention medications are given after a negative pregnancy test result is obtained. Inform the patient of the associated risks and adverse reactions of pregnancy prevention medications. Most hospitals require a signed consent form before administration.

DISCHARGE INSTRUCTIONS

1. Provide the patient with the name of the nurse and doctor in the emergency room.
2. Teach the patient how to take the medication as prescribed and how to manage the common side effects. Instruct the patient not to drive or perform any dangerous tasks while taking narcotic pain medications.
3. Inform the patient that medical personnel testify about the evidence and do not represent either side in court.
4. Provide the patient with the phone number for the National Domestic Violence Hotline 1-800-799-SAFE (7233) if appropriate.
5. Provide the patient with the National Domestic Violence Hotline website address, www.ndvh.org. Advise the patient not to use the website if the patient's computer is monitored and to use the telephone line instead.

6. Recommend a medical provider for follow-up care and provide the name, address, and phone number with a recommendation of when to schedule the care.
7. For sexual assault survivors:
   a. Recommend a follow up examination within 1-2 weeks.
   b. Established medical providers specializing in follow-up for rape victims may be included in the referrals provided by the support team.
   c. Provide the name, address, and phone number of the referral medical provider or agency.
   d. Inform the patient of the expected time the results for the STD tests performed will be available and they remain confidential. Make clear to the patient the results may be released to the local health department due to public health laws and requirements.
   e. Advise the patient of the need for syphilis, HIV and Hepatitis B testing at 6, 12 and 24 weeks after the assault even if the initial results were negative.
   f. The sexual assault team member may also provide written instructions and referral phone numbers.
8. Instruct the patient to call the follow-up medical provider or go directly to the emergency room if any unusual symptoms develop. Encourage the patient NOT to IGNORE WORSENING OR PERSISTENT SYMPTOMS.
9. Ask for verbal confirmation or demonstration of understanding and reinforce teaching as needed.

COMMONLY ORDERED MEDICATIONS

ANTIBIOTICS

Antibiotics for Sexually Transmitted Diseases	
Indications	Prophylactic prevention of gonorrhea, Chlamydia, and trichomoniasis in non-pregnant females
Dose	Ceftriaxone 250 mg IM in a single dose OR Cefixime 400 mg orally in a single dose Plus Metronidazole (Flagyl) 2 gram orally in a single dose (for trichomonas and bacterial vaginosis prevention) plus Azithromycin 1 gram orally in a single dose (for chlamydia prevention) or Doxycycline 100 mg orally twice a day for 7 days

Antibiotics for Sexually Transmitted Diseases	
Note	Flagyl not to be used with pregnant females. Ask for alternative antibiotics. Discuss with the medical provider possible delay of administration of Flagyl if patient indicates recent ETOH ingestion.

OVRAL

Ovral (norgestrel and ethinyl estradiol)	
Indications	Prevention of pregnancy in the sexually assaulted patient. Only effective if taken within 72 hours of unprotected sexual intercourse.
Dose	2 tablets PO
Note	Most hospitals require the patient to sign a consent form for pregnancy prevention medications after being advised of the associated risks and adverse reactions. Pregnancy prevention medications are only given after a negative pregnancy test result is obtained.

PLAN B®

Plan B® (levonorgestrel 0.75 mg.)	
Indications	Prevention of pregnancy in the sexually battered patient. Only effective if taken within 72 hours of unprotected sexual intercourse.
Dose	1 tablet PO and1 tablet PO 12 hours after the first dose. Send home with the patient.
Note	Not to be used for pregnant females.

RELATED CONDITIONS AND INFORMATION

RAPE

The crime of forcing another person to submit to sex acts, especially sexual intercourse.

SEXUAL ASSAULT

Sexual assault is any genital, oral, or anal penetration by a part of the body by an object, using force or without the victim's consent. Acquaintance rape, date rape, statutory rape, child sexual abuse, and incest all qualify under this definition.

RAPE TRAUMA SYNDROME

The acute phase of rape trauma syndrome involves the first 1 to 3 weeks following the event and include shock, numbness, embarrassment, guilt, powerlessness, loss of trust, fear, anxiety, anger, disbelief, shame, depression, denial, disorientation, and multiple physical symptoms including genitourinary discomfort, gastrointestinal irritability, muscle tension, and sleep disturbances. The reorganization phase may have effects up to 4 years following the event and may include changes in lifestyle, residence, and dealing with repetitive nightmares, fears, sexual issues, and phobias.

DOMESTIC VIOLENCE / INTIMATE PARTNER ABUSE

The National Domestic Violence Hotline (NDVH) has a free confidential hotline. The number is 1-800-799-SAFE (7233) with 24-hour support in English and Spanish. Website is http://www.ndvh.org.

According to the NDVH

Abuse is a pattern of coercive controls that one person exercises over another. Battering is a behavior that physically harms, arouses fear, prevents a partner from doing what they wish or forces them to behave in ways they do not want. Battering includes the use of physical and sexual violence, threats and intimidation, emotional abuse, and economic deprivation. Intimate partner violence (also known as domestic violence) is NOT a gender issue. It is a social issue effecting sexes, all ages, races, creeds, sexual orientations, and walks of life.

The quiz below is published by the NDVH to help persons determine if they are abused.

Does your partner:

- Embarrass you with put-downs?
- Look at you or act in ways that scare you?
- Control what you do, who you see or talk to or where you go?
- Stop you from seeing your friends or family members?
- Take your money or Social Security check, make you ask for money, or refuse to give you money?
- Make all of the decisions?
- Tell you that you're a bad parent or threaten to take away or hurt your children?
- Prevent you from working or attending school?
- Act like the abuse is no big deal, it's your fault, or even denies doing it?
- Destroy your property or threaten to kill your pets?
- Intimidate you with guns, knives, or other weapons?
- Shove you, slap you, choke you, or hit you?
- Force you to try and drop charges?
- Threaten to commit suicide?
- Threaten to kill you?

If you answered yes to even one of these questions, you may be in an abusive relationship.

WARNING SIGNS FOR HEALTHCARE PROVIDERS

- Time delays between injury and care
- Responsible party does not participate in post hospital plan of care

- Burns or bruises in various stages of healing
- Multiple fractures
- Frequent emergency room visits
- Noncompliance with prescribed medical interventions
- An intuition that something is not right
- The significant other does not leave the patient's bedside
- History that does not match the injury

INTIMATE PARTNER VIOLENCE SCREENING

Who should be screened?	Everyone presenting to the emergency room
Who should do the screening?	A health care provider who has been educated in the dynamics of intimate partner violence
How should the screening be conducted?	In a private setting with no friends, relatives, or children present Face to face Direct and nonjudgmental
What should they be screened for?	Abuse within the last year Example questions: Have you ever been hurt, threatened, or felt controlled by your partner? Do you ever feel afraid of your partner? Do you feel you are in danger? Is it safe for you to go home? Are you currently or have you ever been in a relationship where you were physically hurt, threatened, or made to feel afraid?

VICTIM SAFETY ASSESSMENT

1. Has the alleged perpetrator recently obtained a weapon?
2. Has there been an increased use of alcohol or drugs?
3. Has the violence become more frequent and/or severe?
4. Has the family dynamics recently changed, e.g., a recent pregnancy, loss of a job?
5. Have threats been made against the child or pets recently?
6. Have threats of suicide or homicide been made?

If the answer to any of these questions is yes, then it may not be safe for the victim to return to the residence. When possible, discuss with the victim developing a safety plan and reinforce that the violence is not the victim's fault.

SPECIAL POPULATIONS

Sexual Assault in Special Populations	
Male	Male victims will routinely not report to law enforcement due to the social stigma of being a victim and not a stereotypical macho male. Reinforce that the violence was not their fault and that they did not cause the event. Remain patient, supportive, and nonjudgmental. Encourage them to seek law enforcement involvement. Reinforce the male victim is not gay after the event. In a male to male sexual battery, explain if the victim experienced an orgasm it does not indicate sexual orientation. Men who are victims of sexual assault or intimate partner violence may experience feelings of depression, isolation, and anxiety. They should be assessed for suicidal ideation.
Sight impaired	Reinforce that the event was not their fault and that they did not cause the event. Remain patient, supportive, and nonjudgmental. Encourage them to report to law enforcement. Provide a quiet, uninterrupted environment. Include the victim in all conversations and identify all persons who are speaking. Explain all aspects of the process in detail. If the victim has a service animal, allow the service animal to remain in the room.

Sexual Assault in Special Populations	
Hearing impaired	Reinforce that the event was not their fault and that they did not cause the event. Remain patient, supportive, and nonjudgmental. Encourage them to report to law enforcement. Ideally, if the victim utilizes sign language, provide a sign language interpreter. If a sign language interpreter is not available, utilize notes. If the victim has a service animal, allow the service animal to remain in the room.
Physical limitations	Reinforce that the event was not their fault and that they did not cause the event. Remain patient, supportive, and nonjudgmental. Encourage them to report to law enforcement. Make provisions for assistance with the examination. Be cognizant of possible pain reactions during the examination even in spinal cord injured victims. If the victim has a service animal, allow the service animal to remain in the room.
Cognitive emotional limitations	Reinforce that the event was not their fault and that they did not cause the event. Remain patient, supportive, and nonjudgmental. Encourage them to report to law enforcement. Allow for an individual trusted by the victim to be in attendance, if not involved with the events. Utilize matter of fact questions and provide simple explanations. If the victim has a service animal, allow the service animal to remain in the room.

Sexual Assault in Special Populations	
Cultural issues	Reinforce that the event was not their fault and that they did not cause the event. Remain patient, supportive, and nonjudgmental. Encourage them to report to law enforcement. Make provisions for an interpreter, if needed. Ethnicity never defines the victim's values or behaviors. Culture is unconscious, a person's behaviors and attitudes are molded by it.
Elder abuse	Reinforce that the event was not their fault and that they did not cause the event. Remain patient, supportive, and nonjudgmental. Encourage them to follow up with law enforcement. Aggressively assess for occult injuries. Respect and dignity are of great importance.
Child abuse	If possible, children should be evaluated by specially trained professionals with experience interviewing and evaluating children. Follow the guidelines established in your area. Reinforce that the event was not their fault and that they did not cause the event. Remain patient, supportive, and nonjudgmental. Encourage them to speak freely with law enforcement. Be supportive of the child's guardian(s) but encourage them to leave the interviewing and evaluation of the child to the experts. Use open-ended and indirect questions to allow them to explain.

DEVELOPMENTAL DIFFERENCES

Developmental Differences	
Preschool Children	Concrete, literal thinkers
	Utilize show-me questions
School Children	Allow narrative explanations. May have difficulty with organization
	Utilize show-me questions

Developmental Differences	
	May have difficulty with time
Adolescents	Can understand abstract ideas
	May have trust issues
	Allow narrative explanations
	May demonstrate egocentric behavior
All Ages	Avoid suggestions and influencing responses. Focus on the child's actual experiences.

TYPES OF CHILD ABUSE SUSPICIOUS SIGNS

Types of Child Abuse Suspicious Signs	
Physical	Child appears afraid of adults and/or demonstrates fear of the guardian.
	Conflicting or unconvincing explanations offered for the injury.
	Guardian describes the child as evil.
	Injuries in varying stages of healing.
	Unexplained injuries.
Emotional	Child demonstrates overtly compliant, passive, aggressive, or demanding behavior.
	Guardian appears disengaged or disinterested in the child's well being
	Guardian constantly belittles and/or blames the child
	Child has physical and emotional developmental delays.
Sexual	Child positive for an STD under 14 years of age
	Child has sudden change in appetite.
	Child has sudden onset of bedwetting.
	Child demonstrates unusual, bizarre, or sophisticated sexual knowledge.
Neglect	Child begs or steals money or food.
	Child lacks needed medical or dental care, immunizations, or glasses
	Child lacks sufficient clothing for the weather.
	Child states no one available to provide care.
	Guardian appears to be indifferent to the child.
	Guardian behaves irrationally or in a bizarre manner.

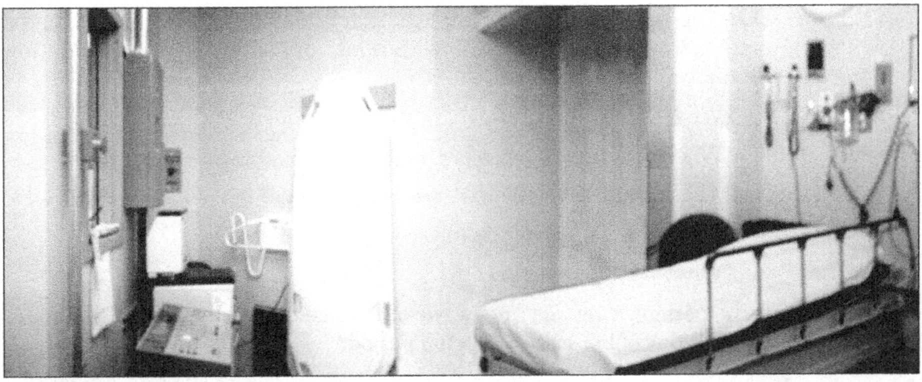

05 BACK PAIN

For details on triage see Chapter 34, Triage in a Nutshell.

PATIENT'S STORY – INTERVIEW QUESTIONS

1. When was the onset of the pain? (Acute < 6 weeks. Subacute 6 to 12 weeks. Chronic >12 weeks.)
2. Where is the pain located and is any radiation present?
3. Is the patient experiencing any sensation or motor deficits below the area of pain?
4. Did anything cause the back pain, e.g., recent trauma, twisting, bending, or lifting a heavy object?
5. How does the pain affect normal function?
    a. Is the patient able to perform daily activities?
    b. Is the pain intermittent or constant?
    c. Is the pain mild, moderate, or severe?
    d. Is the patient able to sleep and rest?
6. Has any treatment been initiated, and has it helped?
7. Does the patient have a history of back problems?
    a. What was the diagnosis and treatment?
    b. Has the patient been treated at a pain management center?
8. Does the patient have any pertinent past history?
9. Does the patient take any routine medications?
    a. What is the name, dosage, route, and frequency of each medication?
    b. When was the last dose?

10. Does the patient take any complementary or alternative therapies, herbal products, over-the-counter medications or supplements, or natural therapies?
    a. What is the name, dosage, route, and frequency of each therapy?
    b. When was the last dose or therapy?
11. Does the patient have allergies to drugs or foods?
    a. What is the name of the allergen?
    b. What was the reaction?
12. If the patient is female and between the ages of 10 to 50 years, when was the first day of her last menstrual period?

NURSING DOMAIN

The nursing domain, nursing diagnosis and plan of care can only be determined after an in-depth interview and consideration of the patient's story.

Domain 12. Comfort. Class 1. Physical comfort.
Domain 4. Activity/Rest Class 2. Activity/Exercise

ANTICIPATED MEDICAL CARE

Review of the Anticipated Medical Care of Back Pain	
Exam	Full body
Urine tests	Urinalysis for suspected UTI and/or pyelonephritis and prostatitis, pregnancy test for women of child-bearing age with no history of a hysterectomy.
Blood tests	ESR (used for screening to help rule out disease)
ECG	None
X-ray	None for chronic or non-traumatic back pain, CT Scan or MRI if neurological deficits noted or unstable vital signs.
Diet	NPO
IV	None
Medications	IM analgesia, steroids, skeletal muscle relaxants
Disposition	Home
Worst-case scenario	Back pain and abdominal pain that mimics renal colic can be a symptom of a ruptured aortic aneurysm. The worst-case scenario is sudden loss of circulatory volume from an unsuspected ruptured aortic aneurysm. Treatment may include STAT surgery, replacement of lost blood volume, type and cross for 20 units of PRBC, and consents for both surgery and anesthesia.

INITIAL CARE PLAN

> Alcohol-based hand sanitizers are the preferred method for cleaning your hands in most clinical situations. Wash your hands with soap and water whenever they are visibly dirty, before eating, and after using the restroom.

1. Ask the patient to undress, remove jewelry that might interfere with the examination, and put on an exam gown. Assist as needed.
2. Notice if the patient is able to undress and don the gown without assistance or if he has limited range of motion. Watch the patient's body posture, ability to move, and fluency of gait. This assessment can be used as a baseline to evaluate effectiveness of treatment.
3. Perform a focused physical examination.
   a. Inspect the back for bruising or deformity.
   b. Palpate the back for areas of tenderness.
4. Place the patient in a comfortable position. The most common is lying on the back with knees flexed and supported.
5. Elevate the siderails and keep the stretcher in the lowest position.
6. Instruct the patient not to eat or drink until evaluated by the medical provider.
7. Keep the patient, family, and caregivers well informed of the plan of care, the remaining time anticipated before disposition, and the rationale for the need to abide by the NPO status.
8. Provide the patient with a device to reach someone for assistance and explain how to use it. Ask the patient to call for help before getting off the stretcher.

ONGOING CARE PLAN

> Inform the medical provider of adverse changes noted during ongoing evaluation. Document that the medical provider was notified of the adverse change. Document if orders were or were not received.

1. Monitor vital signs.
2. Monitor pain therapy closely for the patient's therapeutic response.
   a. The usual time for a medication effectiveness check is 20 to 30 minutes after giving the drug.
   b. If therapy is not effective, ask the medical provider for a repeat dose or an alternative.
3. Evaluate the level of pain control by the patient's body posture, ability to move, and fluency of gait.
4. Monitor closely for the development of adverse reactions to therapy.
   a. Perform interventions to relieve the adverse reaction.

   b. Ask the medical provider for a remedy.

5. If not NPO, provide the patient with food at mealtimes and fluids during the stay.
6. Keep the patient, family, and caregivers well informed of the plan of care and the remaining time anticipated before disposition.
7. Notify the medical provider when all diagnostic results are available for review. Ask for establishment of a diagnosis and disposition.

DISCHARGE INSTRUCTIONS

1. Provide the patient with the name of the nurse and doctor in the emergency room.
2. Inform the patient of their diagnosis or why a definitive diagnosis couldn't be made. Explain what caused the problem if known.
3. Instruct the patient that:
   a. Walking, lifting, and bending may aggravate symptoms of pain and muscle spasm.
   b. Sleeping on a firm mattress is essential to allow healing.
   c. When the symptoms are resolved, slowly increase activity.
   d. Using the prescribed medications and moist heat will help relieve the pain symptoms.
4. Teach the patient how to take the medication as prescribed and how to manage the common side effects. Instruct the patient not to drive or perform any dangerous tasks while taking narcotic pain medications.
5. Recommend a medical provider for follow-up care. Provide the name, address, and phone number with a recommendation of when to schedule the care.
6. Call the follow-up medical provider if shooting pains, weakness or numbness of any of the extremities, bowel or bladder incontinence or trouble urinating develops. If the medical provider is not available, return to the emergency room. Encourage the patient NOT to IGNORE WORSENING SYMPTOMS.
7. Ask for verbal confirmation or demonstration of understanding and reinforce teaching as needed.

COMMONLY ORDERED MEDICATIONS

DILAUDID

Dilaudid (hydromorphone)	
Indications	Moderate to severe pain
Dose	Typical dose 1 to 5 mg IV. Titrate to response. No maximum dose.

Dilaudid (hydromorphone)	
Onset	IV onset rapid, peak 15 to 30 minutes, duration 3 to 4 hours
Side effects	Drowsiness, dizziness, confusion, sedation, increased intracranial pressure, nausea, vomiting, urinary retention, respiratory depression
Monitor	CNS changes, respiratory effectiveness, allergic rash
Note	Dilaudid 5 mg equivalent to Morphine 10 mg IM. Dilute to 4 or 5 ml with NS or sterile water for injection and administer slowly over at least 2 to 3 min. Antidote is naloxone.

TORADOL

Toradol (ketorolac tromethamine)	
Indications	Severe acute pain that requires analgesia at the opioid level
Dose	60 mg IM, reduce the dose to 30 mg IM for a patient >65 years of age, less than 110 pounds, or with renal impairment. 30 mg IV, reduce the dose to 15 mg IV for a patient >65 years of age, less than 110 pounds, or with renal impairment.
Onset	IM onset 10 minutes, peak 50 minutes, duration 4 to 6 hours
Side effects	Nephrotoxicity, dysuria, hematuria, oliguria, azotemia, blood dyscrasia

PHENERGAN

Phenergan (promethazine)	
Indications	Nausea, vomiting
Dose	12.5 to 25 mg IV When used intravenously, promethazine injection should be given in concentration no greater than 25 mg/ml at a rate not to exceed 25 mg/min. Preferably inject through a medication port in IV tubing that is known to be functioning satisfactorily. 25 to 50 mg IM
Pediatric dose	0.25 to 0.5 mg/kg IM or IV every 4 to 6 hours if > 2-year-old
Onset	IM onset 20 min., duration 4 to 6 hours IV onset 3 to 5 min., duration 4 to 6 hours
Side effects	Drowsiness, sedation, hypotension, palpitations, tachycardia
Monitor	Vital signs, sedation, respiratory effectiveness

VALIUM

Valium (diazepam)	
Indications	Muscle spasm

Valium (diazepam)	
Dose	5 to 20 mg IM single dose 5 to 10 mg IV single dose
Onset	IV onset 5 min., peak 15 min., duration 15 min. IM onset 15 min., peak ½ to 1 ½ hours, duration 1 to 1 ½ hours
Side effects	Dizziness, drowsiness, orthostatic hypotension, blurred vision, tachycardia
Monitor	Level of consciousness, respiratory effectiveness

RELATED INFORMATION

ACUTE LOW BACK STRAIN

Acute low back strain is diagnosed by a history that presents clear evidence of a twisting or bending injury. Pain is localized with paraspinal muscular spasm, restriction of movement, and no radiation of pain to the groins or legs. Treatment may include analgesics, skeletal muscle relaxants, and rest.

BACK PAIN

Back Pain Location and Referred Pain	
Pain Location	Can be referred pain from . . .
T10 to 12	Peptic ulcers Tumor of stomach, duodenum, or pancreas
Low back pain	Ulcerative colitis, diverticulitis, PID Cancer of the ovary, uterus, or prostate, or bone disease involving the pelvis
Costovertebral angle	Renal disease
Thoracic-lumbar pain	Aortic dissecting aneurysm
Note	Back pain referred from visceral disease reveals no signs of stiffness and movement of the back does not increase the pain.

CHRONIC LOW BACK PAIN

Chronic low back pain is usually due to degenerative disease of the vertebra with bony spurs, narrowing of the canal, and impingement on nerve roots. Pain is often under treated in the ER because of the medical provider's fear of contributing to addiction. Therefore, patients have a tendency to exaggerate their symptoms. Treatment may include large doses of narcotic pain medications, steroids, and muscle relaxants.

LUMBAR DISC HERNIATION

Lumbar intervertebral disk herniation is most common at L5, S1, less common at L4, L5, and rare at L3, L4 or higher. Findings may include backache, abnormal posture, and limitation of movement. Nerve root involvement is indicated by radiation of the pain unilaterally with sensory disturbances and reflex impairment.

LUMBAR SPINAL STENOSIS

The lumbar spine consists of the five vertebrae in the lower part of the spine between the ribs and the pelvis. Lumbar spinal stenosis is a narrowing in the spinal canal which compresses the nerves traveling through the lower back into the legs. The inflammation of the nerves due to increased pressure causes noticeable symptoms to occur. Degenerative spondylolisthesis and degenerative scoliosis are two conditions associated with lumbar spinal stenosis. Degenerative spondylolisthesis (slippage of one vertebra over another) is caused by osteoarthritis of the facet joints. Typically, it involves the L4 slipping over the L5 vertebra. Degenerative scoliosis (curvature of the spine) occurs most frequently in the lower back. Back pain associated with degenerative scoliosis usually begins gradually and is linked with activity.

VERTEBRAL FRACTURES

Vertebral fractures commonly result from a flexion injury or from a fall with a feet-first landing. Diagnosis is made by x-ray. Vertebral fractures may occur with minimal or no trauma in patients with osteoporosis, multiple myeloma, metastatic bone disease, or Paget's disease.

PEDIATRIC CONSIDERATIONS

BACK PAIN IN CHILDREN

Back Pain in Children	
Disorder	Definition
Scheuermann's Disease (kyphosis)	A common cause of middle (thoracic) back pain in adolescents. Vertebrae become wedged, causing a rounded or hunched back. Pain increases with activity.
Spondylolysis (stress fracture)	May cause lower back pain in adolescents. Pain is usually mild and may radiate to the buttocks and legs. It feels worse with activity and better with rest. A child with spondylolysis may have a stiff-legged walk with short stride length.
Spondylolisthesis	The occurrence of one vertebra shifting forward on the next vertebra below.
Diskitis (disk infection)	Typically affects children aged 1 to 5. Pain in the lower back or abdomen and limited range of motion of the spine, limp or refuse to walk, squat with a straight spine to reach a toy on the floor, rather than bend over
Tumor	Rare. Usually presents in the middle or lower back. Pain is constant, progressive, unrelated to activity, and often at night. Child may have pain, or weakness extending into the legs.

Back Pain in Children	
Backpack syndrome	Backpacks can equal 20% to 40% of the child's own body weight and this may cause strain on the back over time.

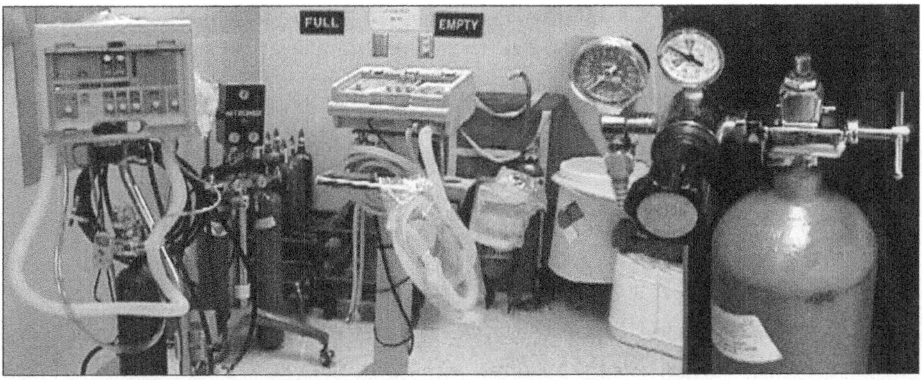

06 BREATHING EMERGENCY

For details on triage see Chapter 34, Triage in a Nutshell.

PATIENT'S STORY – INTERVIEW QUESTIONS

1. When was the onset of the breathing problem?
2. Are any other symptoms associated with the breathing problem?
3. How does the breathing problem affect normal function?
    a. Does the patient have orthopnea (breathing discomfort in all positions except upright, sitting, or standing) or dyspnea (air hunger)?
    b. Is the patient able to sleep and rest?
    c. Is the patient able to tolerate normal activity?
4. Was any treatment started before coming to the hospital and has it helped?
5. Has the patient had similar problems before?
    a. When was the problem?
    b. What was the diagnosis and treatment?
6. Is the patient on oxygen at home?
    a. What is the rate of flow?
    b. How often does the patient use the oxygen?
7. Has the patient ever been on a breathing machine?
8. Does the patient have any pertinent past history?
    a. Does the patient have heart problems?
    b. Does the patient have asthma, COPD, or emphysema?

   c. Does the patient smoke tobacco or have a smoking history? If so, how much? Pack years is the average number of packs per day times the number of years smoked.

9. Does the patient take any routine medications?
   a. What is the name, dosage, route, and frequency of each medication?
   b. When was the last dose?
10. Does the patient take any complementary or alternative therapies, herbal products, over-the-counter medications or supplements, or natural therapies?
    a. What is the name, dosage, route and frequency of each therapy?
    b. When was the last dose or therapy?
11. Does the patient have allergies to drugs or foods?
    a. What is the name of the allergen?
    b. What was the reaction?
12. When was the patient's last tetanus immunization, flu vaccine, and pneumonia vaccine?
13. If the patient is female and between the ages of 10 to 50 years, when was the first day of her last menstrual period?

NURSING DOMAIN

The nursing domain, nursing diagnosis and plan of care can only be determined after an in-depth interview and consideration of the patient's story.

Domain 12. Comfort. Class 1. Physical comfort.
Domain 3. Elimination and Exchange. Class 4. Respiratory Function.

ANTICIPATED MEDICAL CARE

Review of the Anticipated Medical Care of Breathing Emergencies	
Exam	Full body
Urine test	Pregnancy test for women of child-bearing age with no history of a hysterectomy
Blood tests	ABG analysis, CBC, electrolytes, chemistries, drug levels if taking Aminophyllin, blood cultures if febrile
Sputum	Culture, gram stain
ECG	ECG for females and males over 35 years
X-ray	PA and lateral chest x-ray, portable one view at the bedside for unstable patients
Other	Peak expiratory flow rate (PEFR), ventilation perfusion scan

Review of the Anticipated Medical Care of Breathing Emergencies	
Diet	NPO
IV	Hydration with NS or Ringer's solution if patient has COPD without fluid overload. No intravenous infusion if the patient has a fluid overload (CHF or pulmonary edema).
Medications	Diuretics, NTG, and potassium replacements for patients with fluid overload. IV steroids and bronchodilators by hand-held nebulizer for patients with COPD.
Other	Supplemental oxygen by mask, BiPAP, or endotracheal intubation and mechanical ventilation to keep saturation > 94%, an indwelling urinary catheter to monitor urinary output (normal urinary output in a child is 1 to 2 ml/kg per hour and normal adult urinary output is > 30 ml/hr.) Severe COPD patients may be unable to maintain saturation >88% to 92%.
Disposition	Hospital admission may be required if the patient is unable to ventilate effectively (respiratory rate > 30, heart rate >120, PEFR < 120 L/min., FEV < 1000 ml, oxygen sat >88 to 92%).
Worst-case scenario	The worst-case scenario is an unnoticed pCO2 build-up to toxic levels causing coma. Management is mechanical ventilation to correct the acid-base problem.

INITIAL CARE PLAN

> Alcohol-based hand sanitizers are the preferred method for cleaning your hands in most clinical situations. Wash your hands with soap and water whenever they are visibly dirty, before eating, and after using the restroom.

1. Ask the patient to undress, remove necklaces and other jewelry that might interfere with the exam, and put on an exam gown. Assist as needed.
2. Obtain initial vital signs including oxygen saturation. Consider obtaining a rectal temperature if the patient is mouth breathing.
3. Place on oxygen to maintain an oxygen saturation of > 94%. Severe COPD patients may be unable to maintain saturation >88% to 92%.
4. Position the patient to expand lungs and enhance breathing, e.g., sitting with arms supported in an armchair like position.
5. Observe for signs of respiratory distress, e.g., flaring nostrils, the use of accessory muscles, learning forward in a tripod position, head bobbing, and decreased level of alertness. Use these indicators as a quick assessment of the patient's ability to cope with the breathing problem.
6. Perform a focused patient examination
   a. Auscultate the lungs (instruct the patient to take several quick, short, deep breaths).

b. Inspect for peripheral edema.

7. Evaluate the level of consciousness based on the mnemonic **AVPU** or **ACDU** level of consciousness score.
AVPU: **A**lert, **V**erbal, **P**ain, **U**nresponsive.
ACDU: **A**lert, **C**onfused, **D**rowsy, **U**nresponsive.

8. Establish and maintain intravenous access for administration of medications and intravenous fluids.
    a. Hydrate a COPD patient with normal saline
    b. Limit fluids on a patient with CHF, pulmonary edema or renal insufficiency.

9. If the patient is wheezing, initiate treatment with bronchodilators via nebulizer according to hospital policy.

10. Consider placing a urinary indwelling catheter if an accurate output is needed or the patient is activity intolerant.

11. Advise the patient and family if fluids are encouraged or limited. Hydrate a COPD patient and limit fluids on a patient with CHF, pulmonary edema or renal insufficiency. Also, inform the family of the rationale for the need to abide by the NPO status or fluid restrictions.

12. Elevate the siderails and place the stretcher in the lowest position.

13. Inform the patient, family, and caregivers of the usual plan of care. Include time involved for each aspect of the stay and the expected overall time in the ER.

14. Provide the patient with a device to reach someone for assistance and explain how to use it. Ask the patient to call for help before getting off the stretcher.

ONGOING CARE PLAN

> Inform the medical provider of adverse changes noted during ongoing evaluation. Document that the medical provider was notified of the adverse change. Document if orders were or were not received.

1. Monitor vital signs and effectiveness of breathing and circulation.
2. Keep oxygen saturation > 94%. Severe COPD patients may be unable to maintain saturation >88% to 92%.
3. Monitor therapy closely for the patient's therapeutic response to bronchodilators by nebulizer.
    a. Peak flow rates before and after bronchodilator treatments are the most reliable measure of the effectiveness of the bronchodilator.
    b. Onset is rapid. If therapy does not improve the peak flow within 20 minutes, ask the medical provider for a repeat dose or an alternative.
4. Monitor intake and output hourly.
5. Monitor closely for the development of adverse reactions to therapy.

   a. Perform interventions to relieve the adverse reaction.
   b. Ask the medical provider for a remedy.
6. Provide the patient with food at mealtimes.
7. Keep the patient, family, and caregivers well informed of the plan of care and the remaining time anticipated before disposition.
8. Monitor the patient's laboratory and x-ray results. Notify the medical provider of critical abnormalities. Remedy abnormalities as ordered.
9. Notify the medical provider when all diagnostic results are available for review. Ask for establishment of a diagnosis and disposition.

DISCHARGE INSTRUCTIONS

1. Provide the patient with the name of the nurse and doctor in the emergency room.
2. Inform the patient of their diagnosis or why a definitive diagnosis couldn't be made. Explain what caused the problem if known.
3. Instruct the congestive heart failure patient:
   a. To weigh daily and keep a log of the daily weights until seen by the follow-up medical provider. A daily weight gain of a couple of pounds is a sign of fluid buildup and the follow-up medical provider should be notified. An increase in the diuretic medication may be needed.
   b. Notify the follow-up medical provider immediately for shortness of breath, swelling, or chest pain. If the medical provider is not immediately available, return to the ER.
4. Instruct the COPD patient that:
   a. The best treatment is prevention, maintaining adequate hydration, using mediations on a regular basis, avoiding smoke, and seeking early treatment.
   b. Influenza and pneumonia are the most common causes of respiratory infections. Ask the patient to seek medical advice about vaccines for influenza and pneumonia.
   c. Follow-up is essential. Notify the follow-up medical provider immediately for worsening of symptoms. If the medical provider is not immediately available, return to the ER.
5. Instruct the patient with a rib contusion or a minor rib fracture to report fever, dyspnea on exertion, or sputum production to the follow-up medical provider as they may indicate pneumonia.
6. Teach the patient how to take the medication as prescribed and how to manage the common side effects. Instruct the patient not to drive or perform any dangerous tasks while taking narcotic pain medications.
7. Recommend a medical provider for follow-up care. Provide the name, address, and phone number with a recommendation of when to schedule the care.

8. Call the follow-up medical provider immediately or return to the emergency room if the problem worsens or any unusual symptoms develop. Encourage the patient NOT to IGNORE WORSENING OF SYMPTOMS.
9. Ask for verbal confirmation or demonstration of understanding and reinforce teaching as needed.

MEDICATIONS

AMINOPHYLLIN

Aminophyllin	
Indications	Asthma, wheezing, bronchospasm
Adult dose	5 mg/kg IV loading dose over 30 to 45 minutes, maximum loading dose 500 mg 0.7 mg/kg/hr IV maintenance x 12 hours and then 0.5 mg/kg/hr.
Pediatric dose	5.6 mg/kg IV loading dose over ½ hour, maintenance 1 mg/kg/hr
Onset	IV onset immediate, duration 6 to 8 hours
Compatible	Compatible at Y-site with potassium chloride, Bretylium, Dopamine, heparin, Inocor, Lidocaine, Neo-Synephrine, nitroglycerin, Pronestyl
Adverse reaction	Restlessness, insomnia, muscle twitching, tachycardia, nausea, vomiting
Note	Check Theophylline level if patient is on oral medication before giving a loading dose. Theophylline 400 mg equals Aminophyllin 500 mg. Aminophylline brand names include Phyllocontin and Truphylline. Theophylline brand names include Elixophyllin, Quibron-T, Respbid, Slo-Bid Gyrocaps, T-Phyl, Theo-24, Theo-Dur, Theo-X, Theobid, Theochron, Theoclear L.A.-130, Theovent, Truxophyllin, and Uniphyl. Congestive heart failure slows the metabolism of theophylline and can result in toxicity.

BUMEX

Bumex (bumetanide)	
Indications	Fluid overload
Dose	1 to 2 mg IV, maximum 20 mg/day
Onset	IV onset 5 minutes, peak ½ hour, duration 2 to 3 hours
Side effects	Orthostatic hypotension, hypokalemia, hyperglycemia

Bumex (bumetanide)	
Monitor	Urinary output, blood pressure

LASIX

Lasix (furosemide)	
Indications	Peripheral edema, congestive heart failure, pulmonary edema
Dose	0.5 to 1 mg/kg over 1 to 2 min. If no response, double the dose to 2 mg/kg over 1 to 2 min.
Onset	IV onset 5 minutes, peak ½ hour, duration 2 hours
Side effects	Circulatory collapse, hypokalemia, loss of hearing, nausea
Monitor	Output, blood pressure

PROVENTIL

Proventil, Albuterol, Ventolin	
Indications	Bronchospasm, asthma
Adult Dose	2.5 to 5 mg nebulized
Pediatric dose	Nebulized pediatric dose: Age < 1 year .05 to .15 mg/kg Age 1 to 5 years 1.25 to 2.5 mg/dose Age 5 to 12 years 2.5 mg/dose Age > 12 years 2.5 to 5 mg/dose
Onset	Inhaled onset 5 to 15 min., peak 1 to 1 ½ hour, duration 4 to 6 hours
Side effects	Anxiety, tremors, tachycardia
Monitor	Oxygen saturation, heart rate
Other Bronchodilators	
Alupent	Alupent is a long acting bronchodilator. Usual adult nebulized dose is 0.3 ml of a 5% solution of 2.5 ml NS.
Xopenex	Commonly used as a short acting bronchodilator. Usual adult dose is 0.63 mg in 2.5 ml of NS nebulized every 6 to 8 hours in adults and children 6 years and up.

SOLU-MEDROL

Solu-Medrol (methylprednisolone)	
Indications	Severe inflammation, shock, contact dermatitis, pruritus
Dose	100 to 250 mg IV
Pediatric dose	117 mcg to 1.66 mg/kg IV in 3 to 4 divided doses
Onset	IV onset rapid, IM onset unknown, duration 1 to 4 weeks

Solu-Medrol (methylprednisolone)	
Side effects	Circulatory collapse, thrombophlebitis, embolism, thrombocytopenia
Monitor	Hypokalemia and hyperglycemia are adverse effects of long-term therapy.

RELATED INFORMATION

ABG CRITICAL VALUES

Review of ABG Critical Values Requiring Interventions	
pH	Critical value < 7.25 or > 7.55
pCO2	Critical value > 55 and > 60 for COPD patients
O2	Critical value < 55
SpO2	Critical value < 85 (equals a pO2 of 46 to 56)

ABG OXYGEN SATURATION

Review of ABG Oxygen Saturation Levels in Arterial and Venous Blood	
Arterial blood	Oxygen saturation is usually >75%.
Venous blood	Oxygen saturation is usually <75%.
Mixed arterial and venous blood	A specimen of mixed arterial and venous blood commonly has an oxygen saturation level in the eighties. Check the patient's saturation with a pulse oximetry. If oxygen saturation in the ABG result is less than the pulse oximetry saturation, redraw the ABG. The ABG specimen was probably mixed arterial and venous blood.

ACID-BASE IMBALANCE

Review of Acid-Base Imbalance	
Respiratory Acidosis	ABG findings of a pH < 7.35 with a CO2 > 45 are characteristic of respiratory failure. Symptoms may include confusion and lowered level of consciousness. Causes are sedatives, stroke, chronic pulmonary disease, airway obstruction, severe pulmonary edema, and cardiopulmonary arrest. Management is aimed at improvement of ventilation with pulmonary toilet and reversal of bronchospasm. Intubation may be required.

Review of Acid-Base Imbalance	
Respiratory Alkalosis	ABG findings of alkalosis are characteristic of excessive ventilation causing a primary reduction in CO2 and an increase in pH. Symptoms may include seizures, tetany, cardiac arrhythmia, or loss of consciousness. Causes include pneumonia, pulmonary edema, interstitial lung disease, and asthma. Pain and psychogenic causes are common. Other causes include fever, hypoxemia, sepsis, delirium tremens, salicylates, hepatic failure, mechanical hyperventilation, and central nervous system lesions. Management is directed at the underlying disorder. Sedation may be used for psychogenic cases.

ACUTE EPIGLOTTITIS

Acute epiglottitis is a rare life-threatening process in children between the ages of 3 and 7 years. It is associated with a large, cherry-red, edematous epiglottis. The symptoms are drooling, muffled voice sounds or aphonia, dysphagia, and a croaking froglike sound on inspiration. The child may assume the tripod position (sitting forward leaning on both arms) for better air exchange. The child should not be disturbed for fear of worsening the airway obstruction. Vital signs are not taken until the potential of airway obstruction has passed. Parents are asked to stay with the child because separation may increase the child's anxiety and oxygen needs. Visualization of the epiglottis should not be attempted until intubation and tracheotomy equipment are available. Complete airway obstruction can occur suddenly. Bacteremia is present in 50% of cases.

AIRWAY OBSTRUCTIONS

The most common cause of airway obstruction is a relaxed tongue that falls over the back of the throat obstructing the pharynx and larynx. Because the tongue is attached to the lower jaw, performing a head-tilt-chin-lift maneuver forces the tongue away from the back of the throat and restores spontaneous respirations. When a patient goes into respiratory arrest, the first priority is to open the airway with a head-tilt-chin-lift or a jaw-thrust maneuver.

ACUTE MOUNTAIN SICKNESS

Acute mountain sickness (AMS) can start to appear at an altitude of 6,500 feet above sea level. Symptoms often start 6 to 10 hours after ascent and usually subside in 1 to 2 days. They include headache (may be caused by cerebral edema) combined with dizziness, nausea, and fatigue. Exertion aggravates the symptoms. AMS can develop into pulmonary and cerebral edema.

The weight of the air in the atmosphere at sea level is equivalent to 10 meters (32 feet) of water pressing down on us. When the elevation is increased (such as flying or climbing a mountain), there is less air atmosphere and the pressure on the body is less. The important effect of this decrease in pressure is that the percentage of oxygen is exactly the same or 21%. The problem is that there are fewer molecules of oxygen present. The air is referred to as thinner.

ALLEN'S TEST

Before puncturing the radial artery for cannulation, such as drawing ABGs, it is important to evaluate the competency of the ulnar artery should injury to the radial artery occur. An abnormal (positive) Allen's test is suggestive of inadequate collateralization.

Allen's test:

- Both ulnar and radial arteries are manually occluded to prevent arterial flow while the patient repeatedly makes a tight fist to squeeze venous blood out of the hand.
- The patient then extends the fingers, and the examiner observes the blanched hand.
- Compression on the ulnar artery is released, and the examiner observes the hand filling with blood. If filling does not occur within 5 to 10 seconds, radial artery puncture should not be done.

ARTERIAL BLOOD GAS SAMPLING

Under sterile conditions, insert a 22 to 25-gauge needle attached to a heparinized syringe into the radial artery just proximal to the maximal impulse of the radial arterial pulse at an angle. Advance the needle slightly distally into the artery until pulsatile blood is returned. Collect 3 to 5 ml of blood, withdraw the needle quickly, and apply firm pressure to facilitate hemostasis. Place the ABG blood specimen on ice to reduce O_2 consumption and CO_2 production.

ASTHMA

Review of Asthma	
Description	The National Asthma Education Program defines asthma as a disease characterized by airway obstruction that is reversible, airway inflammation, and increased airway responsiveness to a variety of stimuli. Status asthmaticus is obstruction that lasts days or weeks. Extrinsic asthma is asthma due to a known allergen or environmental factor, e.g., pollen, dander, feathers, dust, and foods. Intrinsic asthma is asthma assumed to be due to some endogenous cause because no external cause can be determined.
Symptoms	Symptoms may include bronchospasm with wheezes and a prolonged expiratory phase.
Tests	Chest x-ray may show hilar or basilar infiltrates or be normal.
Management	Medications may include inhaled nebulized bronchodilators every 20 min. for three doses, then every 2 hours until attack subsides. Peak flow rates are essential before and after each bronchodilator treatment to determine the effectiveness of the therapy. Theophylline and Prednisone may be used. Panic and anxiety can be avoided by maintaining a calm reassuring attitude.
Note	An estimated 5% of adults and 10% of children have asthma.

AUTOTRANSFUSION

Autotransfusion is indicated for a patient with hemothorax and hypotension. A basic autotransfusion device is attached to a chest tube and infused intravenously. Autotransfusion from other sites, such as the abdomen, places the patient at an increased risk for bacterial contamination. In the emergency setting, sites other than the chest are not used unless the patient is exsanguinating and no blood products are available.

CLINICAL ASSESSMENT OF LUNGS

Review of Clinical Assessment of Lungs	
Auscultation	Bronchial sounds are normally heard over the bronchus and the manubrium of the sternum (the broad upper division of the sternum with which the clavicle and first two ribs articulate), along the sternal border, and over the trachea. Bronchial sounds heard over the lungs indicate abnormal sound transmission and may be due to consolidation such as atelectasis and pneumonia. Bronchial vesicular sounds are normally heard over the large bronchi below the clavicles and between the scapulae. They are of moderate amplitude, medium to high pitched, and resemble a mixture of bronchial and vesicular sounds. Bronchial vesicular sounds may indicate consolidation or other abnormalities if heard over the lungs. Vesicular sounds are normally produced by the opening of the alveoli on inspiration, the movement of air through the larynx during expiration, heard over the lungs, of low amplitude, medium to low pitch, and described as swishing or rustling. Decreased breath sounds may indicate disruption of alveolar function, consolidation or compression (pulmonary fibrosis, pleural effusion, or COPD).
Palpation	Palpation for tenderness is used in trauma cases to assess for injured areas. Chest excursion is measured by placing the hands parallel to each other over the lower portion of the rib cage on both sides of the spine. The fingers should be 2 inches apart with thumbs pointing toward the spine with fingers spread laterally. On deep inspiration, observe the movement of the thumbs. Chest excursion should separate the thumbs 1 ½ to 3 inches.
Percussion	Percussion is performed over the intercostal spaces following a systemic pattern to compare both sides. The posterior thorax is normally resonant on percussion and the area over the scapula, ribs, and spine is dull. Areas of consolidation are dull.

Review of Clinical Assessment of Lungs	
Adventitious sounds	Crackles (rales) are the most common in dependent lobes and are caused by fluid. Rhonchi are heard over the trachea and bronchi and are caused by fluid in the larger airways. Wheezes can be heard over all lung fields and are caused by bronchospasm that narrows the airways. Pleural friction rub is heard over the lateral lung fields with the patient upright and is caused by inflamed pleura.

BRONCHITIS, ACUTE

Review of Acute Bronchitis	
Description	Bronchitis is an acute inflammation of the bronchus most often caused by viral infectious agents. Secondary bacterial infection also occurs.
Signs and symptoms	Signs and symptoms may include a recent upper respiratory infection and a dry nonproductive cough that is worse at night. Taking a deep breath or talking may initiate coughing. Sputum production occurs in a few days. Scattered wheezes and a mild fever may be present.
Tests	Chest x-ray may be normal.
Management	Management may include humidified oxygen, cough suppressant medications, and antibiotics for bacterial infections.
Prognosis	Prognosis is good. The disease is usually self-limiting.

BRONCHITIS, CHRONIC

Review of Chronic Bronchitis	
Description	Chronic bronchitis occurs frequently in middle-aged men and is uncommon in non-smokers.
Signs and symptoms	Signs and symptoms are excessive mucus production and a cough that occurs for at least 3 consecutive months each year for 2 successive years.
Tests	Chest x-ray may be insignificant. In the late stages, chest x-ray may reveal hyperinflation.
Management	Management may include bronchodilators, nebulized inhalers, and steroids.

CONGESTIVE HEART FAILURE

Review of Congestive Heart Failure

Review of Congestive Heart Failure	
Causes	Congestive heart failure is a fluid overload brought about by an inadequate heart pump. Forward failure causes fluid to accumulate in the lungs and backward failure causes fluid to accumulate in the body. The most common cause of right ventricular failure is left ventricular failure. The increasing pulmonary venous and arterial pressures of the left ventricular failure increase the preload of the right ventricle. Other causes of right ventricular failure are lung disease, valvular disease, and right ventricular infarction. Congestive heart failure slows the metabolism of drugs such as theophylline that are predominant cleared by the liver and can lead to early development of toxicity.
Symptoms	Forward failure (left ventricular failure): Early signs of respiratory failure may include activity intolerance, tachypnea, orthopnea, shortness of breath, and tachycardia. Cyanosis and production of pink frothy sputum are late signs. Impaired ventilation causes hypoxia and hypercapnia. Backward failure (right ventricular failure): Symptoms may include peripheral edema and hepatosplenomegaly from systemic vascular engorgement (with or without tenderness).
Diagnostic findings	ABG findings may include hypoxia and respiratory acidosis. Electrocardiogram may show left ventricular enlargement. Chest x-ray may have findings of infiltrates (pulmonary fluid overload) and an enlarged heart.
Management	The goal of therapy is to maintain sufficient oxygenation to body tissues by increasing oxygenation, decreasing preload, decreasing afterload, and increasing the contractility of the heart. Medical management may include oxygen to keep oxygen saturation > 94%, fluid restriction, diuretics (Lasix, Bumex) to reduce the fluid preload, inotropic medications (digoxin, dobutamine) to increase the pumping action of the heart, morphine to decrease anxiety and the workload placed on the heart, and blood pressure reducing medications (nitroglycerin, nitroprusside) to decrease afterload.

COPD

Review of COPD	
Description	COPD is a group of conditions that include chronic bronchitis and emphysema. Asthma and reactive airway disease are in their own category. These conditions cause hyperplasia, inflammation of goblet cells, and increased production of thick mucus.

Review of COPD	
Facts	Smoking is the most significant factor contributing to the patient's condition. Cessation of smoking may prevent progression. A patient with severe bronchial abnormalities and mild emphysema is commonly called a blue bloater. Hypoventilation leads to hypoxemia and hypercapnia. The patient with severe emphysema and mild bronchitis is commonly called a pink puffer. Hyperventilation assists in adequate oxygenation and cyanosis is absent. Cor pulmonale (hypertrophy or failure of the right ventricle) is a complication of COPD secondary to decreased intravascular blood volume with arterial congestion. A common sign of COPD is a barrel chest that results from hyperinflation and over distention of alveoli. Elastin and collagen, the supporting structures of the lungs, are destroyed and the bronchiolar walls tend to collapse. Air is trapped in the distal alveoli resulting in hyperinflation and over distention of the alveoli. This trapped air causes the barrel chest.
Management	Medical management may include administration of 30% oxygen via mask and bronchodilators by nebulized therapy, steroids, and hydration. Most COPD patients are dependent on the hypoxic drive to maintain adequate ventilation. Uncontrolled or high-flow oxygen therapy may precipitate severe carbon dioxide narcosis and respiratory arrest. Precise oxygen therapy delivered by mask may allow time for medical intervention, thus avoiding intubation and mechanical ventilation. Placing the patient in a high Fowler's position or leaning upright over an over-bed table will ensure optimal ventilation. Pursed lip breathing slows expiration, prevents collapse of lung units, and helps the patient control rate and depth of respirations that decreases dyspnea and feelings of panic.

CROUP

A low-grade fever and a barking or brassy cough with inspiratory stridor caused by partial upper airway obstruction characterize croup. Croup commonly follows an upper respiratory infection by one to two days. The earliest signs of respiratory failure are hypoxemia, restlessness, tachypnea, and tachycardia. A fever can increase respiratory rate by four breaths per minute for each degree rise above normal. Intermediate signs of respiratory failure are accessory respiratory muscle use, retractions, and nasal flaring. Late signs are cyanosis and lethargy. Treatment is directed towards maintaining the airway and adequate respiratory exchange. Aspirin is avoided as an antipyretic because it has been correlated with Reyes syndrome. Medical management of croup may include a cool high-humidity mist, hydration, oxygen, steroids, racemic epinephrine, and intubation for anoxia and airway obstruction. Intravenous hydration is weight based and monitored by skin turgor and urinary output. An initial intravenous fluid bolus of 20 ml/kg can be given based on the child's hemodynamic response. The 4-2-1 rule for maintenance fluids is 4 ml/kg for the first 10 kg of body weight, 2 ml/kg for the next 10 kg of body weight, and 1 ml/kg for the rest of the weight.

Hydration should be provided by the least invasive method possible. The benefit of steroids is clearly demonstrated in clinical research. Racemic epinephrine is the mainstay of treatment because it decreased airway edema. All children who receive racemic epinephrine should also receive steroids. Racemic epinephrine is given by nebulizer commonly 0.25 to 0.5 mL of 2.25% solution diluted in 3 mL of isotonic sodium chloride solution or sterile water and repeated up to 3 times. Monitor the child in the ER for 2 hours post treatment because of the potential of rebound respiratory distress.

ENDOTRACHEAL INTUBATION

Endotracheal intubation is attempted only after other methods of oxygenation have failed. It is not the initial procedure for ventilation in respiratory arrest. Adequate oxygenation is first provided with the use of a bag-valve-mask device. If intubation takes more than 20 to 30 seconds, oxygenation is required with a bag-valve-mask device between attempts. Endotracheal tube placement is confirmed by first listening over the stomach for sounds of rushing air. If nothing is heard, the lungs are then auscultated. If breath sounds are heard, both lungs are auscultated to confirm equality. Final tube placement is confirmed by a portable chest x-ray. The carina is the landmark by which proper depth of endotracheal intubation is measured.

RAPID SEQUENCE INTUBATION (RSI)

Rapid Sequence Intubation (RSI)	
Hospital Policy	Policies vary
Pre-oxygenation	Oxygen at FiO2 100% by mask or ventilate gently if assistance is needed
Pre-medications Wait 3 minutes	Fentanyl 2 to 3 mcg/kg given at a rate of 1 to 2 mcg/kg per minute IV for analgesia if the patient is awake Atropine 0.01 mg/kg IV push for children or adolescents (minimum dose of 0.1 mg) Lidocaine 1.5 to 2.0 mg/kg IV over 30 to 60 seconds (may cause a 2 to 3 min. decrease in intracranial pressure)
Induction and paralysis	Sedation: Etomidate 0.2 to 0.6 mg/kg IV push Paralysis: Succinylcholine 1.5 mg/kg IV push (use 2.0 mg/kg in for infants and small children)

Rapid Sequence Intubation (RSI)	
Mechanical maneuvers	Apply pressure to the cricoid cartilage, pass and position the tube, evaluate breath sounds, ETCO2, CXR, and secure endotracheal tube with commercial holder.
Post intubation medications	MSO4 2 to 4 mg IV Valium 2 to 5 mg IV Pavulon 10 mg IV
Drug onset and duration	Times are approximate Lidocaine onset 45 sec, duration 15 min Pavulon onset 40 sec, duration 50 min Norcuron onset 4 min, duration 50 min Etomidate onset 1 min, duration 4 min Succinylcholine onset 1 min, duration 9 min
Considerations for RSI	Low or high adult respiratory rate <12 >30 Glasgow Coma Scale < 8 or rapidly deteriorating Poor oxygenation or SpO2 <95% Poor ventilation, High pCO2 Inability to control airway Airway obstruction Prolonged transport CPR in progress Blood pressure < 90 SpO2 <95% despite bag value mask support Suspect C-spine fracture Foreign body Inability to open mouth or visualize uvula Laryngeal trauma (needs fiber optic intubation or surgical tracheotomy)

Rapid Sequence Intubation (RSI)	
Sample steps	1. Preparation: Gathering supplies 2. Pre-oxygenation: 100% 3. Pretreatment as indicated 4. Paralysis with induction 5. Positioning 6. Placement 7. Post-intubation management

EXTUBATION

Review of Extubation	
1	Obtain a negative inspiratory force (NIF) of > -20 cm. (normal < -50 to -100)
2	Obtain a forced vital capacity (FVC) of > 10 ml/kg (normal 40 to 70 ml/kg)
3	Suction the tube, suction the mouth, deflate the balloon, have the patient cough, and pull the tube during the cough.
4	Place the patient on supplemental oxygen at the same FiO2 used prior to extubation.
5	Monitor vital signs including oxygen saturation every 5 to 10 minutes for 30 minutes.

HYPERCAPNIA

Hypercapnia is the first change that occurs in severe airway obstruction in a child.

MECHANICAL VENTILATION MODES

Review of Mechanical Ventilation Modes	
BiPAP (Bi-level Positive Airway Pressure)	The BiPAP ventilator regulates flow as needed to maintain desired inspiratory and expiratory pressures. Less effort is needed for the patient to inspire and expire. Fluid in the lungs is lessened due to the positive pressure.
PEEP (Positive End Expiration Pressure)	PEEP is an expiratory ventilator maneuver that limits unimpeded expiratory flow at a preset level of system pressure.
CPAP (Continuous Positive Airway Pressure)	CPAP increases oxygenation by increasing positive airway pressure throughout the respiratory cycle and not just on expiration.
CMV (Controlled Mandatory Ventilation)	CMV delivers tidal volume at a preset rate regardless of the patient's inspiratory efforts.

Review of Mechanical Ventilation Modes	
ACV (Assist Control Ventilation)	ACV augments spontaneous ventilation in patients with normal respiratory drive but weak respiratory musculature.
PSV (Pressure Support Ventilation)	PSV provides positive pressure only in response to a spontaneous breath, so the patient determines rate of delivery.
IMV (Intermittent Mandatory Ventilation)	IMV provides positive pressure breaths at a preset volume and rate independent of the patient's effort.
SIMV (Synchronized Intermittent Mandatory Ventilation)	SIMV synchronizes a mandatory machine delivered breath with the patient's next spontaneous breath.

OXYGEN DELIVERY DEVICES

Oxygen Delivery Devices	Oxygen Delivered
Nasal cannula	4% oxygen per liter
Simple Mask	5 to 8 L/m equals 40% to 50% oxygen
Partial non-rebreather	6 to 8 L/m equals 55% to 70% oxygen
Non-rebreather	6 to 10 L/m equals 100% oxygen
Venturi mask	Variable 24% to 50% oxygen
Nebulizer with aerosol mask, face shield, and T-piece at 8 to 12 L/m	30% to 100% oxygen with controlled moisture and temperature

OXYGEN, HIGH FLOW

High flow oxygen is the first priority when a trauma patient is pale, diaphoretic, and hypoventilating. Long-term high flow oxygen on a COPD patient who is not hypoventilating can decrease the respiratory drive.

OXYGEN, SUPPLEMENTAL

Oxygen delivery systems deliver oxygen that is supplemental to room air. The percentage of supplemental oxygen must be added to the 21% oxygen in room air to equal the total amount delivered to the patient.

PEAK EXPIRATORY FLOW RATES (PEFR)

Peak expiratory flow rates before and after bronchodilator treatments are essential to determine the effectiveness of the bronchodilator therapy. PEFR is how much air is exhaled forcibly from full-lung inflation. Normal range is 400 to 600 L/min. 200 L/min. indicates respiratory fatigue. Oxygen saturation is the indicator for severity.

PETECHIAL RASH

Petechial rash may develop 12 to 96 hours after an injury and is a result of fat globules obstructing the capillaries in the skin and subcutaneous tissue. When a petechial rash is associated with breathing problems, it may be a sign of pulmonary fat embolism.

PNEUMONIA

Review of Pneumonia	
Description	Pneumonia is an acute bacterial, viral, or fungal infection of the pulmonary parenchyma. The most common causal agent is Streptococcus pneumoniae.
Symptoms	Symptoms may include fever, pleuritic chest pain, productive cough, and tachypnea.
Signs	Bronchial breath sounds over the lung area indicate pneumonia.
Tests	Tests may include chest x-ray, hematology, and sputum for gram stain and culture.
Findings	Chest x-ray may show a pattern characteristic of the infecting organism.
Management	Medical management includes identification of the infecting organism and initiation of appropriate antimicrobial therapy.
Note	1% of Americans will have pneumonia during their lifetime.

RESPIRATORY NORMAL VALUES

Review of Normal Respiratory Values	
Tidal volume	Adult male 500 ml. Adult female 400 ml.
Minute ventilation	Respiratory rate times tidal volume
Vital capacity	60 to 70 cc/kg
Peak expiratory flow rate	400 to 600 liters/min.

VENTILATOR SETTINGS, POST ARREST

Review of Post Arrest Ventilator Settings	
FiO2	100%
Inspiratory: Expiratory Ratio (I:E)	1:2
Mode	AC or SIMV
PEEP	Minus 5
Pressure Limits	10 cm H2O higher than pressure generated by the delivered tidal volume

Review of Post Arrest Ventilator Settings	
Rate	10 to 12 breaths per minute
Sensitivity	-2 cm H2O on assist control, not applicable on IMV
Temperature	97 degrees Fahrenheit (Gabriel Daniel Fahrenheit 1686-1736. German-born physicist who invented the mercury thermometer [1714] and devised the Fahrenheit temperature scale).

PULSE OXIMETRY SATURATION AND CORRESPONDING PO2

Pulse Oximetry Saturation and Corresponding pO2	
Saturation	Oxygen levels (pO2)
80% SpO2	40 to 49 pO2
85% SpO2	46 to 56 pO2
87% SpO2	49 to 60 pO2
90% SpO2	55 to 67 pO2
93% SpO2	63 to 78 pO2
95% SpO2	72 to 89 pO2

PULMONARY EDEMA

Review of Pulmonary Edema	
Description	Acute pulmonary edema is a result of an acute event. Inadequate pumping of the left ventricle causes cardiogenic pulmonary edema. Noncardiogenic pulmonary edema or adult respiratory distress syndrome (ARDS) is a result of damage to the alveolar-capillary membrane.
Signs and symptoms	Cardiogenic pulmonary edema may show signs of generalized fluid overload including dyspnea, decreased oxygenation, metabolic acidosis, crackles, wheezes, and productive cough with foamy or pink-tinged sputum.
Tests	Chest x-ray may show bilateral interstitial and alveolar infiltrates.
Management	Medical management may include strict fluid restriction, high-flow oxygen, bronchodilators, BiPAP, diuretics, dobutamine, nitroglycerin, intravenous morphine, and a urinary catheter to monitor output.
Note	Most patients who require mechanical ventilation have a 50% mortality rate. The triad of symptoms in heroin induced pulmonary edema is hypoxia, stupor, and miosis.

PULMONARY EMBOLUS

Review of Pulmonary Embolus	
Description	A pulmonary embolus is an embolus that causes obstruction of arterial pulmonary blood flow to the distal lung commonly resulting in ischemia and infarction of the lung.
Symptoms	Symptoms may include sudden onset of dyspnea, chest pain, and sinus tachycardia.
Tests	Tests may include blood hematology, ABG studies, chest x-ray, ventilation perfusion scan, and pulmonary arteriogram.
Diagnostic findings	Findings may include decreased oxygen on room air (PaO2 < 80 mm Hg) and elevated LDH. An elevated LDH is common in many diseases and alone is not diagnostic of pulmonary embolus. A PaO2 of > 80 is inconsistent with pulmonary embolus. The WBC may be elevated or normal.
Management	Medical management may include intravenous heparin. Heparin reduces the risk of secondary thrombi formation.

RESPIRATORY FAILURE

Respiratory failure is any condition in which the blood oxygen is insufficient to meet the demands of the tissues secondary to decreased lung function. A diagnosis of respiratory failure is based on the patient's history, clinical appearance, and serial changes in the ABG studies. ABG abnormalities alone do not indicate respiratory failure.

RESPIRATORY RATE RATIO TO PULSE

Respiratory rate ratio to pulse is 1:4. An adult with a respiratory rate of 20 will normally have a heart rate of 80.

SODIUM BICARBONATE

Although not commonly used for respiratory acidosis, one ampule of sodium bicarbonate can be given for each -5 of base excess to temporarily correct the pH in respiratory and metabolic acidosis. The acidity of the blood must be kept in a near normal range for medications to be effective.

SMOKE INHALATION

Smoke inhalation is a combination of carbon monoxide intoxication, upper airway obstruction, and chemical injury to the lower airways and lung parenchyma. Carbon monoxide is a killer. Most people that die in fires succumb from the carbon monoxide poisoning and toxic off gassing from the burning material before they are burned. Carbon monoxide links with the hemoglobin replacing the oxygen causing hypoxia and death.

SPONTANEOUS PNEUMOTHORAX

Review of Spontaneous Pneumothorax

Review of Spontaneous Pneumothorax	
Description	Pneumothorax is the collapse of a lung and most commonly occurs in patients between the ages of 20 and 40 years.
Symptoms	Symptoms may include sudden sharp chest pain and dyspnea.
Tests	Chest x-ray
Management	Observation may be indicated for a small pneumothorax area and chest tube insertion for large areas. The typical size chest tube (with or without a trocar) for an adult is#36 or #40 French for hemothorax, and#28 for a pneumothorax. The chest tube is not clamped for any reason including transport. Clamping does not allow the air or fluid to escape and tension may reoccur.
Complications	Complications include hemothorax or cardiovascular compromise from a tension pneumothorax.
Note	50% of the patients who need chest tubes suffer recurrence. A rupture or laceration of the diaphragm can allow the abdominal contents to enter the chest. The movement of the bowel into the thorax creates excessive pressures that compress and shift the thoracic structures and can mimic a pneumothorax.

SPUTUM COLOR

Sputum color may be an indicator of the pathological process. Yellow sputum may signify white blood cells that are the major component of pus. Green sputum may signify production of an enzyme produced by stagnant pus cells. Rust, red, and brown sputum may signify red blood cells in the sputum.

SUBCUTANEOUS EMPHYSEMA

Subcutaneous emphysema results from an increase in intrathoracic pressure that results in alveolar rupture. Air dissects into the tissue and gravitates up to the neck, face, and supraclavicular area. The air can be felt under the skin. A mediastinal air leak can arise from the esophagus or from the lungs. The leak can be heard during auscultation when air is compressed by the contraction of heart (Hamman's sign).

VENOUS CARBON DIOXIDE LEVELS

Elevated venous carbon dioxide levels are an indicator of acidosis.

GERIATRIC CONSIDERATIONS

RESPIRATORY CONSIDERATIONS

Geriatric Respiratory Considerations	
Cilia	Number and effectiveness decrease with age

Geriatric Respiratory Considerations	
Gag Reflex	Decreased due to fewer nerve endings in larynx and increases aspiration risk
Cough Reflex	Blunted with age and increases aspiration risk
Rib Cartilage	Becomes stiffer and may affect respiratory effort
Kyphosis	Bent posture may interfere with respiratory effort
Blood Vessels	Change with age and results in increased resistance in the lungs and lower cardiac output
Muscles	Weaken with age and may contribute to atelectasis

PEDIATRIC CONSIDERATIONS

ANATOMICAL DIFFERENCES

Pediatric Considerations Anatomical Differences	
Nose /Mouth	Smaller and more easily obstructed than adult
Pharynx	Proportionately larger than adult
Trachea	Narrower and more easily obstructed especially by swelling
Cricoid Cartilage	Less developed, less rigid, and narrowest part of the airway in children
Diaphragm	Chest wall softer and children more dependent on diaphragmatic breathing

BRADYCARDIA

Bradycardia is the most common arrhythmia in critically ill children and is usually a symptom of hypoxia.

PEDIATRIC VITAL SIGNS

Age	Respirations Breaths per Minute (BPM)	Pulse Beats per Minute (BPM)	Systolic Blood Pressure
Newborn	30 to 60	100 to 160	50 to 70
1 to 6 Weeks	30 to 60	100 to 160	70 to 95
6 Months	25 to 40	90 to 120	80 to 100
1 Year	20 to 30	90 to 120	80 to 100
3 Years	20 to 30	80 to 120	80 to 110
6 Years	18 to 25	70 to 110	80 to 110

Age	Respirations Breaths per Minute (BPM)	Pulse Beats per Minute (BPM)	Systolic Blood Pressure
10 Years	15 to 20	60 to 90	90 to 120

COMMON CAUSES OF RESPIRATORY EMERGENCIES IN CHILDREN

Disease	Related information
Croup	Acute viral illness causing edema and tracheal narrowing. Caused by Parainfluenza virus, rhinovirus, influenza A, or respiratory syncytial virus (RSV) Usually seen from 6 to 36 months of age Gradual onset cold with barking cough worse at night and low-grade fever. Symptoms may include tachycardia, tachypnea, retractions, inspiratory stridor, and expiratory wheezes. X-ray may show a narrowing of the trachea (Steeple Sign)
Epiglottitis	Acute bacterial illness and may progress to complete airway obstruction Caused by Haemophilus influenza Type B, Streptococcus pneumoniae, or staphylococcus. Acute presentation with high fever Symptoms may include sore throat, difficulty swallowing, muffled voice, drooling and the child may assume a tripod position X-ray may show epiglottic and aryepiglottic swelling. Blood cultures will usually be positive.
Foreign Body Obstruction	Acute obstruction Caused by foreign body Usually seen in children younger than 4 years old Symptoms will vary but may include drooling, stridor, wheezing, chest pain, or unequal breath sounds X-ray or direct visualization may show radiopaque item
Asthma	Chronic inflammatory disorder of the airway Symptoms include inspiratory or expiratory wheezes, prolonged expiratory phase, decreased or unequal breath sounds, tachypnea, and retractions, and coughing in the early morning or night

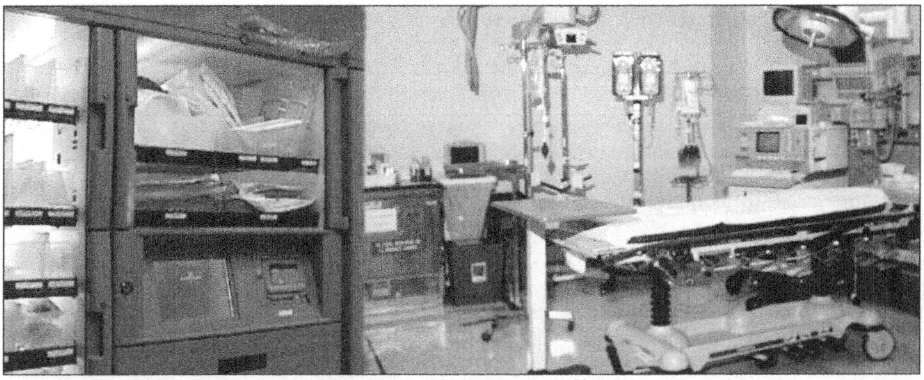

07 BURNS, EXPLOSIONS, AND SUNBURN

For details on triage see Chapter 34, Triage in a Nutshell.

PATIENT'S STORY – INTERVIEW QUESTIONS

1. When was the patient injured?
2. Where are the injuries and are any associated symptoms present, e.g., nausea, vomiting, headache, sweating, or an irregular heartbeat?
3. Does the patient know the cause of the injury, e.g., fire, blast forces, hot water, chemicals, sun?
4. If the cause of the burns is related to a fire, blast or chemicals, does the patient have signs of inhalation burns, e.g. soot in the nares, shortness of breath, coughing, soot in the sputum.
5. Identify the cause and degree of burn.

BURN CLASSIFICATION

Burn Classification	Presence of Pain	Clinical Signs
Superficial-Thickness Burns		
First Degree Epidermis and superficial dermis	Yes	Erythema, minor pain, no blisters
Partial-Thickness Burns		
Second Degree Moderate to deep dermis	Yes	Moderate: Blisters, moderate pain, clear fluid Deep: Whiter appearance, with decreased pain. Difficult to distinguish from full thickness burns

Burn Classification	Presence of Pain	Clinical Signs
Full-Thickness Burns		
Third degree Through the dermis and into subcutaneous fat and muscle	No	White, brown, or black dry leathery tissue (eschar), severe swelling
Fourth degree Through the subcutaneous fat and into the muscle or bone	No	Eschar, muscle and possible bone exposure

6. Calculate Total Body Surface Area (TBSA) of Burn
    a. Wallace's Rule of Nines: The rule of nines is a method for calculating the percentage of total body surface area burned in an adult. To determine the total body surface burned: calculate the head at 9%, front of trunk at 18%, back of trunk at 18%, arms at 9% each, legs at 18% each, and perineum at 1%, and add the percentages together. The rule of nines is not accurate when calculating burns in children.
    b. The Lund and Browder Chart: This chart method is the most accurate method to calculate burn injuries. It accounts for age and body shape differences; and it provides an accurate assessment of burns in both adults and children.
    c. Palmar surface of the hand: A method for calculating the total body surface area burned is to compare the burned area to the size of the patient's palm including the fingers. The palmer surface of the patient's hand equals roughly 1% of their body surface area.
2. For electrical burns:
    a. What was the voltage?
    b. Was it alternating current (AC) or direct current (DC)?

> Homes in the United Stated have AC 110 volt for normal household use and AC 220 volt for stoves, dryers, and other large appliances or tools. DC current is from a battery or an adapter.

    c. What was the duration of contact with the current?
    d. Can entrance, exit, or contact wounds be identified?
    e. Was there an associated flash or thermal burn?
3. Consider the nature of the emergency.
    a. For an eye burn injury, consider #16 Eye Emergency.
    b. For a chemical exposure, consider #08 Carbon Monoxide Inhalation and HAZMAT.
4. Was any treatment applied to the burn, e.g., water, ointment, aloe?

5. Was any treatment started before coming to the hospital and has it helped?
6. Is unlawful activity suspected?
    a. Was law enforcement at the scene?
    b. What agency?
    c. Were drugs or alcohol involved? If so, document what type, quantity, and last time ingested.

Medical personnel are obligated to notify law enforcement if unlawful activity is suspected.

7. Does the patient have any pertinent past history?
8. Does the patient take any routine medications?
    a. What is the name, dosage, route, and frequency of each medication?
    b. When was the last dose?
9. Does the patient take any complementary or alternative therapies, herbal products, over-the-counter medications or supplements, or natural therapies?
    a. What is the name, dosage, route and frequency of each therapy?
    b. When was the last dose or therapy?
10. Does the patient have allergies to drugs or foods?
    a. What is the name of the allergen?
    b. What was the reaction?
11. When was the patient's last tetanus immunization?
12. If the patient is female and between the ages of 10 to 50 years, when was the first day of her last menstrual period?

NURSING DOMAIN

The nursing domain, nursing diagnosis and plan of care can only be determined after an in-depth interview and consideration of the patient's story.

Domain 12. Comfort. Class 1. Physical comfort.
Domain 2. Nutrition Class 5. Hydration.
Domain 11. Safety/Protection Class 1. Infection

ANTICIPATED MEDICAL CARE

Review of the Anticipated Medical Care of Burns, Explosion, and Sunburn

<table>
<tr><th colspan="2">Review of the Anticipated Medical Care of Burns, Explosion, and Sunburn</th></tr>
<tr><td>Medical provider exam</td><td>Local examination of the burned area and full body exam when inhalation or other injuries are suspected</td></tr>
<tr><td>Urine tests</td><td>Urinalysis, pregnancy test in women of reproductive age without history of a hysterectomy</td></tr>
<tr><td>Blood tests</td><td>CBC, electrolytes, BUN, creatinine, blood sugar, alcohol and drug screens, carboxyhemoglobin, arterial blood gas analysis</td></tr>
<tr><td>ECG</td><td>12 lead electrocardiogram</td></tr>
<tr><td>X-ray</td><td>Chest x-ray, CT scan or MRI if involved in explosion or internal injuries suspected</td></tr>
<tr><td>Diet</td><td>NPO</td></tr>
<tr><td>Respiratory</td><td>100% oxygen non-rebreather mask for all significant burn patients. Possible intubation and ventilator management for unconscious patients or any patient exhibiting respiratory compromise such as stridor or increasing hoarseness. If intubation is delayed, the airway may become obliterated and an emergency tracheostomy may need to be performed.</td></tr>
<tr><td>IV</td><td>Anticipate lactated Ringer's solution for fluid resuscitation in the patient with > 10% burns.

The Parkland Formula is the most commonly used fluid resuscitation formula.
<table>
<tr><th>Formula</th><th>First 24 hours</th><th>Next 24 hours</th></tr>
<tr><td>Parkland</td><td>LR 4ml/kg/% one-half in the first 8 hours</td><td>Colloids in amount of 20 to 60% of plasma volume; glucose in water added to maintain urine output 0.5 to 1.0 ml/kg/hr in adults and 1 ml/kg/hr in children.</td></tr>
</table>
Calculate resuscitation fluids from the time burned, not from the time of arrival in the ER

It is important to understand that the formula is a general guide and that adjustments must be made to maintain organ perfusion. Heart rate, blood pressure, level of consciousness, capillary refill, and a urine output of at least 50 ml/hr in adults and 0.5 to 1.0 ml/hr in children estimate organ perfusion.</td></tr>
<tr><td>Urinary output</td><td>In-dwelling urinary catheter to monitor urine output.</td></tr>
<tr><td>Medications</td><td>Morphine dose is based on the relief obtained not by the number of milligrams given.</td></tr>
</table>

Review of the Anticipated Medical Care of Burns, Explosion, and Sunburn	
Burn wound care	Use only sterile gloves, linens, and dry dressings. Cool sterile saline dressings can be used to reduce the burning if the burn is <10% of the TBSA. Burns more than 10% are not cooled because of the risk of hypothermia. Blisters and all non-viable skin are debrided (peeled off or unroofed). All burns except those to the face are cleaned with sterile normal saline, covered with a thick coating of Silvadene and a bulky burn dressing applied. Burns to the face are cleaned with normal saline and covered with Polysporin ointment. A nasogastric tube may also be needed for gastric decompression.

Disposition is Dependent on the Severity of the Burn Injury

Burn Center Referral Criteria

The American Burn Association recommends the following patients be transferred to a burn center.

1. Partial thickness burns of greater than 10% of the total body surface area
2. Burns that involve the face, hands, feet, genitalia, perineum, or major joints
3. Third-degree burns in any age group
4. Electrical burns including lightning injury
5. Chemical burns
6. Inhalation injury
7. Burn injury in patients with preexisting medical disorders that could complicate management, prolong recovery, or affect mortality
8. Any patients with burns and concomitant trauma, such as fractures in which the burn injury poses the greatest risk of morbidity or mortality. In such cases, if the trauma poses the greater immediate risk, the patient's condition may be stabilized initially in a trauma center before transfer to a burn center. Medical provider judgment will be necessary in such situations and should be in concert with the regional medical control plan and triage protocols.
9. Burned children in hospitals without qualified personnel or equipment for the care of children
10. Burn injury in patients who will require special social, emotional, or rehabilitative intervention

Disposition is Dependent on the Severity of the Burn Injury	
Minor burns outpatient or 23-hour observation	• Second degree burns with a body surface area of less than 15% in adults (10% in children) • Third degree burns with a body surface area of less than 2% • Burns not involving eyes, ears, face, hands, feet, or perineum
Moderate burns	• Second degree burns with a body surface area of 15% to 25% in adults (20% in children), • Third degree burns with a body surface of less than 10% • Burns that do not involve eyes, ears, face, hands, feet, or perineum
Major burns	• Second degree burns with a body surface area of 15% to 25% in adults (20% in children) • Third degree burns with a body surface of less than 10% • Burns that do not involve eyes, ears, face, hands, feet, or perineum
Note	Burn centers do not want any ointments applied before transfer. Ask the receiving facility how they want the burns managed prior to transport.
Worst-case scenario	The worst-case scenario is an obstructed airway from an unidentified burned larynx and bronchus. Management is intubation or tracheotomy and mechanical ventilation with PEEP. PEEP is used for any patient who has a potential for developing ARDS (adult respiratory distress syndrome).

INITIAL CARE PLAN

Alcohol-based hand sanitizers are the preferred method for cleaning your hands in most clinical situations. Wash your hands with soap and water whenever they are visibly dirty, before eating, and after using the restroom.

MINOR BURNS

1. Ask the patient to undress, remove all jewelry that might interfere with the examination, and put on an exam gown. Assist as needed.
2. Obtain vital signs including pulse oximetry or test capillary refill.
3. Place on 100% oxygen non-rebreather until respiratory status stabilizes.
4. Insertion of intravenous access for administration of pain medications.
5. Assure the patient that pain relief will be a priority.
   a. Obtain an order for morphine and administer 4 to 10 mg IV every 10 to 20 minutes until the patient obtains relief. Administration of pain

medication should be based on the patient's clinical presentation, not the amount of medication administered.

b. Valium or Versed may be administered for anxiety.

c. Monitor oxygen saturation continuously. If respiratory function becomes ineffective due to decreased level of consciousness from the morphine, reverse the morphine with Narcan. Valium and Versed can be reversed with Romazicon.

6. Perform a focused physical examination.

   a. Auscultate the lungs.

   b. Inspect and document the burns on a Lund and Browder Chart. If this chart is not available, then draw a human figure on a progress note in the chart and indicate the burned areas. Make sure to document the degree of burns. Remember, the patient may have different degrees of burns on their body.

   c. Use only sterile gloves, linens, and dry or moist sterile dressings.

   d. If the burn is <10% of the TBSA, room temperature sterile saline saturated towels or dressings may be placed on the burn to reduce the burning. Do not place moist cool compresses on burns that consist of >10% of the TBSA because of the risk of hypothermia.

   e. Debride non-viable skin and unroof blisters.

   f. Coat with a thick layer of Silvadene or other antibacterial ointment as ordered and apply a bulky burn dressing. Make sure fluffed gauze sponges are placed in the web spaces between the fingers and toes. Do not allow skin surfaces to touch. The dressing must be thick to absorb fluids that will leak from the burn. Explain the rationale for the bulky dressing to the patient.

7. Administer tetanus and diphtheria toxoid if the patient's last immunization was more than ten years ago.

8. Inform the patient, family, and caregivers of the plan of care and the anticipated time before disposition.

9. Provide the patient with a device to reach someone for assistance and explain how to use it. Ask the patient to call for help before getting off the stretcher.

10. Discharge the patient to home with recommendations for outpatient follow-up.

MODERATE AND MAJOR BURNS

1. Remove all clothing, remove all jewelry, and cover the patient with a sterile drape.

2. Obtain vital signs including pulse oximetry or test capillary refill. If possible, attach heart monitor leads to the skin, automatic blood pressure cuff, and pulse oximetry for continuous monitoring. Leads do not have to

be attached to the chest. Document the initial heart monitor strip and document changes of rhythm.

3. Administer oxygen by a 100% non-rebreather mask. Intubation may need to be performed
4. Evaluate any circumferential burns for potential need of an escharotomy to release the tissue tension. Elevate extremities to decrease edema.
5. Assure the patient that pain relief will be a priority.
   a. Obtain an order for morphine and administer 4 to 10 mg IV every 10 to 20 minutes until the patient obtains relief.
   b. Valium or Versed may be administered for anxiety.
   c. Monitor oxygen saturation continuously. If respiratory function becomes ineffective due to decreased level of consciousness from the morphine, reverse the morphine with Narcan. Valium and Versed can be reversed with Romazicon.
6. Place two large bore intravenous cannulas and infuse Lactated Ringer's solution.
   a. Large amounts of intravenous solution are needed.
   b. Infuse intravenous fluids to maintain an hourly urinary output of 0.5 cc/kg/hr for adults and 1.0 cc/kg/hr for children.

Formula	First 24 hours	Next 24 hours
Parkland	LR 4ml/kg/% one-half in the first 8 hours	Colloids in amount of 20 to 60% of plasma volume; glucose in water added to maintain urine output 0.5 to 1.0 ml/kg/hr in adults and 1 ml/kg/hr in children.

7. Perform a focused physical examination.
   a. Inspect the oral cavity for carbonaceous material. Inspect and document the burns on a Lund and Browder Chart. If this chart is not available, then draw a human figure on a progress note in the chart and indicate the burned areas. Make sure to document the degree of burns. Remember, the patient may have different degree of burns on their body.
   b. Evaluate the level of consciousness based on the mnemonic **AVPU** or **ACDU** level of consciousness score.
      AVPU: **A**lert, **V**erbal, **P**ain, **U**nresponsive.
      ACDU: **A**lert, **C**onfused, **D**rowsy, **U**nresponsive.
8. Perform a head-to-toe physical examination.

If two nurses are at the bedside, one can ask the following questions and document the answers of the other who performs the exam. Document positive and negative findings.

a. What is the size and reaction of the pupils?

b. Does the patient have any head pain or injuries to the head?
Is the tongue or mouth injured?
Is any drainage present from the nose or ears?

c. Is the trachea midline?
Is jugular venous distention present? (Patient must be at a 30° angle to accurately assess. It is difficult, if not impossible, to assess under fluorescent lighting).

d. Does the chest expand equally?
Is subcutaneous emphysema present?
Are the heart tones within normal limits?
Are the heart tones diminished?
Are any murmurs present?
Does the patient complain of chest pain?
Is the chest tender to palpation?

e. Are the lung sounds clear on the right and left?
Are wheezes or crackles present?
Are the lung sounds decreased or absent in any area of the lungs?

f. Is the abdomen soft, flat, rigid, or distended?
Are bowel sounds normal, hypoactive, hyperactive, or absent?
Does the patient complain of abdominal pain?
Is the patient's abdomen tender to palpation?

g. Is the patient incontinent?

Examination of the genitalia may be deferred if trauma is not suspected.

h. Do the genitalia appear normal?
Does the patient have bleeding from the urethral meatus or vagina?
Is priapism present?
Does the patient complain of genital pain?
Is the perineal area or genitalia tender to palpation?

i. Does the patient complain of pain when light pressure is applied to the iliac crests?
Is the pelvis stable or unstable?

j. Does the patient have normal motion and sensation in the upper and lower extremities?
Are distal pulses present in the upper and lower extremities?

k. Does the patient have normal movement of his back?
Does the patient complain of back pain?
While keeping the back immobilized, turn the patient.
Inspect the posterior surfaces.
Does the patient have obvious back injuries?
Is the back tender to palpation?

l. Does skin inspection reveal any damage to the skin, e.g., abrasions, lacerations, bruises, needle tracks, or petechiae?

9. If the patient has a significant burn, he has lost some of his ability for temperature regulation.
    a. Warm the intravenous and the irrigation fluids.
    b. Increase the temperature in the room.
    c. Keep the patient covered with warmed blankets.
10. Administer medications covered by hospital protocol, e.g., diphtheria - tetanus toxoid booster.
11. If debris is present, remove if possible, without irrigating with normal saline as this could place the patient at risk for hypovolemia.
12. Place an indwelling urinary catheter.

> Accurate intake and output is essential. Burns in the genitalia can cause swelling that will make voiding and catheterization impossible later.

13. Order diagnostic tests as approved by hospital protocol.
14. Obtain arterial blood gas analysis.
15. Elevate the siderails and keep the stretcher in the lowest position.
16. Inform the patient not to eat or drink and teach the patient and family the rationale for the NPO status.
17. Inform the patient, family, and caregivers of the plan of care and the anticipated time before disposition.
18. Provide the patient with a device to reach someone for assistance and explain how to use it. Ask the patient to call for help before getting off the stretcher.

ONGOING CARE PLAN

> Inform the medical provider of adverse changes noted during ongoing evaluation. Document that the medical provider (by name) was notified of the adverse change and what orders, if any, were received.

1. Monitor vital signs, effectiveness of breathing, and temperature.
2. Observe for restlessness, difficulty swallowing, dyspnea, and hoarseness that might represent compromise of the airway and breathing.
3. Monitor pain management therapy closely for the patient's therapeutic response. If therapy is not effective, ask the medical provider for a repeat dose or an alternative.
    a. Burn patients need pain medication frequently. The usual time for a medication effectiveness check is every 10 to 20 minutes. Morphine is the drug of choice.
    b. Regional blocks can be used for extremity burns.
4. Monitor closely for the development of adverse reactions to therapy.
    a. Perform interventions to relieve the adverse reaction.

   b. Inform medical provider of adverse reaction and ask for a remedy.

5. Keep the patient, family, and caregivers well informed of the plan of care and the remaining time anticipated before disposition.
6. Monitor the patient's laboratory and radiographic results and notify the medical provider of critical abnormalities. Remedy abnormalities as ordered.
7. Notify the medical provider when all diagnostic results are available for review. Ask for establishment of a diagnosis and disposition.

DISCHARGE INSTRUCTIONS

1. Provide the patient with the name of the nurse and medical provider in the emergency room.
2. Inform the patient of their diagnosis or why a definitive diagnosis couldn't be made. Explain what caused the problem if known.
3. Teach the common side effects of the medications and what to do if any of these occur. Instruct the patient not to drive or perform any dangerous tasks while taking narcotic pain medications.
4. Inform the patient that:
   a. Any burn is a potential serious injury to the skin.
   b. Minor burns are treated with pain medications and elevation of the burned area. Wash the burned area daily and apply the burn cream as prescribed.
   c. Serious burns require outpatient dressing changes and treatment by a medical professional possibly at a regional burn center.
5. Recommend a medical provider for follow-up care. Provide the name, address, and phone number with a recommendation of when to schedule the care.
6. Instruct the patient to notify the follow-up medical provider immediately if fever or purulent drainage develops. If the medical provider is not available in a reasonable amount of time, return to the emergency room. Encourage the patient NOT to IGNORE WORSENING OR PERSISTENT SYMPTOMS.
7. Ask for verbal confirmation or demonstration of understanding and reinforce teaching as needed.

COMMONLY ORDERED MEDICATIONS

MORPHINE

Morphine sulfate (MSO4)	
Indications	Moderate to severe pain
Dose	4 to 10 mg IV administered over 5 min.
Pediatric dose	50 to 100 mcg/kg IV, maximum 10 mg/dose

Morphine sulfate (MSO4)	
Onset	IV onset rapid, peak 20 minutes, duration 4 to 5 hours
Side effects	Confusion, sedation, hypotension, respiratory depression
Monitor	Effectiveness of respirations

NARCAN

Narcan (naloxone)	
Indications	Opioid overdose
Dose	0.4 to 2 mg IV every 2 to 3 min. A maximum dose has not been established. However, if the patient does not respond after 10 mg of Narcan, the diagnosis of an opioid overdose must be questioned.
Pediatric dose	0.01 mg/kg IV every 2 to 3 min.
Onset	IV onset 1 minute, duration 45 minutes.
Side effects	Nervousness, ventricular tachycardia, increased systolic blood pressure in high doses
Monitor	Monitor the patient's level of responsiveness. Anticipate a return of the narcotic state. The duration of Narcan is 45 min. and the duration of morphine is 4 to 6 hours.

SILVADENE

Silvadene (silver sulfadiazine topical cream)	
Indications	Prophylactic broad spectrum anti-infective
Adult and child dose	Apply 1% cream topically once or twice a day 1.5 mm thick to all burned areas. DO NOT use on a child < 2 months old or on the face.
Onset	Topical onset rapid
Side effects	Reversible leukopenia, rash, urticaria, itching

RELATED CONDITIONS AND INFORMATION

BLAST FORCES

Blast forces cause tissue damage resulting from the body's contact with light, heat, and pressure resulting in burns, blunt trauma, and penetrating wounds. The amount of injury sustained is dependent on the velocity that strikes the victim. Blunt trauma causes crushing injuries to the body and widespread damage. Penetrating injuries disrupt the skin and cause trauma along the path of projection. Early head-to-toe physical examination coordinated with diagnostic intervention is essential to determine the need for transfer to a trauma center.

General Indicators for Transfer to a Trauma Center

General Indicators for Transfer to a Trauma Center
Glasgow coma scale < 13; or systolic blood pressure <90; or respiratory rate < 10 or >29
Penetrating injury to trunk or head, flail chest
Two or more long bone fractures
Burns > 15% total body surface area or to the face or airway
Evidence of high impact and vehicle deformity, passenger compartment intrusion
Ejection from vehicle
Rollover
Death of same car occupant
Pedestrian struck at speeds of 20 miles per hour or more
Age < 5 or > 55 years suffering multiple trauma
Known history of cardiac or respiratory disease associated with multiple trauma
When in doubt, call the trauma center and speak with the trauma surgeon. Level 1 trauma centers are staffed 24 hours a day and serve as an educational resource for emergency personnel.
Do not send the parents to the receiving hospital until the child has left the transferring facility.
Appropriate inter facility transfer includes the following: • Acceptance by the receiving facility • Copies of the medical record • Qualified personnel with the level of skill and equipment needed to care for the patient in transport

COMMON CAUSES OF BURNS IN THE HOUSEHOLD

Common Causes of Burns in the Household
Barbecue grills
Clothing iron
Curling and flat irons
Fireplaces
Radiators
Ovens
Hot pots on the stove
Coffee
Hot water
Steam from microwaved food

DOPPLER PULSE

Christian Johann Doppler, 1803-1853, was an Austrian physicist and mathematician who first enunciated the principle known as the Doppler Effect in 1842. A pulse audible by Doppler distal to the burn is the best indicator of circulation. A pulse ox can be used to find pulses distal to the burn on a digit.

ELECTRICAL BURNS

Electrical burns are caused by electricity as it passes through the body and meets resistance from body tissue. The heat it causes is proportional to the amperage of the current and the electrical resistance of the body. External burns are usually caused at the entry and exit sites. Nerves, blood vessels, and muscles are less resistant and more easily damaged than fat or bone. Organs, such as the brain, heart, and lungs are damaged quickly and easily. The smaller the body part the more intense the heat. Considerable damage can occur in the extremities. Electrical current can cause the heart to fibrillate. AC current can cause tetany and intensify the patient's grip on the electrical source increasing the time of exposure. The electrical current in homes in the United States is AC, 110 and 220 volt. The patient of a suspected electrical injury should be evaluated for entrance and exit wounds. The exit wound would be detected where the patient was grounded. Exit wounds may be misleading since it is a deep wound and the magnitude can be underestimated by the appearance on the surface.

ESCHAR

Dead tissue at the site of third- and fourth-degree burns.

ESCHAROTOMY

Escharotomy is a surgical incision made with a scalpel or Bovie through the eschar of a circumferential third- or fourth-degree burn. The purpose of this procedure is to relieve pressure and improve circulation to the extremity.

FASCIOTOMY

Fasciotomy is a surgical incision made with a scalpel or Bovie through the eschar and into the fascia of a circumferential third- or fourth-degree burn. The purpose of this procedure is to relieve pressure and improve circulation to the extremity.

FLAME BURNS

Flame burns are the most common type of burns. In the past, most flame burns occurred in structure fires. It is reported that smoke detectors have actually decreased the number of house fires. Most burns are now caused by smoking while intoxicated, motor vehicle crashes, and ignited clothing. Flame burns in the outdoors are often caused by kerosene, gasoline, and the fuel used to ignite charcoal.

FLASH BURNS

Flash burns are caused by explosion of gases, flammable liquids, and/or electrical arcs. Flash burns are often associated with airway damage.

FLUID REPLACEMENT

Fluid replacement recommended by the American Burn Association is 2 to 4 ml of intravenous fluid for every kilogram of body weight and for each percent of body surface area burned (2 or 4 ml times body weight in kilograms times the percentage of body surface burned). Of the calculated amount, one-half is to be infused in the first 8 hours after the burn. If the patient is in shock, more fluids may be needed.

LIGHTNING

Lightning flows electrical current around or through the body capable of severe damage. People surviving lightning strikes describe temporary paresthesias and paralysis.

THERMAL BURNS

Thermal burns make up 60% of all burns and result from flames, flashes, steam, and scalding liquids.

SCALD BURNS

Scald burns are caused by exposure to hot liquids. Water at 140 degrees can cause a deep partial-thickness burn in 3 seconds. Water at 156 degrees can burn in one second. The thicker the liquid and the longer it remains in contact with the skin, the more increases the likelihood of serious burns. Cooking oils and grease can reach 400 degrees.

STOP THE BURNING

For all burns, stopping the burning process is a top priority. Immediately remove any clothing or jewelry that may cause continued burning to the skin. These items include charred or saturated clothing, shoes, wedding rings, bracelets and necklaces. Once clothing and jewelry are removed, aseptic technique is used to apply sterile gauze compresses of sterile normal saline to the burned areas. If the patient has >10% TBSA burned, he has lost some of his ability for temperature regulation and cool compresses are not used because of the risk of hypothermia.

SUNBURN

Sunburn is a burn to the skin caused by ultraviolet radiation from the sun and tanning lamps. Ultraviolet radiation comes in two different wavelengths, UVA and UVB. Although UVB is thought to be more damaging to the skin in respect to skin cancer, both UVA and UVB are causative agents for sunburns. The degree of the burn sustained depends on the wavelength and length of exposure. Symptoms, such as erythema occur 2 to 6 hours after exposure with peak effects manifesting 12 to 24 hours after exposure. Although most sunburns are not serious, rare cases of life-threatening sun poisoning have occurred.

Eye burns cause photophobia, vision loss, corneal irregularity, and cataracts. Management for minor sunburns may include analgesia and topical anesthetic ointments. Second- and third-degree burns are treated the same as other thermal burns. Management for serious sunburn may include Lactated Ringers intravenous fluids, analgesics, steroids, and sterile dressings with antibiotic ointments.

FACTORS AFFECTING QUANTITY OF ULTRAVIOLET RADIATION STRIKING THE EARTH

Factors Affecting Quantity of Radiation Striking the Earth	
Atmosphere	Clouds and pollution
Time	At noon the distance from the sun is the shortest.
Season	The angle of the sun is closest to the earth in the summer close to 90 degrees.

Factors Affecting Quantity of Radiation Striking the Earth	
Latitude	The distance from the sun is shortest at the equator.

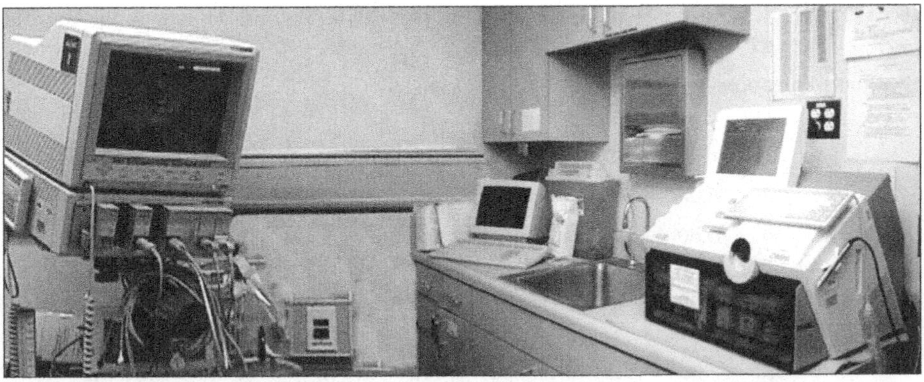

08 Carbon Monoxide Inhalation and Hazardous Material

For details on triage see Chapter 34, Triage in a Nutshell.

Patient's Story – Interview Questions

Carbon Monoxide Inhalation

1. When did the incident occur?
2. Are the symptoms confined to the respiratory system?
3. What were the circumstances of the exposure?

If the inhalation was a suicide attempt, incorporate appropriate aspects from chapter #27 Psychiatric Emergency and Suicide Attempt.

4. How does the incident affect the patient's normal function?
5. Has any treatment been initiated, and has it helped?

Hazardous Material Exposure

1. When was the exposure?
2. When did the patient first notice any symptoms?
3. Where are the injuries or what body system is involved and are any associated symptoms present?
4. What caused the injury?
   a. What chemicals were involved?
   b. Do the patient or emergency personnel know the warning placard number or the chemical ID number?
5. How does the injury or symptoms affect the patient's normal function?
   a. Is neurovascular function normal distal to the injuries?
   b. Does the patient have normal use of the injured area?

6. Was the patient decontaminated at the scene and what was the process, e.g., water rinse or a soap and water scrub?

STANDARD QUESTIONS FOR HISTORY OF PRESENT ILLNESS

1. Does the patient have any pertinent past history?
2. Does the patient take any routine medications?
    a. What is the name, dosage, route, and frequency of each medication?
    b. When was the last dose?
3. Does the patient take any complementary or alternative therapies, herbal products, over-the-counter medications or supplements, or natural therapies?
    a. What is the name, dosage, route and frequency of each therapy?
    b. When was the last dose or therapy?
4. Does the patient have allergies to drugs or foods?
    a. What is the name of the allergen?
    b. What was the reaction?
5. When was the patient's last tetanus immunization?
6. If the patient is female and between the ages of 10 to 50 years, when was the first day of her last menstrual period?

NURSING DOMAIN

The nursing domain, nursing diagnosis and plan of care can only be determined after an in-depth interview and consideration of the patient's story.

Domain 12. Comfort. Class 1. Physical comfort.
Domain 11. Safety/Protection Class 4. Environmental Hazards.

ANTICIPATED MEDICAL CARE

Review of the Anticipated Medical Care of Carbon Monoxide Inhalation and HAZMAT	
Exam	Full body
Urine	Pregnancy test for women of reproductive age without history of a hysterectomy
Blood	STAT ABG for carbon monoxide poisoning Hematology, chemistries, coagulation studies, type and screen for a hazardous material exposure
ECG	ECG for females and males over 35 years, all ages with a cardiac history
X-ray	Chest

Review of the Anticipated Medical Care of Carbon Monoxide Inhalation and HAZMAT	
Other	Strict adherence to the institution's HAZMAT policy
Diet	NPO
IV	Normal saline or Ringer's solution
Medications	Morphine
Other	Treatment as outlined on the chemical ID placard in the institution's HAZMAT protocol manual
Worst-case scenario	The worst-case scenario is an unsuspected airway compromise from a chemically burned larynx, bronchus, or lung. Treatment may include intubation or tracheotomy and mechanical ventilation with PEEP.

INITIAL ASSESSMENTS AND INTERVENTIONS

> Alcohol-based hand sanitizers are the preferred method for cleaning your hands in most clinical situations. Wash your hands with soap and water whenever they are visibly dirty, before eating, and after using the restroom.

CARBON MONOXIDE INHALATION

1. Ask the patient to undress, remove jewelry that might interfere with the examination, and put on an exam gown. Assist as needed.
2. Obtain vital signs and an arterial blood gas analysis.

> The SpO2 on pulse oximetry may be misleading. On arterial blood gases, the patient will have a below normal SaO2 and the PaO2 will remain normal. Since the PaO2 is normal, the patient does not increase ventilation and the patient sustains tissue hypoxia. The carbon monoxide (CO) is excreted by the lungs with a half-life of four to six hours once the patient is removed from the exposure, the half-life decreases to 40 to 80 minutes with 100% oxygen therapy and to 15 to 30 minutes with hyperbaric oxygen. The patient may present with the characteristic cherry-red skin and mucous membranes.
>
> Treatment includes administration of oxygen by tight-fitting mask until CO levels are less than 10% and all symptoms have resolved. Hyperbaric oxygen therapy (HBOT) is recommended by most practitioners for patients with CO levels of > 40% with coma and for patients with CO levels of > 25% with seizures, arrhythmias, or other sequelae.

3. Place the patient on 100% oxygen by a non-rebreather mask or use hyperbaric oxygen therapy.

COHb Levels	Symptoms and Treatment
5 to 10%	No symptoms to mild headache and vertigo Oxygen therapy at 100% with a tight-fitting mask
10 to 20%	Symptoms include headache, nausea, vomiting, and loss of coordination Oxygen therapy at 100% with a tight-fitting mask.
20 to 30%	Symptoms include confusion, ST depression, and visual disturbances Oxygen therapy at 100% with a tight-fitting mask
40 to 60%	Symptoms include coma, seizures, and cardiac arrhythmias Hyperbaric oxygen therapy recommended
> 60%	Death

4. Perform a focused physical examination.
   a. Auscultate the lungs.
   b. Listen to heart sounds.
   c. Evaluate the level of consciousness based on the mnemonic **AVPU** or **ACDU** level of consciousness score.
   AVPU: **A**lert, **V**erbal, **P**ain, **U**nresponsive.
   ACDU: **A**lert, **C**onfused, **D**rowsy, **U**nresponsive.

HAZARDOUS MATERIAL EXPOSURE

1. Remove ALL clothes and ALL jewelry. Place in a biohazard bag.
2. Decontaminate the patient as outlined in the hospital's HAZMAT policy. After the patient is decontaminated, place the patient in a hospital gown.
3. Obtain vital signs; attach heart monitor leads, automatic blood pressure cuff, and pulse oximetry for continuous monitoring. Document the initial heart monitor strip and document changes of rhythm.
4. Administer oxygen if saturation is < 94%. Severe COPD patients may be unable to maintain saturation >88% to 92%.
5. Evaluate the level of consciousness based on the mnemonic **AVPU** or **ACDU** level of consciousness score.
   AVPU: **A**lert, **V**erbal, **P**ain, **U**nresponsive.
   ACDU: **A**lert, **C**onfused, **D**rowsy, **U**nresponsive.
6. Perform a head-to-toe physical examination.

> If two nurses are at the bedside, one can ask the following questions and document the answers of the other who performs the exam. Document positive and negative findings.

   a. What is the size and reaction of the pupils?

b. Does the patient have any head pain or injuries to the head?
Is the tongue or mouth injured?
Is any drainage present from the nose or ears?

c. Is the trachea midline?
Is jugular venous distention present (unable to detect under fluorescent light)?

d. Does the chest expand equally?
Is subcutaneous emphysema present?
Are the heart tones within normal limits?
Are the heart tones diminished?
Are any murmurs present?
Does the patient complain of chest pain?
Is the chest tender to palpation?

e. Are the lung sounds clear on the right and left?
Are wheezes or crackles present?
Are the lung sounds decreased or absent in any area of the lungs?

f. Is the abdomen soft, flat, rigid, or distended?
Are bowel sounds normal, hypoactive, hyperactive, or absent?
Does the patient complain of abdominal pain?
Is the patient's abdomen tender to palpation?

g. Is the patient incontinent?
Examination of the genitalia may be deferred if trauma is not suspected.
Do the genitalia appear normal?
Does the patient have bleeding from the urethral meatus or vagina?
Is priapism present?
Does the patient complain of genital pain?
Is the perineal area or genitalia tender to palpation?

h. Does the patient complain of pain when light pressure is applied to the iliac crests?
Is the pelvis stable or unstable?

i. Does the patient have normal motion and sensation in the upper and lower extremities?
Are distal pulses present in the upper and lower extremities?

j. Does the patient have normal movement of his back?
Does the patient complain of back pain?
While keeping the back immobilized, turn the patient.
Inspect the posterior surfaces.
Does the patient have obvious back injuries?
Is the back tender to palpation?

k. Does skin inspection reveal any damage to the skin, e.g., abrasions, lacerations, bruises, needle tracks, or petechiae?

7. For burns from a chemical exposure, draw a human figure on the chart, document the areas of burn, and classify them.

BURN CLASSIFICATION

Burn Classification	Presence of Pain	Clinical Signs
Superficial-Thickness Burns		
First Degree Epidermis and superficial dermis	Yes	Erythema, minor pain, no blisters
Partial-Thickness Burns		
Second Degree Moderate to deep dermis	Yes	Moderate: Blisters, moderate pain, clear fluid Deep: Whiter appearance, with decreased pain. Difficult to distinguish from full thickness burns
Full-Thickness Burns		
Third degree Through the dermis and into subcutaneous fat and muscle	No	White, brown, or black dry leathery tissue (eschar), severe swelling
Fourth degree Through the subcutaneous fat and into the muscle or bone	No	Eschar, muscle and possible bone exposure

STANDARD INTERVENTIONS

1. Establish intravenous access and draw laboratory blood specimens.
2. Draw a variety of tubes that will allow the lab to perform hematology, chemistry, and coagulation studies. Patients on anticoagulants need a prothrombin time. Consider drawing other labs, e.g., type and screen, blood cultures.
3. Administer medications covered by hospital protocols, e.g., diphtheria and tetanus toxoid.
4. Inform the patient not to eat or drink and teach the patient and family the rationale for the NPO status.
5. Elevate the siderails and place the stretcher in the lowest position.
6. Inform the patient, family, and caregivers of the plan of care and the anticipated time until disposition. Also, inform the family of the rationale for the need to abide by the NPO status.
7. Provide the patient with a device to reach someone for assistance and explain how to use it. Ask the patient to call for help before getting off the stretcher.

ONGOING CARE PLAN

Inform the medical provider of adverse changes noted during ongoing evaluation. Document that the medical provider was notified of the adverse change. Document if orders were or were not received.

1. Monitor vital signs and effectiveness of breathing.
2. Monitor for signs and symptoms of worsening. Observe for restlessness, difficulty swallowing, dyspnea, and hoarseness that indicate airway compromise.
3. Monitor ABG results for patients with carbon monoxide inhalation. Consider placing an arterial line for frequent blood draws.

COHb Levels	Symptoms and Treatment
5 to 10%	No symptoms to mild headache and vertigo Oxygen therapy at 100% with a tight-fitting mask
10 to 20%	Symptoms include headache, nausea, vomiting, and loss of coordination. Oxygen therapy at 100% with a tight-fitting mask
20 to 30%	Symptoms include confusion, ST depression, and visual disturbances. Oxygen therapy at 100% with a tight-fitting mask
40 to 60%	Symptoms include coma, seizures, and cardiac arrhythmias. Hyperbaric oxygen therapy recommended
> 60%	Death

4. Monitor pain management therapy closely for burned patients to assess therapeutic response.
    a. Burn patients need pain medication frequently. The usual time for a medication effectiveness check is every 10 to 20 minutes.
    b. Morphine is the drug of choice.
    c. Regional blocks can be used for extremity burns.
    d. If therapy is not effective, ask the medical provider for a repeat dose or an alternative.
5. Monitor closely for the development of adverse reactions to therapy.
    a. Perform interventions to relieve the adverse reaction.
    b. Ask the medical provider for a remedy.
6. If not NPO, provide the patient with food at mealtimes and fluids during the stay.
7. Keep the patient, family, and caregivers well informed of the plan of care and the remaining time anticipated before disposition.

8. Monitor the patient's laboratory and x-ray results and notify the medical provider of critical abnormalities. Remedy abnormalities as ordered.
9. Notify the medical provider when all diagnostic results are available for review. Ask for establishment of a diagnosis and disposition.

DISCHARGE INSTRUCTIONS

1. Provide the patient with the name of the nurse and doctor in the emergency room.
2. Inform the patient of their diagnosis or why a definitive diagnosis couldn't be made. Explain what caused the problem if known.
3. Teach the common side effects or adverse effects of the prescribed medications and what to do if any of these occur. Instruct the patient not to drive or perform any dangerous tasks while taking narcotic pain medications.
4. Recommend a medical provider for follow-up care. Provide the name, address, and phone number with a recommendation of when to schedule the care.
5. Instruct the patient to call the follow-up medical provider immediately or return to the emergency room if problems persist for over eight hours, worsen in any way, or any unusual symptoms develop. ENCOURAGE the patient NOT to IGNORE WORSENING OR PERSISTENT SYMPTOMS.
6. Ask for verbal confirmation or demonstration of understanding and reinforce teaching as needed.

MEDICATIONS

MORPHINE

Morphine sulfate (MSO4)	
Indications	Moderate to severe pain
Dose	4 to 10 mg IV over 5 min.
Pediatric dose	50 to 100 mcg/kg IV, maximum 10 mg/dose
Onset	IV onset rapid, peak 20 minutes, duration 4 to 5 hours
Side effects	Confusion, sedation, hypotension, respiratory depression
Monitor	CNS changes, sedation level, effectiveness of respirations

NARCAN

Narcan (naloxone)	
Indications	Opioid overdose
Dose	0.4 to 2 mg IV every 2 to 3 min. A maximum dose has not been established. However, if the patient does not respond after 10 mg of Narcan, the diagnosis of an opioid overdose must be questioned.

Narcan (naloxone)	
Pediatric dose	0.01 mg/kg IV every 2 to 3 min.
Onset	IV onset 1 min., duration 45 min.
Side effects	Nervousness, ventricular tachycardia, increased systolic blood pressure in high doses
Monitor	Anticipate the return of the narcotic sedation level. The life of the morphine is 4 to 5 hours and the life of the Narcan is 45 minutes.

RELATED CONDITIONS AND INFORMATION

CARBON MONOXIDE COHB LEVELS

COHb Levels	Symptoms and Treatment
5 to 10%	No symptoms to mild headache and vertigo Oxygen therapy at 100% with a tight-fitting mask
10 to 20%	Symptoms include headache, nausea, vomiting, and loss of coordination. Oxygen therapy at 100% with a tight-fitting mask
20 to 30%	Symptoms include confusion, ST depression, and visual disturbances. Oxygen therapy at 100% with a tight-fitting mask.
40 to 60%	Symptoms include coma, seizures, and cardiac arrhythmias. Hyperbaric oxygen therapy is recommended.
> 60%	Death

CARBON MONOXIDE POISONING

Carbon monoxide (CO) is a tasteless, odorless, and colorless gas that is present in the smoke from organic materials such as wood, coal, and gasoline. When inhaled, it binds to the oxygen binding sides on the hemoglobin molecule and the oxygen is reduced. The amount of oxygen left is not readily available to the tissues and hypoxia results. The SpO2 on pulse oximetry may be misleading. On arterial blood gases, the patient will have a below normal SaO2 and the PaO2 will remain normal. Since the PaO2 is normal, the patient does not increase ventilation and the patient sustains tissue hypoxia. The carbon monoxide (CO) is excreted by the lungs with a half-life of four to six hours once the patient is removed from the exposure. The half-life decreases to 40 to 80 minutes with 100% oxygen therapy and to 15 to 30 minutes with hyperbaric oxygen. The patient may present with the characteristic cherry-red skin and mucous membranes. Treatment includes administration of oxygen by tight-fitting mask until CO levels are less than 10% and all symptoms have resolved. Hyperbaric oxygen is recommended for patients with CO levels of > 40% with coma and for patients with CO levels of > 25% with seizures, arrhythmias, or other sequelae.

CHEMICAL BURNS

Chemical burns are caused when the body comes into direct contact with caustic chemicals (hazardous material). The chemical causes a denaturing of protein within the tissues or a desiccation (drying out) of the cells. The damage to the tissue is directly related to the time of exposure and the concentration of the chemical. Alkaline products (pH > 7) such as soda and anhydrous ammonia cause more tissue damage than acids. Successful treatment requires fast removal of the chemical. Not all chemicals are removed successfully with water, some require soap, and others are intensified with soap and water. Every hospital is required to have a HAZMAT (hazardous material) manual that covers decontamination procedures for most chemicals. The patient and staff are in danger as long as the chemicals are present. The medical care of burns from chemicals is managed by the same techniques as thermal burns. If no information exists for a particular chemical, call the poison control center for instructions.

HYDROFLUORIC ACID (HF)

One of the strongest inorganic acids and used mainly for industrial purposes including glass etching, metal cleaning, electronics manufacturing, but it also may be found in home rust removers. Tissue damage is caused by corrosive burns from the free hydrogen ions and chemical burns from tissue penetration of the fluoride ions. Fluoride ions penetrate and form insoluble salts with calcium and magnesium. Soluble salts also are formed with other cations but dissociate rapidly. Consequently, fluoride ions release, and further tissue destruction occurs. Hypocalcemia may result. Burns will present in varying grades:

- Grade 1: white burn and/or erythema and pain
- Grade 2: white burn and/or erythema and pain, plus edema and blistering
- Grade 3: white burn and/or erythema and pain, edema, blistering, and necrosis

Treatment includes:

Treatment of Hydrofluoric Acid (HF)	
Evidence of hypocalcemia	IV 10% Calcium Gluconate
Topical	2.5% Calcium Gluconate gel to affected area
Subcutaneous infiltration	0.5 mL of a 10% solution per square centimeter of surface burn extending 0.5 cm beyond the margin of involved tissue

Treatment of Hydrofluoric Acid (HF)	
Burns to digits	IV regional calcium gluconate: 10 to 15 mL of 10% calcium gluconate plus 5000 units of heparin diluted up to 40 mL in 5% dextrose. Use an ischemic arm block technique to infuse the solution intravenously. Release the cuff when any of the following conditions first occur: • pain from the digits resolves • the cuff becomes more painful than the burn • 20 minutes of ischemic time elapses. Treatment can be repeated after 4 hours if needed. Continuous ECG and clinical monitoring are essential during this procedure.
Or	Intra-arterial calcium gluconate: • Place an arterial catheter in the radial or brachial artery to perfuse the digits. • Infuse a solution of 10 mL of 10% calcium gluconate in 40 mL of 5% dextrose over a 4-hour period. Further infusions can be administered after 4 to 8 hours. Several treatments may be needed. • Ensure that the catheter is appropriately placed intravascularly by continuous waveform analysis. Tissue necrosis and digit loss have occurred following extravasation of calcium salts. • Continuous ECG and clinical monitoring are essential during this procedure.
Inhalation burns	Provide 100% oxygen by mask, 2.5% calcium gluconate by nebulizer with 100% oxygen, continuous pulse oximetry, ECG, and clinical monitoring.
Ingestion	Consider gastric lavage with calcium chloride, e.g. 20 mmol calcium in 1000 mL normal saline solution early in overdose.
Note	Marked pain in the absence of significant surface dermal injury should raise suspicion of HF acid burns.

RADIATION EXPOSURE

Visit the Center for Disease Control and Prevention (CDC) website at http://www.cdc.gov/ and search for radiation for more details. The radiation toolkit is especially helpful.

Ionizing radiation has the ability to penetrate cells and randomly deposit energy within them. It is unaffected by the usual cellular barriers. When sufficiently intense, the energy kills cells by inhibiting their division. The United States Energy

Research and Development Administration has regional offices for information and assistance on radiation emergencies.

According to the CDC most scientists in the international community measure radiation using the Systems International (SI), a uniform system of weights and measures that evolved from the metric system. In the United States, however, the conventional system of measurement is still widely used.

The CDC relates that different units of measure are used depending on what aspect of radiation is being measured. For example, the amount of radiation being given off, or emitted, by a radioactive material is measured using the conventional unit curie (Ci), named for the famed scientist Marie Curie, or the SI unit Becquerel (Bq). The radiation dose absorbed by a person (that is, the amount of energy deposited in human tissue by radiation) is measured using the conventional unit rads or the SI unit gray (Gy). The biological risk of exposure to radiation is measured using the conventional unit rem or the SI unit sievert (Sv). Visit the CDC website at http://www.cdc.gov for more details.

RADIATION EXPOSURE STANDARD EMERGENCY PROCESS

Review of Standard Emergency Process for Radiation Exposure
Notify administrative personnel and refer to HAZMAT policy.
Notify trained health physicists from the nuclear medicine department.
Obtain the necessary survey meter (Geiger counter) to measure the intensity of the radiation.
Notify the law enforcement agency with jurisdiction.
Prepare a room that is lead lined and lends itself to washing, such as the morgue or x-ray.
Turn off air circulation to the area to avoid spread of the contamination.
Check the patient, stretcher, and EMS personnel for contamination with the survey meter on arrival to the hospital. Record the measurements. Mild to severe nausea and vomiting are associated with most cases of radiation exposure. Seizures and death are associated with severe contamination (exposure to > 2,000 rads).
Give lifesaving measures as needed. Emergency personnel need to wear protective clothing, e.g., gown, gloves, cap, and mask.
SAVE ALL LIQUID USED IN WASHING. DO NOT ALLOW CONTAMINATED LIQUID TO ENTER THE SEWERAGE. Save all materials including clothing contaminated with blood, urine, stool, vomitus, and all metal objects such as glasses, jewelry and dental plates. Label with name, date, and time. Mark clearly RADIOACTIVE — DO NOT DISCARD.

Review of Standard Emergency Process for Radiation Exposure
Start decontamination by cleansing and scrubbing the patient with soap and warm water. Showering may be necessary. Provide extra friction to hair-covered areas, nares, ears, body orifices, and body folds. Wounds can be decontaminated with irrigation, débridement, and covered with a self-adhering drape during the rest of the scrubbing process. Remove contact lenses and flush eyes with clean water.
Re-measure radiation contamination and record measurements after each washing or showering. If the radiation is not reduced after external decontamination, internal contamination must be suspected.
Gastric lavage, cathartics, and chelating or blocking agents that prevent the uptake of the radioactive iodine manages internal contamination.
Leukopenia and thrombocytopenia occur in patients exposed to radiation. The onset of symptoms is dependent on the amount of exposure. Symptoms manifest themselves 4 to 5 weeks after an exposure of 100 to 300 rads, 3 weeks after an exposure of 300 to 600 rads, and 1 to 3 weeks after an exposure of more than 600 rads.

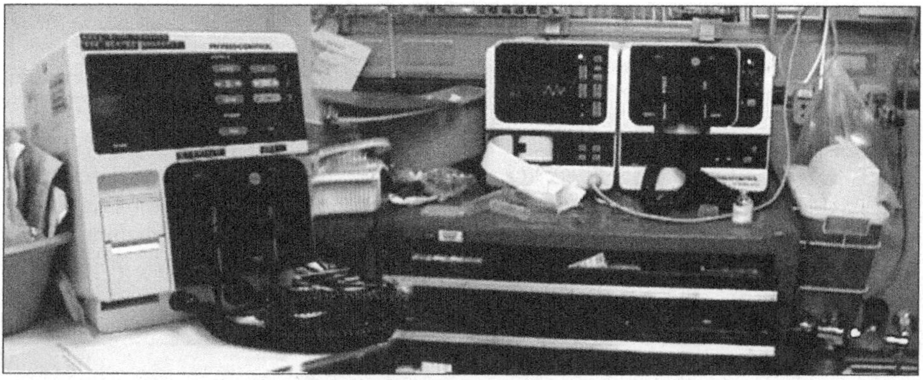

09 CARDIOPULMONARY ARREST

For details on triage see Chapter 34, Triage in a Nutshell.

ADVANCED LIFE PROTOCOL

The primary CABD assessment should take no more than 30 seconds. Tap and shout something like, are you all right. The time taken may in fact increase the time before compressions are started and decrease the patient's change for survival. Check for responsiveness and pulse for not more than 10 seconds.

Then immediately begin advanced life support.

Action priorities in advanced life support

1. Defibrillation
2. Intubation
3. IV/IO access
4. Medications

VENTRICULAR FIBRILLATION AND PULSELESS V-TACH

Review of the Algorithm for Ventricular Fibrillation and Pulseless V-Tach
Call for help, begin CPR, give oxygen if available, and attach monitor/defibrillator when available. Intubate and establish IV/IO access when possible.
Perform continuous CPR throughout resuscitation.
If shockable rhythm, give 1 shock (first) at 360 J (monophasic) or 120 to 200 J (biphasic) (if phase unknown use 200 J), resume CPR (2 minutes), and check rhythm. If shockable rhythm, give 1 shock (second).
Administer epinephrine 1 mg IV/IO, repeat every 3 to 5 minutes or vasopressin 40 units IV/IO push, single dose, one time only to replace first and second dose of epinephrine.
Check rhythm. If shockable rhythm, give 1 shock (third).

Review of the Algorithm for Ventricular Fibrillation and Pulseless V-Tach
Consider antiarrhythmic medications: **Amiodarone**: 300 mg IV/IO push. Consider repeating 150 mg IV/IO once. Maximum 3 doses. **Lidocaine**: 1.0 to 1.5 mg/kg IV/IO. For refractory ventricular fibrillation may give additional 0.5 to 0.75 mg/kg IV/IO push. Repeat in 5 to 10 min. Maximum total 3 mg/kg. If the rhythm is converted follow with an IV/IO 1 to 4 mg/min.
Consider magnesium sulfate 1 to 2 gm IV/IO diluted in 10 ml D5W IV/IO push
After 5 cycles of CPR, check rhythm, defibrillate if indicated
Consider sodium bicarbonate 1 mEq/kg IV/IO
If spontaneous circulation returns, ventilate and treat the underlying cause.

PULSELESS ELECTRICAL ACTIVITY (PEA)

Review of the Algorithm for Pulseless Electrical Activity
Call for help, begin CPR, give oxygen if available, and attach monitor/defibrillator when available. Intubate and establish IV/IO access when possible.
Perform continuous CPR throughout resuscitation.
Administer epinephrine 1 mg IV/IO and repeat every 3 to 5 minutes or vasopressin 40 units IV/IO to replace first or second dose of epinephrine.
If rate is slow, consider atropine 1 mg IV/IO every 3 to 5 minutes up to a maximum of four doses.
Check rhythm. If shockable rhythm, give 1 shock.
Consider hypovolemia, hypoxia, hydrogen ion (acidosis), hypo- or hyperkalemia, hypoglycemia, hypothermia, toxins (drug overdose), tamponade (cardiac), tension pneumothorax, thrombosis (coronary or pulmonary), trauma
If spontaneous circulation returns, ventilate and treat the underlying cause.

ASYSTOLE

Review of the Algorithm for Asystole
Call for help, begin CPR, give oxygen if available, and attach monitor/defibrillator when available. Intubate and establish IV/IO access when possible.
Perform continuous CPR during resuscitation.
Confirm asystole in more than one lead.
Administer epinephrine 1 mg IV/IO. Repeat every 3 to 5 minutes or may give 1 dose vasopressin 40 units IV/IO to replace first or second dose of epinephrine.

Review of the Algorithm for Asystole
For asystole or slow PEA rate, consider atropine 1 mg IV/IO repeat every 3 minutes up to three doses.
Check rhythm. If shockable rhythm, give 1 shock.
Consider hypovolemia, hypoxia, hydrogen ion (acidosis), hypo- or hyperkalemia, hypoglycemia, hypothermia, toxins (drug overdose), tamponade (cardiac) tension pneumothorax, thrombosis (coronary or pulmonary), trauma
If spontaneous circulation returns, ventilate and treat the underlying cause.

BRADYCARDIA

Review of the Algorithm for Bradycardia
HR < 60 beats per minute with inadequate perfusion
Call for help, give oxygen if available, and attach monitor/defibrillator when available. Intubate and establish IV/IO access when possible.
Prepare for transcutaneous (external) pacing.
Administer atropine 0.5 mg IV/IO to a maximum dose of 3 mg. If ineffective begin pacing.
Consider dopamine 2 to 10 mcg/kg/min IV/IO infusion
Consider epinephrine 2 to 10 mcg/min IV/IO infusion
If spontaneous circulation returns, ventilate and treat the underlying cause.

COMMONLY ORDERED MEDICATIONS

ATROPINE

Atropine	
Indications	Symptomatic bradycardia, pulseless arrest
Adult dose	1 mg IV/IO bolus every 3 to 5 minutes, maximum of 3 doses. 2 to 3 mg via ET diluted with 10 ml NS
Pediatric dose	0.02 mg/kg IV/IO minimum 0.1 mg IV/IO, maximum single dose 0.5 mg for a child and 1.0 mg for an adolescent
Onset	IV/IO onset 2 to 4 minutes, duration 4 to 6 hours
Compatibility	Compatible at Y-site with KCl, Tagamet, dobutamine, epinephrine, Heparin, Pronestyl
Side effects	Tachycardia
Note	May be administered undiluted IV/IO. Use cautiously with myocardial ischemia. Doses less than 0.5 mg can cause paradoxical tachycardia.

CALCIUM CHLORIDE

Calcium Chloride	
Indications	Known or suspected hyperkalemia, hypocalcemia, antidote for toxic effects of calcium channel blocker overdose
Adult dose	500 mg to 1000 mg (5 to 10 ml of a 10% solution) IV/IO slow push
Pediatric dose	20 mg/kg IV/IO slow push
Onset	IV/IO onset immediate, duration ½ to 1½ hours
Side effects	Cardiac arrest, hypercalcemia
Note	Administer undiluted or dilute in equal amounts of NS for injection. Do no administer with sodium bicarbonate.

DOPAMINE

Dopamine	
Indications	Pump problems. Hypotension with signs and symptoms of shock, second line drug for symptomatic bradycardia
Adult dose	Usual infusion rate 2 to 20 mcg/kg/min IV/IO.
Pediatric dose	Usual infusion rate 2 to 20 mcg/kg/min IV/IO
Onset	IV/IO onset 5 minutes, half-life 2 minutes, duration less than 10 minutes
Side effects	Tachycardia, arrhythmias
Note	Increase and decrease by 1 to 2 mcg/kg/min. Swan Ganz catheter or central line is recommended. For extravasations, use Regitine. Do not mix with sodium bicarbonate or other alkaline solutions.

EPINEPHRINE IN CARDIAC ARREST

Epinephrine in Cardiac Arrest	
Indications	Cardiac arrest, V Fib, asystole, PEA, cardiac decompensation not responsive to other drugs
Adult dose	1 mg (10 ml. of 1:10,000 solution) IV/IO bolus over 1 minute. Administer every 3 to 5 minutes during cardiac arrest. Follow each dose with a 20 ml flush and elevate the site for 10 to 20 seconds after dose.
Pediatric dose	0.01 mg/kg IV/IO (0.1 ml/kg of the 1:10,000 solution) every 3 to 5 minutes during cardiac arrest
Onset	IV/IO onset immediate
Compatibility	Do not mix in alkaline solutions
Side effects	Tachycardia, severe anxiety, arrhythmias, hypertension

EPINEPHRINE IV/IO INFUSION

Epinephrine IV/IO Infusion	
Indications	Profound shock
Adult dose	Begin with rapid infusion and then titrate to response. Usual initial infusion 0.1 to 1 mcg/min IV/IO. Higher doses may be effective.
Pediatric dose	Begin with rapid infusion and then titrate to response. Usual initial infusion 0.1 mcg/kg IV/IO
Onset	IV/IO onset immediate
Side effects	Tachycardia, severe anxiety, arrhythmias, hypertension

ISUPREL IV/IO INFUSION

Isuprel IV/IO Infusion (isoproterenol)	
Indications	Bradycardia unresponsive to atropine and refractory Torsade de pointes
Adult dose	2 mcg to 10 mcg/min. IV/IO
Onset	IV/IO onset rapid, duration 10 min.
Compatibility	Compatible at Y-site with potassium chloride, dobutamine, Heparin, Inocor, Lidocaine.
Side effects	Tachycardia
Note	Contraindicated in cardiac arrest, use pacing first, use Isuprel only if external pacer not available

LIDOCAINE BOLUS

Lidocaine Bolus	
Indications	Ventricular arrhythmias
Adult dose	1 to 1.5 mg/kg rapid IV/IO push. May give an additional 0.5 to 0.75 mg/kg IV/IO push and repeat in 5 to 10 minutes for a maximum of 3 doses or a total of 3 mg/kg. Endotracheal dose is 2 to 4 mg/kg.
Pediatric dose	1 mg/kg rapid IV/IO push. Maximum dose 100 mg
Onset	IV/IO onset immediate
Compatibility	Compatible at Y-site with Aminophylline, Bretylium, dobutamine, Dopamine, epinephrine, Heparin, Inocor, Isuprel, Neo-Synephrine, Nitroglycerin, Pronestyl
Side effects	Nausea, vomiting, confusion
Note	Follow bolus with IV/IO infusion

LIDOCAINE IV/IO INFUSION

Lidocaine IV/IO Infusion

Lidocaine IV/IO Infusion	
Indications	Ventricular ectopy
Adult dose	1 to 4 mg/min. IV/IO, for a bolus of 1 mg/kg use an IV/IO rate of 2 mg/min; for a 2 mg/kg bolus use a 3 mg/min rate; for a 3 mg/kg bolus use a 4 mg/min. rate
Onset	IV/IO onset 2 min., duration 20 min.
Compatibility	Compatible at Y-site with heparin, streptokinase, potassium chloride
Side effects	Nausea, vomiting, confusion, seizures, toxicity
Note	Do not use in heart block or slow rhythms. The patient may need the ventricular rhythm to sustain circulation.

MAGNESIUM SULFATE

Magnesium Sulfate	
Indications	Hypomagnesemia
Adult dose	1 to 2 grams (diluted in 10 ml D5W) IV/IO over 5 to 20 min. For Torsade de pointes give a loading dose of 1 to 2 grams IV/IO mixed with 50 to 100 ml of D5W over 5 to 60 min. and follow with a 0.5 to 1 gram/hr Titrate to control Torsade de pointes
Onset	IV/IO onset 1 to 5 minutes, duration ½ hour
Compatibility	Compatible at Y-site with dobutamine, Heparin, morphine, potassium chloride
Side effects	Hypotension, circulatory collapse, heart block
Note	Prophylactic use in all AMI patients is not recommended. Can be given via ETT.

SODIUM BICARBONATE

Sodium Bicarbonate	
Indications	Cardiac arrest with suspected acidosis
Adult	8.4% solution 1st dose 1 mEq/kg IV/IO 2nd dose 0.5 mEq/kg IV/IO every 10 min. 3rd and subsequent doses determined by ABG analysis results (acid-base balance). ABG results are not reliable during cardiac arrest.
Pediatric dose	1 mEq/kg per dose IV/IO. Infuse slowly.
Onset	IV/IO onset rapid, peak rapid
Side effects	Circulatory collapse

Sodium Bicarbonate	
Note	A 50 ml syringe of 8.4% solution provides 50 mEq of sodium bicarbonate is commercially available. Sodium bicarbonate is also available in a 4.2% solution for infant resuscitation.

RELATED CONDITIONS AND INFORMATION

CARDIAC ARREST

Cardiac arrest is a non-traumatic, non-violent, and unexpected sudden cessation of effective heart action causing loss of functional circulation. Common causes are ventricular tachycardia and ventricular fibrillation.

CARDIOPULMONARY ARREST

Cardiopulmonary arrest is a sudden cessation of functional ventilation and circulation causing functional collapse of both the respiratory and circulatory system.

DRUG ADMINISTRATION CONSIDERATIONS

- Drugs that can be administered IV can be administered IO (intraosseous) at the same dose.
- IV drugs administered peripherally should be followed by a flush of at least 5 ml.
- IO drugs should be followed by a flush of at least 5 ml.
- Endotracheal drugs require a higher dose and are unreliable. IV/IO is the preferred route. Dilute endotracheal drugs with NS to a volume of 3 to 5 ml and instill in the endotracheal tube. Follow with 3 to 5 ml. NS and provide 5 positive pressure breaths.

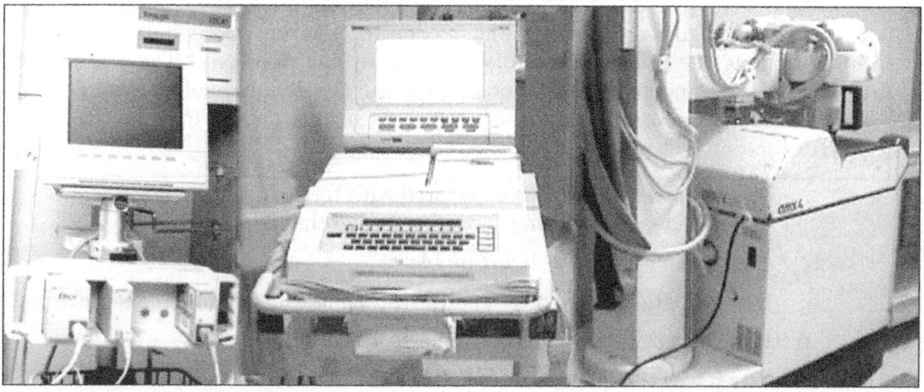

10 CHEST PAIN

> For details on triage see Chapter 34, Triage in a Nutshell.

PATIENT'S STORY – INTERVIEW QUESTIONS

1. When did the chest pain begin?
2. Is the chest pain active or resolved?
3. For active chest pain:
   a. When did the pain begin?
   b. What was the patient doing when the pain began?
   c. Did any event or activity cause the pain?
4. For resolved or intermittent chest pain:
   a. For how many days, weeks, or months has the pain been present?
   b. How often do the episodes of pain occur?
   c. How long do the episodes of pain last?
   d. Does any event or activity cause the pain?
5. How does the patient describe the pain?
   a. What is the character of the pain, e.g., sharp, burning, crushing, or a heavy feeling?
   b. Does anything make the pain better or worse?
6. In what region of the chest is the pain located?
   a. Does it radiate to another region of the body, e.g., jaw, arms, neck?
   b. What is the severity of the pain?

> It is appropriate to use the terms mild, moderate, or severe and equally appropriate to use a scale of 0 to 10. Zero typically means no pain. The meaning of a 10 is not the same for all nurses or all patients. The definition of 10 must be determined, documented, and consistently used for that patient to be an effective pain evaluation tool.

7. Are any other symptoms associated with the pain; e.g., shortness of breath, nausea, vomiting, sweating, or lightheadedness?
8. Does the patient have heart problems?
9. Did the patient have recent chest trauma or exertion involving the arms?
10. Has the patient taken NTG and if so, did it help?
11. When was the last dose?
12. Did the patient ingest any recreational drugs in the past 12 hours, e.g., cocaine or narcotics?
13. Has any treatment been initiated, and has it helped?
14. Has the patient had similar problems before?
    a. When was the problem?
    b. What was the diagnosis and treatment?
15. Does the patient have any pertinent past history?
16. Does the patient take any routine medications?
    a. What is the name, dosage, route, and frequency of each medication?
    b. When was the last dose?
17. Does the patient take any complementary or alternative therapies, herbal products, over-the-counter medications or supplements, or natural therapies?
    a. What is the name, dosage, route and frequency of each therapy?
    b. When was the last dose or therapy?
18. Does the patient have allergies to drugs or foods?
    a. What is the name of the allergen?
    b. What was the reaction?
19. If the patient is female and between the ages of 12 to 50 years, when was the first day of her last menstrual period?

NURSING DOMAIN

The nursing domain, nursing diagnosis and plan of care can only be determined after an in-depth interview and consideration of the patient's story.

> Domain 12. Comfort.
> Class 1. Physical comfort.

Domain 4. Elimination and Exchange. Class 4. Cardiovascular/pulmonary response.
Domain 11. Physical Injury. Class 2. Rick for physical injury.
Domain 4. Activity/Rest Class 4. Cardiovascular/Pulmonary responses.

ANTICIPATED MEDICAL CARE

Review of the Anticipated Medical Care of Chest Pain	
Protocol	Acute Coronary Syndrome Algorithm. Goals are door-to-needle (fibrinolysis) 30 minutes and door-to-balloon of 90 minutes.
Exam	Full body
Urine tests	None
Blood tests	Hematology, electrolytes, renal function studies, coagulation studies, cardiac markers, e.g., CK-MB, myoglobin, troponin
ECG	12 lead electrocardiogram, echocardiogram, stress echocardiogram
X-ray	Portable chest x-ray
Diet	NPO
IV	Saline locked intravenous access
Medications	Practice the mnemonic **MONA**. Put the patient on oxygen and administer aspirin. Use nitroglycerin first and then morphine to relieve chest pain as needed. **M**orphine 2 to 4 mg IV **O**xygen via nasal cannula at 4 L/min. **N**itroglycerin SL, spray, topical, or IV **A**spirin 160 to 325 mg Heparin and thrombolytics If a patient is allergic to aspirin, the alternative antithrombotic agent is Ticlid (ticlopidine hydrochloride) 250 mg orally.
ECG changes of injury (ST elevation or new BBB)	STEMI stand for ST-elevation MI Drugs: Beta-blockers, clopidogrel (oral antiplatelet agent, such as Plavix), heparin (unfractionated abbreviated UFH or low molecular weight heparin abbreviated LMWH)

Review of the Anticipated Medical Care of Chest Pain	
ECG changes of ischemia (ST depression or T-wave inversion)	UA/NSTEMI stands for unstable angina non-ST elevation MI Drugs: Beta-blockers, nitroglycerin, clopidogrel (oral antiplatelet agent, such as Plavix), heparin, nitroglycerin, and glycoprotein IIb/IIIa inhibitors ((ReoPro, Integrilin, Aggrastat)
Disposition	Admission may be required for continued workup. Cardiac decision unit may handle cardiac stress testing on an outpatient basis as part of the ER admission.
Worst-case scenario	The worst-case scenario is sudden loss of cardiac circulation from a blocked left main coronary artery. Management may include preparation for STAT cardiac catheterization and open-heart surgery. Obtain consent for catheterization, surgery, and anesthesia.

INITIAL CARE PLAN

> Alcohol-based hand sanitizers are the preferred method for cleaning your hands in most clinical situations. Wash your hands with soap and water whenever they are visibly dirty, before eating, and after using the restroom.

1. Ask the patient to undress, take off jewelry that might interfere with the examination, and put on an exam gown. Assist as needed.

> The primary goal is to reduce the patient's oxygen needs.

2. Elevate the head of the stretcher.
3. Obtain vital signs including a pulse oximetry. Attach heart monitor leads and automatic blood pressure cuff for continuous monitoring. Document the initial heart monitor strip and document changes of rhythm.
4. Obtain a 12-lead electrocardiogram within 10 minutes of admission
5. Establish an intravenous access line and draw laboratory specimens. Draw a variety of tubes that will allow the lab to perform hematology, chemistry, and coagulation studies.

> Commonly ordered tests include hemogram, electrolytes, blood sugar, BUN, creatinine, coagulation studies, and cardiac markers; e.g., CK-MB, myoglobin, and troponin.

1. Administer medications covered by hospital protocol, e.g., consider implementing the mnemonic **MONA**. All patients are greeted with a smile from Mona. The mnemonic is used as a reminder of each medication and not practiced in the order given. Put the patient on oxygen and administer aspirin. Use nitroglycerin first and then morphine to relieve chest pain as needed.
   Morphine 2 to 4 mg IV to reduce preload with peripheral vasodilation, reduce sympathetic activity, and thereby decrease the myocardial workload.
   Oxygen nasal cannula at 4 L/min. to enrich oxygen supply.
   Nitroglycerin SL to dilate the coronary arteries, improve blood flow to the heart muscle, and decrease preload and afterload.
   Aspirin 160 to 325 mg to reduce the risk of clot formation. If a patient is allergic to aspirin, the alternative antithrombotic agent is Ticlid (ticlopidine hydrochloride) 250 mg orally.

6. Perform a focused physical assessment.
   a. Auscultate lung sounds to evaluate for fluid in the lungs as an indicator of left ventricular failure.
   b. Auscultate heart sounds to evaluate for murmurs and rubs.
   c. Inspect for peripheral edema as an indicator of right ventricular failure.

7. Obtain a brief targeted history for eligibility of thrombolytics.
   a. If the patient has experienced chest pain for more than 15 minutes and less than 12 hours. If the answer is no, do not go any further with your questions. The patient is not eligible.
   b. Does the ECG show a STEMI or new BBBB? If yes continue.
   c. If any of the following questions are answered yes, fibrinolysis may be contraindicated.
      i. Is the systolic BP greater than 180?
      ii. Is the diastolic BP greater than 110?
      iii. Right versus left arm systolic BP difference greater than 15?
      iv. History of structural central nervous system disease?
      v. Significant closed head or facial trauma within the past 3 months?
      vi. Recent (within 6 weeks) major trauma, surgery, GI or GU bleed.
      vii. Bleeding or clotting problem or on blood thinners?
      viii. CPR greater than 10 minutes
      ix. Pregnant female?
      x. Serious systemic disease, such as advanced or terminal cancer, severe liver or kidney disease?

d. Is the patient at high risk? If any of the questions below are yes and the hospital is not capable of angioplasty, consider transfer to a facility capable of percutaneous cardiac interventions or angioplasty.
   i. Heart rate more than or equal to 100 beats per minute and systolic BP less than 100 mm Hg?
   ii. Signs of pulmonary edema?
   iii. Signs of shock?
   iv. Contraindications to fibrinolytic therapy?

8. Instruct the patient not to eat or drink and teach the patient and family the rationale for the NPO status.
9. Place and maintain the bed siderails up with the stretcher in the lowest position.
10. Inform the patient, family, and caregivers of the usual plan of care and the expected overall time before disposition.
11. Provide the patient with a device to reach someone for assistance and explain how to use it. Ask the patient to call for help before getting off the stretcher.

ONGOING CARE PLAN

> Inform the medical provider of adverse changes noted during ongoing evaluation. Document that the medical provider was notified of the adverse change. Document if orders were or were not received.

1. Monitor heart rate, rhythm, and ST segment changes. If the patient has heart damage or ischemia, monitor the affected lead.
   a. V1, V2, V3 for anterior heart ischemia or damage
   b. II, III, aVF for inferior heart ischemia or damage
   c. I, V4, V5, V6 for lateral heart ischemia or damage
2. Monitor vital signs and effectiveness of breathing every 15 to 30 minutes.
3. Perform focused ongoing assessments.
4. Assess pain intensity, location, and duration. Administer NTG and morphine as needed.

> If the patient is allergic to morphine, Demerol can be used. Demerol 75 to 100 mg is equal to approximately 10 mg of morphine. Morphine is ten times more potent than Demerol mg for mg.

5. Monitor the therapeutic effect of the medications. Most acceptable to cardiac staff for evaluation of effectiveness is a scale of 0 to 10.

> Zero typically means no pain. The meaning of a 10 is not the same for all nurses or all patients. The definition of 10 must be determined, documented, and consistently used for that patient to be an effective pain evaluation tool.

6. Auscultate lungs and heart sounds during angina.

A transient abnormal point of maximal impulse, pulsus alternans (a weak pulse alternating with a strong one), or an atrial gallop (S4) may be detected during an angina attack.

7. Monitor closely for the development of adverse reactions to therapy and remedy.
8. If not NPO, provide the patient with food at mealtimes and fluids during the stay.
9. Keep the patient, family, and caregivers well informed of the plan of care and the remaining time anticipated before disposition.
10. Monitor the patient's laboratory and radiographic results and notify the medical provider of critical abnormalities. Remedy abnormalities as ordered.
11. Notify the medical provider when all diagnostic results are available for review. Ask for establishment of a diagnosis and disposition.

DISCHARGE INSTRUCTIONS

1. Provide the patient with the name of the nurse and doctor in the emergency room.
2. Inform the patient of their diagnosis or why a definitive diagnosis couldn't be made. Explain what caused the problem if known.
3. For chest wall or pleuritic pain, inform the patient that the problem was minor, of a stable nature, and the probability of a heart attack was low.
4. Instruct the patient with angina to achieve his ideal body weight, avoid smoking, and reduce high blood pressure if present. Avoid activities that increase the symptoms and take NTG as prescribed.
5. Teach the patient how to take the medication as prescribed and how to manage the common side effects. Instruct the patient not to drive or perform any dangerous tasks while taking narcotic pain medications.
6. Recommend a medical provider for follow-up care. Provide the name, address, and phone number with a recommendation of when to schedule the care.
7. Instruct the patient to call 911 if chest pain is unrelieved by nitroglycerin, becomes severe, radiates to the arms, neck, jaw, or is associated with sweating or nausea. Encourage the patient NOT to IGNORE WORSENING OR PERSISTENT SYMPTOMS.
8. Ask for verbal confirmation or demonstration of understanding and reinforce teaching as needed.

COMMONLY ORDERED MEDICATIONS

HEPARIN

Heparin

Heparin	
Indications	Adjunctive therapy in ACS (unstable angina/NSTEMI) and STEMI, anticoagulant therapy for prophylaxis and treatment of venous thrombosis, pulmonary embolus, to reduce the risk of embolus in atrial fibrillation
Adult dose	Generic weight-based protocol: Initial bolus 60 U/kg IV (maximum 4000 U) Continue 12 U/kg per hour IV Adjust every 6 hours to maintain the aPTT 1 ½ to 2 ½ times the control value
Onset	IV onset 5 min., peak 10 min., duration 2 to 6 hours
Compatibility	Compatible at Y-site with potassium chloride, Aminophylline, Dopamine, Isuprel, Lidocaine, Neo-Synephrine, Levophed Not compatible at Y site with dobutamine
Side effects	Bleeding

LOPRESSOR

Lopressor (metoprolol)	
Indications	PSVT, hypertension
Adult dose	5 mg IV slowly every 5 min., maximum 15 mg IV
Onset	IV onset immediate, peak 20 minutes, duration 5 to 8 hours
Compatibility	Compatible at Y-site with Activase, Demerol, morphine, nitroglycerin, Heparin
Side effects	Bronchospasm, bradycardia <40, heart block > 1st degree, systolic blood pressure <90
Note	Lopressor is a second line agent after adenosine, Diltiazem, and digoxin. Lopressor is contraindicated in heart block, CHF, and asthma.

MORPHINE

Morphine sulfate (MSO4)	
Indications	Moderate to severe pain
Dose	1 to 4 mg IV administered over 1 to 5 min. every 5 to 30 min. for chest pain
Pediatric dose	50 to 100 mcg/kg IV, maximum 10 mg/dose
Onset	IV onset rapid, peak 20 minutes, duration 4 to 5 hours
Compatibility	Incompatible with Lasix, compatible with most other solutions
Side effects	Confusion, sedation, hypotension, respiratory depression
Note	May reverse with Narcan 0.4 to 2 mg IV.

Morphine sulfate (MSO4)	
Monitor	Effectiveness of respirations

NITROGLYCERIN SL

Nitroglycerin SL	
Indications	Suspected cardiac ischemia
Adult dose	0.3, 0.4, or 0.6 mg SL every 5 min., maximum 3 tablets
Onset	SL onset 1 to 3 min., duration ½ hour, half-life 1 to 4 min.
Side effects	Headache, flushing, dizziness, postural hypotension
Note	Do not administer NTG with a systolic blood pressure of <90. Tablets should be kept under the tongue for 1 to 2 minutes until dissolved and nothing taken by mouth.
Monitor	Blood pressure

NITROGLYCERIN OINTMENT

Nitroglycerin Ointment	
Indications	Suspected cardiac ischemia
Adult dose	½ inch to 2 inches topically to the anterior chest
Onset	Topical onset ½ to 1 hour, duration 2 to 12 hours
Side effects	Headache, flushing, dizziness, postural hypotension
Note	Ointment is applied to the anterior chest. Avoid areas of potential heart monitor or electrocardiogram lead placement. DO NOT apply to extremities to decrease the side effects; the therapeutic actions are also decreased.
Monitor	Blood pressure

NITROGLYCERIN

Nitroglycerin IV	
Indications	Suspected heart ischemia, acute MI, left ventricular failure, hypertension
Adult dose	5 mcg/min. and increase by 5 mcg/minute every 5 min. to the desired effect
Onset	IV onset immediate, duration variable
Compatibility	Compatible at Y-site with Aminophylline, Bretylium, dobutamine, Dopamine, Inocor, Lidocaine, potassium chloride, diltiazem, famotidine, haloperidol, Lidocaine, nitroprusside, pancuronium, ranitidine, streptokinase, vecuronium
Side effects	Headache, hypotension

Nitroglycerin IV	
Note	Use glass bottle or non-latex bag with special tubing to prevent absorption of medicine into the tubing and bag. Some hospital's protocol allows the nurse to increase the NTG to relief of pain, but not to decease unless an order to wean is received from the medical provider. Some protocols require the nurse to check with the medical provider if over 200 mcg/min. is required.

PLAVIX

Plavix PO	
Indications	Acute ST segment elevation MI (STEMI)
Adult dose	300 mg PO loading dose, then 75 mg PO once daily in combination with aspirin
Onset	Within 24 hours, peak 3 to 7 days, duration 5 days.
Side effects	GI bleeding, neutropenia, thrombotic thrombocytopenic purpura
Note	Inhibits platelet aggregation

THROMBOLYTICS

Thrombolytics	
Activase (tPA)	
Indications	Acute MI
Adult dose	Accelerated infusion 1st dose: 15 mg IV bolus 2nd dose: 0.75 mg/kg IV over the next 30 min., max 50 mg 3rd dose: 0.5 mg/kg IV over the next 60 min., max 35 mg
Retavase	
Adult dose	1st dose: 10-unit IV bolus over 2 min. 2nd dose: (30 minutes later) 10 units IV bolus over 2 min.
Streptokinase	
Indications	Acute MI
Adult dose	1.5 million IV in a one-hour infusion
Tenecteplase (TNKase)	
Indications	Acute MI
Adult dose	Bolus 30 to 50 mg weight adjusted. One single dose is push over 5 seconds intravenously

RELATED CONDITIONS AND INFORMATION

ACUTE MYOCARDIAL INFARCTION

Review of Acute Myocardial Infarction (AMI)	
Causes	When the coronary arteries are unable to provide enough oxygen carrying blood to meet the oxygen requirements of the heart muscle, the heart muscle becomes ischemic and infarcts.
Symptoms	Symptoms may include chest pain not relieved with NTG or rest, usually lasting more than 30 minutes, many times occurring at rest, and usually associated with nausea, vomiting, diaphoresis, and weakness. Twenty percent of AMI patients do not experience chest pain. Patients with diabetes mellitus are prone to neuropathy and many have a silent AMI sustaining heart muscle injury without pain. In patients over 85 years, the presenting symptom is often shortness of breath. Patients with heart transplants do not experience pain because the pain receptors are cut during the transplant.
ECG diagnostic findings	First, the initial T wave inversion signifies an area of ischemic heart muscle from decreased blood supply. The cells are not yet actively dying. Second, the ST segment elevation of more than 2 mm in the affected area signifies an area of the heart muscle is infracting. The cells are actively in the process of dying. Third, Q wave formation signifies an area of cellular death.
Diet	NPO
IV	NS TKO or a saline locked intravenous access
Medications	Morphine IV Oxygen nasal cannula at 4 L/min Nitroglycerin SL or spray one every five min., maximum three Aspirin 160 to 325 mg PO Heparin IV, beta blockers IV or PO, nitroglycerin IV
Monitor	Monitor for arrhythmia, CHF, ventricular failure, circulatory collapse, pulmonary edema, and cardiogenic shock.
Diagnostic workup	Diagnostic workup may include cardiac stress testing and cardiac catheterization.
Disposition	Hospital admission may be required for definitive treatment.
Note	Denial is the first response to a MI. Reality orientation is not appropriate in the ER. Education includes definition of diagnosis and treatment, effect on lifestyle, and how to eliminate risk factors. Healing takes from six to eight weeks.
Expected outcome	Relief of chest pain is the primary focus of interventions to minimize or abort damage to the heart.

ANGINA

Review of Angina	
Cause of pain	Chest pain is a result of an imbalance between the oxygen supply to the heart and the demand. When the demand for oxygen is greater than the supply, severe paroxysmal chest pain occurs. The pain is caused by an insufficient supply of blood to the heart causing a temporary ischemia of the myocardium (inadequate oxygen for the myocardium to meet its metabolic needs). The coronary arteries are unable to provide enough oxygen carrying blood to meet the oxygen requirements of the heart muscle.
Signs and symptoms	Signs and symptoms may include severe paroxysmal chest pain, diaphoresis, cold and clammy skin, nausea, vomiting, indigestion, shortness of breath (dyspnea), lightheadedness, anxiety, and increased heart rate. During an angina attack, a transient abnormal point of maximal impulse, pulsus alternans (a weak pulse alternating with a strong one), and an atrial gallop (S4) may be detected.
Stable angina	Stable angina occurs as a predictable event after exercise or increased activity.
Unstable angina	Unstable angina occurs after exercise and at rest, is prolonged, and frequently worsens with each episode. It is associated with left main and proximal LAD coronary artery disease with 70% to 100% stenosis.
Prinzmetal's unstable angina	Prinzmetal's unstable angina occurs at rest and usually at the same time of day. Prognosis is poor with a 50% mortality rate in the first year.
Management	Management includes monitoring of vital signs and oxygen saturation, establishing an intravenous access, and drawing blood specimens. Tests may include hematology, chemistry, coagulation studies, cardiac markers (CK-MB, myoglobin, and troponin), a 12-lead electrocardiogram, and a targeted history of eligibility for thrombolytics. Medical management may include administering oxygen, aspirin, nitroglycerin, and morphine to relieve chest pain. Diagnostic workup may include cardiac stress testing and cardiac catheterization.
Expected outcome	Relief of chest pain is the primary focus of interventions to minimize or abort damage to the heart.

ASPIRIN ALLERGY

If a patient is allergic to aspirin, the alternative antithrombotic agent is Ticlid (ticlopidine hydrochloride) 250 mg orally.

CARDIAC MARKERS

CK/MB levels usually remain elevated for up to 72 hours.

Troponin levels remain elevated for up to 7 days.

Myoglobin usually normalized 8 hours after an injury.

CHEST PAIN

Esophagitis mimics heart pain. Chest pain can also be caused by cholelithiasis, hiatal hernia, gastric ulcer, peptic ulcer, and pancreatitis.

CHEST WALL PAIN

Review of Chest Wall Pain	
Causes	Chest wall pain is due to strain of muscles or ligaments commonly from excessive exercise.
Symptoms	Symptoms may include point tenderness and pain aggravated by cough or deep breathing.
Management	Medical management includes ruling out cardiac disease, analgesics, and anti-inflammatory medications.
Discharge Instructions	Instructions include the use of anti-inflammatory medications and to avoid lifting, straining, or exertion. Inform the patient to expect slow gradual improvement over the next one to three days and not to ignore new symptoms.

ACUTE CORONARY SYNDROME (ACS)

A term sometimes used to describe patients who have either an acute myocardial infarction (AMI) or unstable angina. It includes both Q-wave and non-Q-wave AMI. Patient symptoms are shortness of breath, discomfort in one or more arms, neck, jaw, or stomach; gastrointestinal distress (described as nausea or indigestion), and lightheadedness.

COSTOCHONDRITIS

Review of Costochondritis	
Causes	Costochondritis is an inflammation of the cartilages of the costochondral and costosternal junction.
Symptoms	Symptoms may include pain in the anterior chest that is usually sharp and localized but may be brief and darting or a persistent ache.
Management	Medical management includes ruling out cardiac disease, analgesics, and anti-inflammatory medications.
Discharge Instructions	Instructions include how to take anti-inflammatory medications and to avoid lifting, straining, or exertion. Inform the patient to expect slow gradual improvement over the next one to three days and not to ignore new symptoms.

HYPOTHERMIA AND RESUSCITATION

When a core temperature is below 28° C (82.4° F), electrical defibrillation is generally unsuccessful. Begin CPR, control and maintain the airway, and monitor cardiac rhythm and temperature while warming the patient.

Hypothermia is a common problem in patients with myxedema coma due to the slowed metabolism. Temperature is usually above 35° (95° F).

INFERIOR MI COMPLICATIONS

Inferior MI complications may include compromise of the sinus node circulation. In 55% of all people, the right coronary artery provides circulation to the sinus node and when compromised causes sinus bradycardia. Atropine is contraindicated. Atropine speeds up the heart and consumes oxygen. Treatment is to lay the patient down and elevate the legs.

Circulation to the AV node by the right coronary artery is present in 90% of people. When circulation to the AV node is compromised, it causes heart block. A Mobitz I block is of little consequence. A pacemaker needs to be placed for third heart block.

Circulation to the mitral valve is from the right coronary artery and when compromised a blowing murmur develops. Thirty percent of people with an inferior MI develop right ventricle infarction. A right ventricle infarction can be proven with right V leads. Intravenous normal saline will increase volume and stretch the right ventricle. D5W is contraindicated. It goes into the cell, decreases volume, increases vasoconstriction, and increases the afterload.

Demerol is the drug of choice for right ventricle MI pain. MSO4 decreases blood flow to the right ventricle by pooling blood as it vasodilates. Nitroglycerin is contraindicated because it causes vasodilation and decreases volume.

ANTEROSEPTAL MI COMPLICATIONS

An anteroseptal MI can compromise the blood flow of the lateral anterior descending coronary artery compromising circulation to the Bundle of HIS and bundle branches causing heart block. Mobitz II has a 44% to 94% mortality risk. The mortality is reduced to 14% when a pacemaker is inserted. A pacemaker is needed for a patient with an anteroseptal MI and a RBBB whether the block is old or new.

CONSIDER ALTERNATIVES

When a patient presents with chest pain, consider myocardial infarction, pulmonary edema, congestive heart failure, acute pulmonary embolus, pneumothorax, pneumonia, and bronchitis.

ARRHYTHMIA

An arrhythmia is an irregularity in the force or rhythm of the heartbeat. Cardiac ischemia can cause arrhythmias. Careful evaluation and documentation are needed. Treat immediately with ACLS protocols.

ENZYMES CARDIAC MARKERS

Test	Initial Elevation	Peak	Return to normal

Test	Initial Elevation	Peak	Return to normal
CK Creatine kinase	2 to 6 hours	18 to 36 hours	3 to 6 days
CK-MB Creatine kinase-MB	2 to 3 hours	24 hours	2 to 3 days
LDH Lactic dehydrogenase	12 to 24 hours	24 to 48 hours	5 to 6 days
Myoglobin	1 to 2 hours	4 to 6 hours	24 hours
Troponin	4 to 8 hours	14 to 18 hours	< 10 days

EXERCISE

Exercise can cause chest pain (angina) when oxygen supply is inadequate to meet the increased myocardial metabolic needs. The coronary arteries are unable to meet the oxygen requirements of the myocardium during exercise. It is a problem of supply and demand.

ELECTROCARDIOGRAM QRS COMPLEX AND T-WAVE CHANGES

Review of Electrocardiogram Changes	
T-wave inversion	T-wave inversion is indicative of ischemic heart muscle from decreased blood supply. Ischemia means the heart muscle needs more blood supply and oxygen but is not actively in the process of dying. Inverted T waves can quickly change to ST segment changes as the myocardium begins to die.
Elevated and depressed ST segments	ST segments can be normally elevated 1 mm above the baseline in limb leads and as much as 2 mm in precordial leads; but, can never be normally depressed more than 0.5 mm in any lead. Elevation and depression of the ST segment show that an area of the heart muscle is infarcting, actively in the process of dying. Infarcting heart muscle can be resuscitated and the damage reversed by returning the blood flow to adequate levels. Infarcting heart muscle presents a true EMERGENT situation. Time lost is muscle lost.
Q-waves	Q waves show that an area of the heart is infarcted. Infarcted means dead. Q waves usually occur 24 hours after the injury. Dead muscle cells cannot be resuscitated. Formation of stable scar tissue in the area of the dead cells takes six to eight weeks.
V1, V2, V3	Shows anterior damage
II, III, aVF	Shows inferior damage
I, V4, V5, V6	Shows lateral heart damage

HOT OFFLOAD

Hot offload means there is a need to run under the blades to get a very critical patient out of a rotor wing (helicopter) air ambulance. Personnel approach the nose of the helicopter in a crouched position at 12 o'clock directly or from not more than 45° to the right or left of the nose.

NITROGLYCERIN

Nitroglycerin must be given immediately at the onset of chest pain to reduce the risk of continuing ischemia.

OXYGEN HUMIDIFIERS

Review of Oxygen Humidifiers	
Low flow nasal cannula or simple mask	Able to humidify
High flow Ventimask	Unable to humidify because it restricts flow, alters FiO2, and whistles
Reservoir systems, non-rebreather, partial rebreather	Unable to humidify because it restricts flow and increases bottle pressure

PLEURISY

Review of Pleurisy	
Definition	Pleurisy is an inflammation of the pleura (the outside of the lung). It may be primary or secondary, usually unilateral, and can be acute or chronic.
Symptoms	Symptoms may include fever, chills, and knifelike pain on the affected side aggravated by deep breathing or coughing. Pain can be referred to the abdomen.
Management	Medical diagnostic workup may include CBC and chest x-ray. Negative physical and x-ray findings suggest epidemic pleurodynia (viral inflammation). Hemoptysis and parenchymal involvement on chest x-ray suggest infection or infarction. Medicines may include analgesic and anti-inflammatory medications for pain control and antibiotics if signs of infection are present.
Disposition	Pleurisy is usually followed as an outpatient. Admission may be required if infarction is suspected.
Discharge Instructions	Instructions include how to take the medications prescribed and to drink lots of water. If SOB, chest pain of a different character, or worsening of the present symptoms occur, call the follow-up medical provider.

PERICARDITIS

Review of Pericarditis	
Definition	Pericarditis is infection of the pericardium.

Review of Pericarditis	
Cause	The cause of pericarditis is a microorganism infection secondary to viral infections, acute MI, metastatic neoplasm, radiation therapy (up to 20 years earlier), chronic renal failure, rheumatoid arthritis, or heart surgery (up to months earlier).
Symptoms	Symptoms may include intense chest pain. It is characteristically sharp, pleuritic, positional (relieved by leaning forward), and associated with fever and palpitations. Pericarditis can imitate the pain of an acute myocardial infarction.
Diagnostic findings	Electrocardiogram reveals diffuse ST elevation, concave upward, usually in all leads except aVR and V1. Chest x-ray shows increased heart size. If a large pericardial effusion is present, there is a water bottle configuration. Echocardiogram is the most specific test.
Management	Medical management includes aspirin and analgesic medicine. Anticoagulants are generally contraindicated because of the risk of pericardial hemorrhage. Hospitalization may be required for a detailed cardiac workup and possible pericardiectomy.
Note	Pericarditis is most readily identified by the auscultation of a pericardial friction rub best heard along the left sternal border. Cardiac tamponade leading to ventricular fibrillation is a life-threatening complication of pericarditis. Invasive diagnostic procedures such as heart catheterization procedures can result in the development of infective endocarditis.

TIME IS MUSCLE

Time lost is heart muscle lost. Infarcted heart muscle cannot be revived. Drug to door goal is thirty minutes.

THROMBOLYTIC CONTRAINDICATIONS

Review of Thrombolytic Contraindications
Absolute: • Prior intracranial hemorrhage • Known structural cerebral vascular lesion • Know malignant intracranial neoplasm • Ischemic stroke within 3 months • Suspected aortic dissection • Active bleeding (excluding menses) or bleeding diathesis • Significant closed head or facial trauma within 3 months

Review of Thrombolytic Contraindications
Relative: • History of chronic, severe, poorly controlled hypertension • History of prior ischemic stroke greater than 3 months ago, dementia, know intracranial pathology • Traumatic or prolonged (> 10 minutes) CPR or major surgery in the past 3 weeks • Recent (past 2 to 4 weeks) internal bleeding • Non-compressible vascular punctures • Prior allergic reaction to streptokinase or anistreplase or prior exposure (more than 5 days ago) • Pregnancy • Active peptic ulcer • Current use of anticoagulants

THROMBOLYTIC INDICATIONS

Review of Indications for Thrombolytics
ST elevation (1 mm or more in at least two contiguous leads)
New BBB, strongly suspicious of injury
Signs and symptoms of acute myocardial infarction
Time of symptom onset < 12 hours

TRANSFER LEGISLATION

Transfer legislation mandates that the transfer personnel and equipment are appropriate for the needs of each patient. If the patient is receiving intensive level care, such as multiple titratable IV drips, assisted ventilation, and/or intra-aortic balloon pump, a nurse or medical provider who is experienced in this type of intensive care may be required. Paramedics typically do not have the expertise needed to provide the care needed. If the receiving facility is some distance away and the patient is critical, a rotor wing air ambulance (helicopter) may be necessary.

STEMI

STEMI stands for ST segment elevation myocardial infraction.

PEDIATRIC CONSIDERATIONS

BROSELOW-LUTEN SYSTEM

This color-coded system for use with pediatric patients was derived in the early eighties. The zones have been color coded and incorporated into the Broselow tape™ for emergency drug dosing and equipment selection and has become standard of care. A reference at each color bar on the tape informs you of estimated weight, equipment sizes, and drug dosages to perform emergency resuscitation on a child.

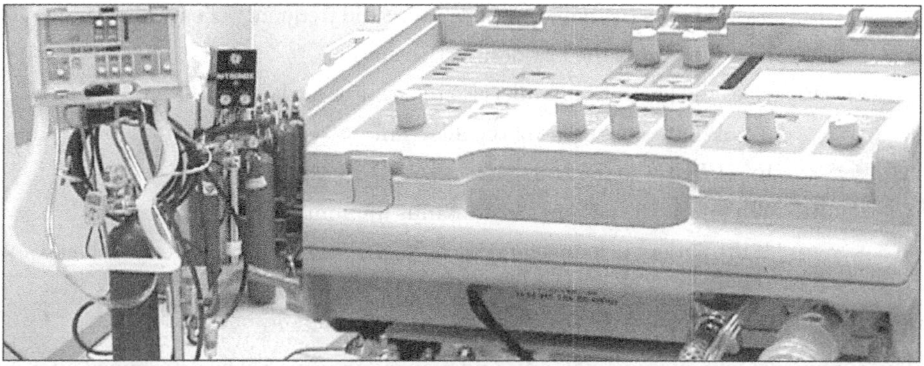

11 CHOKING AND AIRWAY OBSTRUCTION

For details on triage see Chapter 34, Triage in a Nutshell.

PATIENT'S STORY – INTERVIEW QUESTIONS

1. When was the onset of the choking?
2. Where is the obstruction (airway or esophagus)?
3. Why did the patient choke?
4. How does the obstruction affect normal function now?
   a. Is the patient able to speak clearly?
   b. Is the patient breathing effectively?
   c. Is the patient able to swallow?

Choking may result from spasm of the larynx induced by an irritating gas. Not all choking victims inhale food or foreign bodies. Irritation of the larynx can cause airway obstruction from spasm.

5. Did anyone try any maneuvers to stop the choking and did they help?
6. Has the patient had similar problems before?
   a. When was the problem?
   b. What was the diagnosis and treatment?
7. Does the patient have any pertinent past history?
8. Does the patient take any routine medications?
   a. What is the name, dose, route, and frequency of the medication?
   b. When was the last dose?
9. Does the patient take any complementary or alternative therapies, herbal products, over-the-counter medications or supplements, or natural therapies?

   a. What is the name, dosage, route and frequency of each therapy?
   b. When was the last dose or therapy?
10. Does the patient have allergies to drugs or foods?
   a. What is the name of the allergen?
   b. What was the reaction?
11. When was the patient's last tetanus immunization?
12. If the patient is female and between the ages of 10 to 50 years, when was the first day of her last menstrual period?

NURSING DOMAIN

The nursing domain, nursing diagnosis and plan of care can only be determined after an in-depth interview and consideration of the patient's story.

Domain 3. Elimination and Exchange. Class 4. Respiratory function.
Domain 11. Safety/Protection Class 2. Physical injury.

ANTICIPATED MEDICAL CARE

Review of the Anticipated Medical Care of Choking and Airway Obstructions	
Exam	Full body
X-ray	Chest x-ray, soft tissue neck x-ray
Diet	NPO
IV	None
Medications	Glucagon
Other	Direct laryngoscopy, bronchoscopy
Disposition	Hospital observation may be required if edema of the throat is suspected.
Worst-case scenario	The worst-case scenario is a compromised airway with inability to ventilate. Management is STAT bronchoscopy with removal of foreign body.

INITIAL CARE PLAN

> Alcohol-based hand sanitizers are the preferred method for cleaning your hands in most clinical situations. Wash your hands with soap and water whenever they are visibly dirty, before eating, and after using the restroom.

1. Ask the patient to undress, remove all jewelry that might interfere with the examination, and put on an exam gown. Assist as needed.
2. Position the patient in a high Fowler's position.

3. Obtain vital signs; attach heart monitor leads, automatic blood pressure cuff, and pulse oximetry for continuous monitoring. Document the initial heart monitor strip and document changes of rhythm.
4. Assure the patient that he is safe.
5. Perform a focused physical examination.
    a. Auscultate the lungs.
    b. Listen to the sounds of breathing at the neck.
    c. Evaluate the level of consciousness based on the mnemonic **AVPU** or **ACDU** level of consciousness score.
    AVPU: Alert, **V**erbal, **P**ain, **U**nresponsive.
    ACDU: Alert, **C**onfused, **D**rowsy, **U**nresponsive.
6. Establish an intravenous access if obstruction is still present and draw blood specimens. Draw a variety of tubes that will allow the lab to perform hematology, chemistry, and coagulation studies and hold for medical provider order.
7. Administer medications covered by hospital protocol.
8. Inform the patient not to eat or drink and teach the patient and family the rationale for the NPO status.
9. Elevate the siderails and place the stretcher in the lowest position.
10. Inform the patient, family, and caregivers of the usual plan of care and the expected overall time before disposition.
11. Provide the patient with a device to reach someone for assistance and explain how to use it. Ask the patient to call for help before getting off the stretcher.

ONGOING CARE PLAN

> Inform the medical provider of adverse changes noted during ongoing evaluation. Document that the medical provider was notified of the adverse change. Document if orders were or were not received.

1. Monitor vital signs and effectiveness of breathing.
2. Monitor for signs of worsening, e.g., restlessness, difficulty swallowing, dyspnea, and hoarseness.

> Airway obstruction can occur after a foreign body is removed. Swelling and laryngeal spasm can cause airway compromise leading to airway obstruction later in the ER course.

3. Monitor therapy closely for the patient's therapeutic response.
    a. The usual time for a medication effectiveness check is 20 to 30 minutes after giving the drug.
    b. If therapy is not effective, ask the medical provider for a repeat dose or an alternative.

4. Monitor closely for the development of adverse reactions to therapy.
    a. Perform interventions to relieve the adverse reaction.
    b. Ask the medical provider for a remedy.
5. If not NPO, provide the patient with food at mealtimes and fluids during the stay.
6. Keep the patient, family, and caregivers well informed of the plan of care and the remaining time anticipated before disposition.
7. Monitor the patient's laboratory and x-ray results and notify the medical provider of critical abnormalities. Remedy abnormalities as ordered.
8. Notify the medical provider when all diagnostic results are available for review. Ask for establishment of a diagnosis and disposition.

DISCHARGE INSTRUCTIONS

1. Provide the patient with the name of the nurse and doctor in the emergency room.
2. Inform the patient of their diagnosis or why a definitive diagnosis couldn't be made. Explain what caused the problem if known.
3. Teach the patient how to take the medication as prescribed and how to manage the common side effects. Instruct the patient not to drive or perform any dangerous tasks while taking narcotic pain medications.
4. Recommend a medical provider for follow-up care. Provide the name, address, and phone number with a recommendation of when to schedule the care. Encourage the patient to follow-up to assure no injury is present on repeat examination.
5. Instruct the patient that the airway or breathing passages may be injured or inflamed to a minor degree. Any airway problems or worsening are not expected. Return to the emergency room for difficulty breathing, swallowing, hoarseness, or fever. Encourage the patient NOT to IGNORE WORSENING OR PERSISTENT SYMPTOMS.
6. Ask for verbal confirmation or demonstration of understanding and reinforce teaching as needed.

MEDICATIONS

GLUCAGON

Glucagon	
Indications	Esophageal foreign body obstruction
Adult dose	1 to 5 mg SC or IV
Pediatric dose	1 mg SC or IV
Onset	IV onset 1 min., duration 9 to 17 min.
Side effects	Nausea
Note	Use immediately after reconstitution.

Glucagon	
Monitor	Blood sugar levels

VALIUM

Valium (diazepam)	
Indications	Conscious sedation
Dose	5 to 10 mg IV single dose 5 to 20 mg IM single dose
Onset	IV onset 5 min., peak 15 min., duration 15 min. IM onset 15 min., peak ½ to 1 ½ hours
Side effects	Decreased respiratory effectiveness, dizziness, drowsiness, orthostatic hypotension, blurred vision, tachycardia
Monitor	Level of consciousness, respiratory effectiveness

VERSED

Versed (midazolam hydrochloride)	
Indications	Conscious sedation
Adult dose	1 to 2.5 mg IV over at least 2 min., every 2 min., maximum 5 mg IV. If narcotic medications were administered before the Versed, use approximately 30% less Versed.
Pediatric dose	Pediatric patients 12 to 16 years old should be dosed as adults. 0.05 to 0.2 mg/kg IV loading dose over 2 to 3 min Versed is used with caution in child who are not intubated.
Onset	IV onset 3 to 5 min.
Compatibility	Use NS to flush IV line before and after dose
Side effects	Serious life threatening decreased respiratory tidal volume and respiratory rate
Monitor	Effectiveness of breathing
Note	Versed is a potent sedative that requires slow administration and individualized dosage. Versed is 3 to 4 times as potent as Valium. The reversing agent is Romazicon (flumazenil).

RELATED CONDITIONS AND INFORMATION

ASSESSMENT OF VERSED AFFECT

Sedation Level	Facial Expression	Response
Alert	Normal, eyelids open	Readily responds to voice
Drowsy	Mild relaxation, eyelids < ½ closed	Lethargic response to normal voice

Sedation Level	Facial Expression	Response
Asleep	Marked relaxation, jaw slack, eyelids > ½ closed	Responds only to prodding or shaking
Deep sleep	Eyelids closed	Does not respond to prodding or shaking

BRONCHOSCOPY

A bronchoscopy is an examination of the bronchi commonly done under conscious sedation with Valium or Versed through a bronchoscope. The scope is designed to pass through the trachea and allow visualization of the tracheal bronchial tree. The instrument can be used for tissue biopsy and removal of foreign body.

FOREIGN BODY AIRWAY OBSTRUCTION IN CHILDREN

The National Safety Council reports more than 90% of the deaths from foreign body aspiration occur in children younger than 5 years and 65% of the victims are infants. Since safety standards have regulated the size of toys and their parts for young children, the incidence of foreign body aspiration of toys has decreased.

Food size has not changed, and hot dogs, grapes, and nuts are among the leading foods aspirated. Foreign body aspiration should be immediately suspected in infants and children who have a sudden onset of coughing, gagging, and stridor or wheezing. The Heimlich maneuver is recommended for removal of an upper airway obstruction in children.

HEIMLICH MANEUVER

MANUAL BLIND FINGER SWEEPS ARE NOT PERFORMED IN INFANTS AND CHILDREN DUE TO THE RISK OF PUSHING THE FOREIGN BODY FURTHER INTO THE AIRWAY.

Infants

The Heimlich maneuver for age <1 year

1. With the patient face down, deliver up to five back blows with the heel of the hand.
2. Turn the patient over and alternately deliver five abdominal thrusts with two fingers placed on the lower half of the sternum. Repeat alternating back and abdominal blows until the object is expelled or it is determined that the patient needs an artificial airway.

Children

The Heimlich maneuver procedure for age >1 year

1. Perform abdominal thrusts in a conscious victim.
2. Continue until the object is expelled or it is determined that the patient needs an artificial airway.

Adults

The Heimlich maneuver procedure for patients > 8 years (adults)

1. Deliver abdominal thrusts for a conscious victim until the object is expelled or the patient losses consciousness.

2. For victims who are unconscious, lay supine, and place hands just below the rib cage at the distal end of the sternum. Perform abdominal thrusts until the object is expelled or it is determined the patient needs an artificial airway.

COMMON CAUSES OF CHOKING

Review of Common Causes of Choking		
Pediatric	Food: • chewing gum • chewy candy (caramels) • chucks of meat • food in the mouth while running and playing • fruit seeds • fruits with skins (grapes) • hard candy • hotdogs • marshmallows • nuts • poorly chewed food • popcorn • raw vegetables (carrots) • sausages	Non-Food: • arts and crafts materials • balloons • balls, small • buttons • coins • jewelry • marbles • pen tops • plastic wrappings • toys with small parts • watch batteries
Adult	Food: • food ingested in large pieces • food poorly chewed Cause may be contributed to ingestion of alcohol before or during a meal	

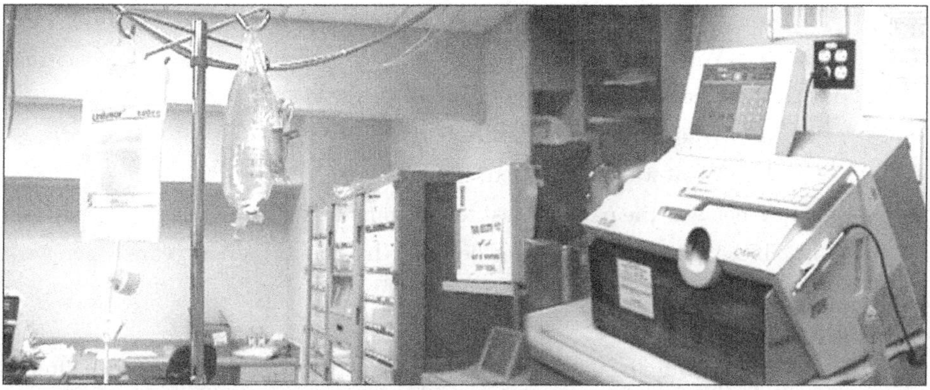

12 DIABETIC EMERGENCY

For details on triage see Chapter 34, Triage in a Nutshell.

PATIENT'S STORY – INTERVIEW QUESTIONS

1. Have you had a recent injury?
2. When did the symptoms begin?
3. Does the patient take diabetic medications?
    a. What is the name of the medication?
    b. What is the prescribed dose and frequency?
    c. When was the last dose?
    d. When was the patient's last food?
4. Did anything cause the symptoms, e.g., vomiting, inability to eat, no available medications, overdose of insulin or hypoglycemic agents?
5. Has any treatment been initiated, and has it helped?
6. When was the last finger stick blood sugar and what was the result?
7. Has the patient had similar problems before?
    a. When was the problem?
    b. What was the diagnosis and treatment?
8. Does the patient have any pertinent past history?
9. Does the patient take any routine medications?
    a. What is the name, dosage, route, and frequency of each medication?
    b. When was the last dose?
10. Does the patient take any complementary or alternative therapies, herbal products, over-the-counter medications or supplements, or natural therapies?

  a. What is the name, dosage, route and frequency of each therapy?
  b. When was the last dose or therapy?

11. Does the patient have allergies to drugs or foods?
  a. What is the name of the allergen?
  b. What was the reaction?
12. When was the patient's last tetanus immunization?
13. If the patient is female and between the ages of 10 to 50 years, when was the first day of her last menstrual period?

NURSING DOMAIN

The nursing domain, nursing diagnosis and plan of care can only be determined after an in-depth interview and consideration of the patient's story.

Domain 2. Nutrition. Class 4. Metabolism.

ANTICIPATED MEDICAL CARE

Review of the Anticipated Medical Care of Diabetic Emergencies	
Exam	Full body
Urine	Urinalysis; pregnancy test for women of reproductive age unless they have had a hysterectomy
Blood	Rapid bedside blood glucose, CBC, chemistries, electrolytes, ABG analysis
ECG	None
X-Ray	Chest x-ray
Diet	If alert, American Diabetic Association diet, otherwise NPO
IV	NS initially. When blood sugar reaches 250 mg/dl, anticipate a change of intravenous fluids to D5 1/2NS until the patient is able to eat.
Medications	For hypoglycemia, administer D50 followed by food. For hyperglycemia > 400 associated with acidosis, anticipate treatment with intravenous insulin, potassium replacement, and replacements of fluid deficient until the patient's urinary flow is adequate.
Other	Urinary catheter to monitor hourly urine output
Disposition	Hospital admission may be required for the patient with hyperglycemia.
Worst-case scenario	The worst-case scenario is unsuspected severe hypoglycemia that returns unnoticed when the duration of the causal injected insulin lasts longer then the intravenous glucose treatment.

INITIAL CARE PLAN

> Alcohol-based hand sanitizers are the preferred method for cleaning your hands in most clinical situations. Wash your hands with soap and water whenever they are visibly dirty, before eating, and after using the restroom.

1. Ask the patient to undress, remove all jewelry that interfere with the examination, and put on an exam gown. Assist as needed.
2. Obtain vital signs.
    a. Attach heart monitor leads, automatic blood pressure cuff, and pulse oximetry for continuous monitoring. Document the initial heart monitor strip and document changes of rhythm.
    b. Obtain a rectal temperature if patient is obtunded or unconscious.
3. Place on oxygen if saturation is < 94%. Severe COPD patients may be unable to maintain saturation >88% to 92%.
4. Perform a focused physical examination.
    a. Auscultate lungs.
    b. Evaluate the level of consciousness based on the mnemonic **AVPU** or **ACDU** level of consciousness score.
    AVPU: **A**lert, **V**erbal, **P**ain, **U**nresponsive.
    ACDU: **A**lert, **C**onfused, **D**rowsy, **U**nresponsive.
5. Establish intravenous access with normal saline or Ringer's solution.
6. Draw laboratory blood specimens. Draw a variety of tubes to allow the lab to do hematology, chemistries, and coagulation studies. Draw blood cultures if the patient is febrile or other signs of systemic infection are present.
7. Perform a point of care finger stick blood sugar (FSBS).
8. For severe hyperglycemia:
    a. Hold all subcutaneous insulin.
    b. Perform a FSBS every hour.
    c. Use an intravenous solution of NS as a primary line until FSBS is 250 mg/dL to 300 mg/dL.
    d. The current therapy of choice is regular insulin infused at 0.1 units/kg/hr up to 5 to 10 units/kg/hr mixed with IV fluids.
    e. Mix 100 units of regular insulin in 100 ml NS and piggyback into primary line.
    f. Do not give IV insulin bolus or start insulin drip if serum K is <3.3. Adjust rate every hour according to the following sliding scale.

Review of Generic Intravenous Insulin Sliding Scale	
FSBS mg/dl	Insulin intravenous rate

Review of Generic Intravenous Insulin Sliding Scale	
< 80	• Stop infusion • Give ½ amp (25ml) D50 • Recheck FSBS in 30 minutes • Restart infusion at reduced rate when glucose is over 80.
80 to 99	Decrease insulin drip by 1.0 units/hr. Recheck FSBS in 30 minutes
100 to 149	Decrease by 0.5 units/hr
150 to 199	Maintain current rate
200 to 300	Increase by 0.5 units/hr
>300	Increase by 1.0 unit/hr

g. Anticipate fluid replacement of 1 to 2 liters of NS over the first 1 to 2 hours and a total of 8 to 10 liters over the first 6 to 8 hours. When plasma glucose falls below 250mg/dL change IV fluids to D5 ½ NS at 125ml/hr.

h. Obtain an ABG to evaluate acid-base balance.

i. If blood draws are expected to be frequent, establish an arterial access line.

9. For hypoglycemia:

   a. If the patient is unconscious, administer Gvoke HypoPen, nasal glucagon (Baqsimi), or D50 IV. Repeat FSBS in 15 minutes. If < 70mg/dL, repeat treatment. Patient may require an IV drip of a D5 or D10 solution if hypoglycemia persists.

   b. If the patient is alert, give 15 grams of carbohydrates (3-4 glucose tablets, 1 glucose gel, or 4 oz of juice). Repeat FSBS in 15 minutes. If <70mg/dL, repeat treatment.

   c. Follow with a small meal.

10. Initiate diagnostic tests covered by hospital protocol.

11. Consider placing an indwelling urinary catheter for close monitoring of urine output.

12. Elevate the siderails and place the stretcher in the lowest position.

13. Inform the patient, family, and caregivers of the usual plan of care. Include time involved for each aspect of the stay and the expected overall time before disposition and the rationales.

14. Provide the patient with a device to reach someone for assistance and explain how to use it. Ask the patient to call for help before getting off the stretcher.

ONGOING CARE PLAN

Inform the medical provider of adverse changes noted during ongoing evaluation. Document that the medical provider was notified of the adverse change. Document if orders were or were not received.

1. Monitor vital signs frequently.
2. Monitor for signs and symptoms of worsening.
3. Perform hourly blood sugars.
4. Investigate when the last hypoglycemic medication was taken pre-hospital to determine when a hypoglycemic attack might occur.
5. Monitor therapy closely for the patient's therapeutic response.
6. Monitor closely for the development of adverse reactions to therapy.
    a. Perform interventions to relieve the adverse reaction.
    b. Ask the medical provider for a remedy.
7. If the patient is not NPO, provide food at mealtimes and fluids during the stay.
8. Keep the patient, family, and caregivers well informed of the plan of care and the remaining time anticipated before disposition.
9. Monitor the patient's laboratory and radiographic results and notify the medical provider of critical abnormalities. Remedy abnormalities as ordered.
10. Notify the medical provider when all diagnostic results are available for review. Ask for establishment of a diagnosis and disposition.

DISCHARGE INSTRUCTIONS

1. Provide the patient with the name of the nurse and doctor in the emergency room.
2. Inform the patient of their diagnosis or why a definitive diagnosis couldn't be made. Explain what caused the problem if known.
3. Evaluate the patient's knowledge of carbohydrates and refer to a dietician if indicated.
4. Teach the patient how to take the medication as prescribed and how to manage the common side effects. Instruct the patient not to drive or perform any dangerous tasks while taking narcotic pain medications.
5. Teach the patient how to maintain adequate blood sugar levels.
6. Instruct the patient that:
    a. If they are unable to eat for any reason, call their medical provider. Advise them a dangerous low blood sugar can result if they are unable to eat while taking their medications for diabetes.
    b. Symptoms of a low blood sugar are sweating, palpitations, and lightheadedness.

c. They should treat symptoms of low blood sugar by taking carbohydrates. A snack of 10 to 15 grams of carbohydrate is recommended, e.g., 4 to 6 ounces of orange juice, apple juice, or ginger ale; 8 ounces of milk; four graham crackers or five saltine crackers squares.

7. Inform the patient the American Diabetes Association has information available on the Internet, by phone, and at most doctors' offices.
8. Recommend that the patient check a glucose level with a home blood glucose testing machine and test urine daily for ketones.
9. Recommend a medical provider for follow-up care. Provide the name, address, and phone number. Recommend when to schedule the follow-up care.
10. Instruct the patient to call the follow-up medical provider immediately or return to the emergency room if the problem worsens in any way or any unusual symptoms develop. Encourage the patient NOT to IGNORE WORSENING OR PERSISTENT SYMPTOMS.
11. Ask for verbal confirmation or demonstration of understanding and reinforce teaching as needed.

COMMONLY ORDERED MEDICATIONS

GLUCAGON

Glucagon	
Indications	Hypoglycemia when IV route is not available
Adult dose	1 mg IV, IM, SC, or intranasally.
Pediatric dose	0.5 mg < 20kg or 1 mg > 20kg
Onset	IV onset 5-20 min, IM 30 min, SC 30-34min, duration 30 to 90 min
Side effects	Nausea
Note	Should be used immediately after reconstitution.
Monitor	Blood sugar levels. IV dextrose should be administered as soon as available.

DEXTROSE

Dextrose (glucose)	
Indications	Hypoglycemia
Adult dose	50% dextrose 50 ml IV or PO
Pediatric dose	25% dextrose 0.5 to 1 gram/kg IV or IO
Onset	IV onset immediate, PO rapid
Compatibility	May be mixed with normal saline or Ringer's solution

Dextrose (glucose)	
Side effects	Hyperglycemia, peripheral vein irritation with high concentration solutions
Note	The solution is hypertonic and can cause sclerosis of peripheral veins. A 50 ml syringe of D50 can be diluted with 50 ml NS to make D25 or with 150 ml to make D12.5. A maximum concentration of 25% dextrose in water should be infused in a peripheral vein. The concentration for neonates is 12.5%.
Monitor	Blood sugar levels

INSULIN

Type	Onset	Peak	Duration
Long acting (Lantus, Levemir) Intermediate Acting (Humulin N, Novolin N)	1.1 hours 1 to 2 hours	Almost peakless 6 to 14 hrs	Approximately 24 hours 16 to 24 hours
Ultra-long acting insulin (Toujeo, Tresiba)	6 hours	None	Approximately 36 hours
Regular SC (Humulin R, Novolin R) Regular IV Regular Insulin is the only approved insulin for IV use	30 to 60 min 10 to 30 min	1 to 5 hours 30 to 60 min	6 to 10 hours ½ to 1 hour
Rapid acting (Apidra, Humalog, NovoLog)	5 to 30 min	½ to 3 hrs	3 to 6 hours
Mixed insulin Combination NPH and regular insulin (Humulin 70/30 and 50/50, Novolin 70/30) Combination of intermediate and rapid acting insulin (Humalog 75/25 and 50/50, NovoLog 70/30)	30 to 60 min 5 to 30 min	1.5 hrs and 6 to 14 hours ½ to 3 hrs and 6 to 14 hours	10 to 16 hours 3 to 16 hours

INSULIN IV INFUSION

Insulin IV Infusion	
Indications	Diabetic ketoacidosis, hyperglycemia
Adult dose	Usual infusion rates are 1.5 to 10 units/kg/hour IV with sliding scale parameters to cover two-hour blood glucose levels. Goal is to reduce serum glucose slowly at a rate of 50 to 75 mg/dL/hr.
Onset	IV onset 10 to 30 min., peak 30 to 60 min., duration ½ to 1 hour. Do not give IV insulin bolus or start insulin drip until potassium is 3.3 or greater.
Side effects	As blood sugar drops, the potassium drops sharply.
Note	The fact that the plastic of the bag and intravenous tubing may absorb some of the insulin is not clinically significant because the dose is titrated to the patient's response (blood sugar level) and not dosed by a fixed unit dose.

POTASSIUM CHLORIDE

Potassium Chloride	
Indications	Potassium deficiency
Adult dose	For K+ >2.5 administer up to 200 mEq/day IV not to exceed 20 mEq/hr IV. For K+ < 2.5 administer up to 400 mEq/day IV not to exceed 40 mEq/hr IV. Maximum in a central line is 1 mEq/min IV.
Onset	IV onset rapid
Note	Blood bank blood may contain up to 30 mEq per liter. Hemolyzed lab blood specimens show high potassium levels as the potassium leaks from the ruptured cells into the serum. K-Phos 15 mm = KCl 22 mEq (5 ml=4.4 mEq)

RELATED CONDITIONS AND INFORMATION

ACID-BASE ABNORMALITIES

Review of Metabolic Acidosis	
Characteristics	Low HCO3 resulting from the addition of acids or loss of HCO3 is characteristic of metabolic acidosis.
Symptoms	Symptoms may include hyperventilation, cardiovascular collapse, and nonspecific symptoms ranging from anorexia to coma.
Causes	Causes of metabolic acidosis include ketoacidosis (diabetes mellitus, starvation, alcohol), lactic acidosis, poisoning (salicylates, ethylene glycol, and ethanol), and renal failure.

Review of Metabolic Acidosis	
Laboratory studies	Tests may include BUN, creatinine, glucose, lactate, serum ketones, serum osmolality, and a toxicology screen.
Management	Look at the anion gap, normal is 9 to 14. Causes of an increased gap are starvation acidosis, diabetic ketoacidosis, lactic acidosis, alcoholic ketoacidosis, uremic acidosis, and ingestions of toxins, e.g., salicylates. Causes of metabolic acidosis with normal gap are acid gain; e.g., hyperalimentation fluids, early renal failure, Spirolactone, bicarbonate loss in renal tubular acidosis, acetazolamide, cholestyramine, pancreatic drainage, jejunoileal bypass, ureterosigmoidostomy, ileal conduit, diarrhea, and laxative abuse.

METABOLIC ALKALOSIS

Review of Metabolic Alkalosis	
Characteristics	Metabolic alkalosis is a primary increase in serum HCO3.
Causes	Most cases originate with volume concentration and loss of acid from the stomach (vomiting and nasogastric drainage) and the kidney (diuretics). Severe K+ depletion also causes metabolic alkalosis by increasing HCO3 reabsorption. Patients with chronic pulmonary disease, high PCO2, and high serum HCO3 levels may develop alkalosis when ventilation is acutely improved.
Management	Medical management is aimed towards correction of the underlying cause. The diuretic Diamox is sometimes used with COPD patients because it causes the kidneys to release bicarbonate.

MIXED DISORDERS

Review of Mixed Disorders	
Characteristics	A mixed disorder is when more than a single acid-base disturbance exists.
Causes	Causes of mixed disorders include combined metabolic and respiratory acidosis with cardiogenic shock, metabolic alkalosis and acidosis in patients with vomiting and diabetic ketoacidosis, and metabolic acidosis with respiratory alkalosis in patients with sepsis.
Management	Medical management is aimed at correcting the underlying cause.

CARBOHYDRATES IN SNACKS

Review of Snacks with 10 to 15 Grams of Carbohydrate

Review of Snacks with 10 to 15 Grams of Carbohydrate
4 to 6 ounces of orange juice, apple juice, or one-half can of regular soda
4 graham crackers squares
5 saltine crackers squares

DIABETES INSIPIDUS

Review of Diabetes Insipidus	
Definition	Diabetes insipidus is polyuria and polydipsia caused by inadequate secretion of vasopressin (antidiuretic hormone) and is more common in young patients than in older patients.
Symptoms	Symptoms may include a urine output of 5 to 10 liters in 24 hours, specific gravity 1.001 to 1.005, signs of dehydration with thirst, and dry skin.
Cause	The cause is unknown in half the cases; and in the others, the cause is trauma to the pituitary gland or a tumor.
Treatment	Treatment may include vasopressin replacement therapy by injection or nasal spray and removal of the tumor if present.
Note	Monitor the patient's fluid intake and output. Look for signs and symptoms of dehydration and hypovolemic shock.

DIABETES MELLITUS

Diabetes Mellitus	
Definition	Diabetes mellitus is a disorder of carbohydrate metabolism.
Symptoms	Symptoms may include hyperglycemia, glycosuria, polyuria, polydipsia, and polyphagia. Type 2 diabetes (non-insulin dependent) is the most common type of diabetes.
Cause	The cause is failure of the pancreas to produce insulin. The reason the beta cells of the pancreas fail is unknown.
Complications	Complications may include acidosis due to excessive production of ketone bodies, ulcerations of the lower extremities, low resistance to infections, cardiovascular and renal disorders, electrolyte imbalance, eye disorders, blindness, and neuropathies.
Treatment	Medical treatment includes a consistent carbohydrate intake (45 to 60 grams of carbohydrate per meal), insulin, exercise, and exceptional hygiene.
Note	Diabetes is a chronic incurable disease. Since the isolation and production of insulin in 1921, a diabetic's symptoms can be ameliorated and life prolonged with proper therapy.

FINGER STICK BLOOD SUGAR

Base the frequency of point of care finger stick blood sugar analysis on the onset, peak, and duration of type of insulin used.

HYPEROSMOLAR HYPERGLYCEMIC STATE (HHS)

Hyperglycemia, hyperosmolarity, and sensorium changes are more common in older adults with non-insulin-dependent diabetes who have become severely dehydrated. Blood sugar levels are exceedingly high >1000 mg/dl. The severe hyperglycemia leads to osmotic diuresis and decreased renal excretion that compounds existing hyperglycemia and hyperosmolality to >320 mOsm/L (normal 290 to 300 mOsm/L). Treatment includes intravenous fluid resuscitation and insulin administration. When the serum glucose falls between 250 to 300 mg/dl, the insulin is discontinued, and the fluids are changed to a hypertonic solution containing glucose (D5 ½ NS) to reduce the risk of hypoglycemia, hypokalemia, and cerebral edema. A typical pattern of serum potassium levels is initial elevation followed by gradually decreasing levels. The potassium is elevated in response to the acidosis that shifts the cellular potassium into the intravascular space. Over time, diuresis causes loss of potassium and the potassium is further depleted as the potassium shifts into the intracellular compartment in response to the insulin therapy and correction of the acidosis. Anticipate fluid replacement of 1 to 2 liters of normal saline over the first 1 to 2 hours. Potassium replacement starts with the first intravenous fluids. Anticipate 8 to 10 liters for lost volume replacement. Fluid replacement dilutes serum potassium levels. Acidosis is not commonly treated with sodium bicarbonate unless the pH is 7.1 or below. When the blood sugar is lowered the pH is increased. If sodium bicarbonate was given, a rebound could occur.

DIABETIC KETOACIDOSIS (DKA) COMPARED TO HYPEROSMOLAR HYPERGLYCEMIC STATE (HHS)

	HHS	DKA
Natural Insulin Production	Enough to prevent ketoacidosis but not enough to prevent hyperglycemia	None
Precipitating factors	Omission of or resistance to hypoglycemia agents, surgery, trauma, pancreatitis, infections, or emotional stress	Omission of or resistance to insulin, surgery, trauma, pancreatitis, infections, or emotional stress

	HHS	DKA
Signs and symptoms	Dehydration, elevated blood sugar commonly >600, pH normal, comatose, hyperglycemia promotes osmotic diuresis and an elevated serum osmolarity causing the brain cells to become dehydrated altering the level of consciousness, normal ventilation, fluid volume deficit with profound dehydration	Less dehydrated, elevated blood sugar commonly <600, pH < 7.35, rarely comatose, hyperventilation, hyperglycemia promotes osmotic diuresis and an elevated serum osmolarity causing the brain cells to become dehydrated altering the level of consciousness, hyperventilation, Kussmaul respiration, to blow off carbon dioxide and compensate for acidosis
Age	Over 50 years	Young
Previous history	Known diabetes in 50% of the cases	Is often initial presentation of new onset diabetes
Mortality	20% to 50%	1% to 10%
Home Treatment	Diet or oral agents	Insulin

HYPOGLYCEMIA TREATMENT

Dextrose 50% solution or 25 grams of carbohydrate is the treatment for hypoglycemia. The IV onset is immediate. Dextrose may be given PO if the patient is alert and no IV is available. Onset is rapid. Glucagon may be given 1 mg IM, SC, IV, or nasally. Pediatric dose of D25 is 0.5 to 1 gram/kg of D25.

INSULIN PUMPS

Patients with subcutaneous insulin pumps are usually very knowledgeable about their pump. If the patient is unconscious, suicidal, disoriented, or an MRI or CT is required, removal of the insulin pump may be necessary. Basal and bolus insulin will be needed to prevent ketoacidosis.

INSULIN RESISTANCE

Insulin resistance occurs naturally in humans from 4 a.m. to 9 a.m. as a reaction to a secretion of a growth hormone. This is also referred to as the Dawn Phenomenon.

PEDIATRIC HYPOGLYCEMIA

Children and infants have limited glycogen stores that can be rapidly depleted during episodes of physical stress. Clinical signs of hypoglycemia are poor perfusion, diaphoresis, tachycardia, hypothermia, irritability, and hypotension. An initial intravenous fluid bolus of 20 ml/kg can be given based on the child's hemodynamic response. The 4-2-1 rule for maintenance fluids is 4 ml/kg for the first 10 kg of body weight, 2 ml/kg for the next 10 kg of weight, and 1 ml/kg for the rest of the body weight. A point-of-care finger stick blood sugar test should be performed on any critically ill infant or child and glucose administration considered for hypoglycemia.

POTASSIUM

The serum potassium drops sharply as the blood sugar drops. Monitor serum potassium and replace as needed.

SOMOGYI EFFECT

Somogyi effect includes hyperglycemia associated with nightmares, fluctuating blood glucose levels, and morning headache as a response to unperceived nocturnal hypoglycemia. Also called the dawn phenomenon and brittle diabetes.

PEDIATRIC CONSIDERATIONS

TYPE 1 DIABETES IN CHILDREN

Review of Type 1 Diabetes in Children	
Age of Onset	Usually < 20 years of age
Incidence	10%
Links	Family history Human leukocyte antigen (HLA) gene present Triggered by autoimmune response Caucasian No lifestyle link
Insulin requirement	Always
Oral medication	Not effective
Diet	Controlled balance of nutrition and activity
Presenting symptoms	Polyuria, polyphagia, polydipsia, fatigue, weight loss
Ketoacidosis	Common and is often the first presentation of type 1 diabetes

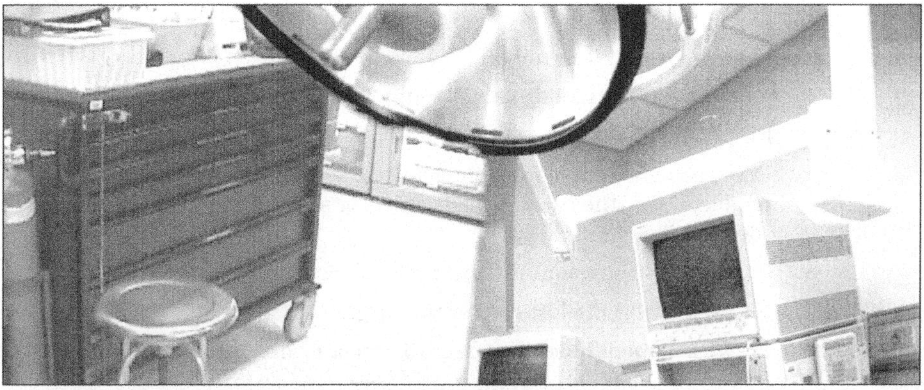

13 DROWNING AND NEAR DROWNING

For details on triage see Chapter 34, Triage in a Nutshell.

PATIENT'S STORY – INTERVIEW QUESTIONS

1. When did the incident take place?
2. Where are the injuries?
   a. Consider placing the patient in cervical spine immobilization if neck pain or tenderness is present.
   b. Are any associated symptoms present?
3. Why did the incident happen, e.g., heart attack, seizure, trauma, fatigue, or suicide attempt?
4. How is the patient's normal function affected?
   a. How long was the patient submerged?
   b. How long was the patient apneic?
   c. Was CPR initiated and by whom?
   d. Is neurovascular function normal distal to injury sites?
   e. Does the patient have normal use of injured areas?
5. Has any treatment been initiated, e.g., oxygen, and has it helped?
6. Where did the incident take place, e.g., at the beach in saltwater, at a lake in fresh water, or in a swimming pool?
7. Is unlawful activity suspected?
   a. Was law enforcement at the scene?
   b. What agency?

Medical personnel are obligated to notify law enforcement if unlawful activity is suspected.

8. Does the patient have any pertinent past history?
9. Does the patient take any routine medications?
   a. What is the name, dosage, route, and frequency of each medication?
   b. When was the last dose?
10. Does the patient take any complementary or alternative therapies, herbal products, over-the-counter medications or supplements, or natural therapies?
    a. What is the name, dosage, route and frequency of each therapy?
    b. When was the last dose or therapy?
11. Does the patient have allergies to drugs or foods?
    a. What is the name of the allergen?
    b. What was the reaction?
12. When was the patient's last tetanus immunization?
13. If the patient is female and between the ages of 10 to 50 years, when was the first day of her last menstrual period?

NURSING DOMAIN

The nursing domain, nursing diagnosis and plan of care can only be determined after an in-depth interview and consideration of the patient's story.

Domain 3. Elimination and Exchange. Class 4. Respiratory function.
Domain 11. Safety/Protection. Class 6. Thermoregulation. Class 1. Infection.

ANTICIPATED MEDICAL CARE

Review of the Anticipated Medical Care of Drowning and Near Drowning	
Exam	Full body
Urine tests	None
Blood tests	CBC, electrolytes, renal function studies, ABG
X-ray	Chest x-ray
ECG	ECG for females and males over 35 years
Diet	NPO
IV	Normal saline or Ringer's solution
Medications	Diuretics, bronchodilators, antibiotics, steroids

Review of the Anticipated Medical Care of Drowning and Near Drowning	
Other	Anticipate C-spine immobilization until the cervical spine is cleared by x-ray, respiratory support may include hyperventilation with mechanical ventilation and PEEP or BiPAP, warming, irrigation of eyes and instillation of prophylactic antibiotic ointment, irrigation of ears, and irrigation of body orifices where debris is present.
Disposition	A hospital admission may be required.
Worst-case scenario	The worst-case scenario is partial or total vision loss due to severe eye damage from debris or infection that could have been avoided with irrigation and prophylactic antibiotics

INITIAL CARE PLAN

Alcohol-based hand sanitizers are the preferred method for cleaning your hands in most clinical situations. Wash your hands with soap and water whenever they are visibly dirty, before eating, and after using the restroom.

1. Ask the patient to undress, remove all jewelry that might interfere with the examination, and put on an exam gown. Assist as needed.
2. Position to improve ventilation, e.g., a reclining-chair position (laying on stretcher with the head of the stretcher elevated, arms supported at sides, foot of stretcher slightly elevated to prevent sliding down and to allow the patient's back to be supported against the back of the stretcher thus expanding the chest).
3. Obtain initial vital signs including pulse saturation or test capillary refill.
    a. Attach heart monitor leads, automatic blood pressure cuff, and pulse oximetry for continuous monitoring. Document the initial heart monitor strip and document changes of rhythm.
    b. Consider obtaining a rectal temperature if hypothermia is suspected or the patient is unable to cooperate.
4. Place on oxygen. Consider administering high flow 100% oxygen by non-rebreather mask even if pulse oximetry saturation is within normal limits.
5. Perform a physical examination focused on the respiratory system.
    a. Auscultate the lungs.
    b. Perform a cursory head-to-toe inspection and look for evidence of injuries.
    c. Evaluate the level of consciousness based on the mnemonic **AVPU** or **ACDU** level of consciousness score.
    AVPU: Alert, **V**erbal, **P**ain, **U**nresponsive.
    ACDU: Alert, **C**onfused, **D**rowsy, **U**nresponsive.

6. Clean and dress any wounds. Consider obtaining routine and marine (saline medium) cultures.
7. Irrigate the eyes if debris is present. Consider instillation of prophylactic antibiotic eye ointment. Consider irrigation of ears and body orifices if debris is present.
8. Keep the patient warm.
    a. Use warming techniques, e.g., warmed oxygen, warmed intravenous fluids, and heated blankets to reduce the risk of hypothermia.
    b. Place warmed blanket around the head, neck, and shoulders like a shawl. Place another blanket over the body and tightly tuck it around the patient.
    c. Consider the use of warming lights or a mechanical warming blanket.
9. Establish intravenous access. Draw laboratory blood specimens. Draw a variety of tubes that will allow the lab to perform hematology, chemistries, and coagulation studies if the patient is on anticoagulants or is cirrhotic. Consider blood cultures.
10. Obtain an arterial blood gas and consider placement of an arterial line if frequent blood draws are expected. Correct acid-base imbalances.
11. Consider placement of a Swan Ganz catheter to monitor fluid resuscitation.
12. Consider placing an indwelling Foley catheter to hourly monitor urinary output.
13. Consider placing a nasogastric tube to reduce the risk of gastric dilation, vomiting, and aspiration.
14. Inform the patient not to eat or drink and teach the patient and family the rationale for the NPO status.
15. Elevate the siderails and place the stretcher in the lowest position.
16. Inform the patient, family, and caregivers of the usual plan of care. Include time involved for each aspect of the stay and the anticipated time before disposition.
17. Provide the patient with a device to reach someone for assistance and explain how to use it. Ask the patient to call for help before getting off the stretcher.

ONGOING CARE PLAN

> Inform the medical provider of adverse changes noted during ongoing evaluation. Document that the medical provider was notified of the adverse change. Document if orders were or were not received.

1. Monitor heart rate and rhythm, blood pressure, effectiveness of breathing, and core temperature.

2. Monitor the level of consciousness using the AVPU mnemonic.
3. Monitor therapy closely for the patient's therapeutic response.
    a. The usual time for a medication effectiveness check is 20 to 30 minutes after giving the drug.
    b. If therapy is not effective, ask the medical provider for a repeat dose or an alternative.
4. Monitor closely for the development of adverse reactions to therapy.
    a. Perform interventions to relieve the adverse reaction.
    b. Ask the medical provider for a remedy.
5. If not NPO, provide the patient with food at mealtimes and fluids during the stay.
6. Keep the patient, family, and caregivers well informed of the plan of care and the remaining time anticipated before disposition.
7. Monitor the patient's laboratory and x-ray results and notify the medical provider of critical abnormalities. Remedy abnormalities as ordered.
8. Notify the medical provider when all diagnostic results are available for review. Ask for establishment of a diagnosis and disposition.

DISCHARGE INSTRUCTIONS

1. Provide the patient with the name of the nurse and doctor in the emergency room.
2. Inform the patient of their diagnosis or why a definitive diagnosis couldn't be made. Explain what caused the problem if known.
3. Teach the patient how to take the medication as prescribed and how to manage the common side effects. Instruct the patient not to drive or perform any dangerous tasks while taking narcotic pain medications.
4. Recommend a medical provider for follow-up care. Provide the name, address, and phone number with a recommendation of when to schedule the care.
5. Instruct the patient to call the follow-up medical provider immediately or return to the emergency room if breathing problems or any unusual symptoms develop. Encourage the patient NOT to IGNORE WORSENING OR PERSISTENT SYMPTOMS.
6. Ask for verbal confirmation or demonstration of understanding and reinforce teaching as needed.

COMMONLY ORDERED MEDICATIONS

BUMEX

Bumex (bumetanide)	
Indications	Fluid overload

Bumex (bumetanide)	
Dose	1 to 2 mg IV, maximum 20 mg/day
Onset	IV onset 5 min., peak ½ hour, duration 2 to 3 hours
Side effects	Orthostatic hypotension, hypokalemia, hyperglycemia
9Monitor	Urinary output, blood pressure

DOPAMINE

Dopamine	
Indications	Hypotension with signs and symptoms of shock, secondary drug for symptomatic bradycardia
Adult dose	IV Titration Dopaminergic: 1 to 3 mcg/kg/min. IV Inotropic: 3 to 10 mcg/kg/min. IV Alpha adrenergic: >10 mcg/kg/min., maximum 20 mcg/kg/min. IV
Pediatric dose	2 to 20 mcg/kg IV
Onset	IV onset 5 minutes, ½ life 2 minutes, duration less than 10 minutes
Side effects	Tachycardia, arrhythmias
Note	Increase and decrease by 1 to 2 mcg/kg/min. Swan Ganz or central line is recommended. For extravasations, use Regitine. Do not mix with alkaline solutions.

DOBUTREX

Dobutrex (dobutamine)	
Indications	Cardiac decompensation from pump (heart) problems
Adult dose	2.5 to 15 mcg/kg/min. IV, maximum of 40 mcg/kg/min. IV
Pediatric dose	2 to 20 mcg/kg per min. IV, titrate to the desired effect
Compatibility	Compatible at Y-site with Dopamine, epinephrine, Inocor, Isuprel, Lidocaine, Neo-Synephrine, Nitroglycerin, Levophed, Pronestyl, NOT compatible with KCl
Note	Increase by 2 to 3 mcg/kg/min. A Swan Ganz is recommended to monitor cardiac output and PCWP. Do not mix in alkaline solutions. Use with extreme caution post MI. Correct volume depletion before use.

LASIX

Lasix (furosemide)	
Indications	Fluid overload with systolic blood pressure >90 without signs and symptoms of shock

Lasix (furosemide)	
Dose	0.5 to 1 mg/kg IV over 1 to 2 min, if no response, double the dose to 2 mg/kg IV over 1 to 2 min
Onset	IV onset 5 minutes, peak ½ hour, duration 2 hours
Side effects	Circulatory collapse, hypokalemia, loss of hearing, nausea
Monitor	Urinary output, blood pressure

MORPHINE

Morphine sulfate (MSO4)	
Indications	Moderate to severe pain
Dose	1 to 10 mg IV given over 1 to 5 min., every 5 to 30 min.
Pediatric dose	50 to 100 mcg/kg IV, maximum 10 mg/dose IV
Onset	IV onset rapid, peak 20 minutes, duration 4 to 5 hours
Side effects	Confusion, sedation, hypotension, respiratory depression
Note	May reverse with Narcan 0.4 to 2 mg IV. If more than 10 mg is needed, the diagnosis of a narcotic overdose must be questioned.
Monitor	CNS changes, sedation level, effectiveness of respirations

NITROGLYCERIN

Nitroglycerin	
Indications	Chest pain, acute myocardial infarction, left ventricular failure, hypertension
Adult dose	Titration, the usual dose is 10 mcg/min. to 20 mcg/min. IV, increase by 5 mcg/min. every 5 minutes. No maximum dose has been established. The dose is limited by the onset of adverse reactions such as hypotension.
Onset	IV onset immediate, duration is variable
Compatibility	Compatible at Y-site with Aminophylline, Bretylium, dobutamine, Dopamine, Inocor, Lidocaine, potassium chloride
Side effects	Headache, hypotension

Nitroglycerin	
Note	Non-latex or glass bottle with special tubing is recommended to avoid absorption of the medicine into the bag and tubing. The fact that the latex absorbs the nitroglycerine (NTG) has no clinical significance because the dose is titrated to effect and not given as a fixed dose. Some hospital protocols allow the nurse to increase the NTG to relief of pain, but not to decease unless an order to wean is received from the medical provider. Some hospital protocols require the nurse to check with the medical provider if a dose of over 200 mcg/min. is required for pain relief.

PROVENTIL, ALBUTEROL, VENTOLIN

Proventil, Albuterol, Ventolin	
Indications	Bronchospasm, asthma
Adult Dose	2.5 to 5 mg nebulized
Pediatric dose	Nebulized Age < 1 year .05 to .15 mg/kg/dose Age 1 to 5 years 1.25 to 2.5 mg/dose Age 5 to 12 years 2.5 mg/dose Age > 12 years 2.5 to 5 mg/dose
Onset	Inhaled onset 5 to 15 minutes, peak 1 to 1 ½ hour, duration 4 to 6 hours
Side effects	Anxiety, tremors, tachycardia
Monitor	Oxygen saturation, heart rate
Other Bronchodilators	
Alupent	A long acting bronchodilator. Usual adult nebulized dose is 0.3 ml of a 5% solution in 2.5 ml NS.

RELATED CONDITIONS AND INFORMATION

ABG CRITICAL VALUES

ABG Critical Values	
pH	< 7.25 or > 7.55
pCO2	> 55
O2	< 55
SpO2	< 85 (equals a pO2 of 46 to 56)

ABG OXYGEN SATURATION

ABG Oxygen Saturation	
Arterial blood	Oxygen saturation >75%

Venous blood	Oxygen saturation <75%
Mixed arterial and venous blood	For oxygen saturation percent in the eighties on an ABG, check patient's saturation with pulse oximetry and if ABG saturation is less than the pulse oximetry saturation, redraw the ABG. It is probably mixed arterial and venous blood.

ASPHYXIATION

Asphyxiation is a condition in which an extreme decrease of oxygen in the body accompanied by an increase of carbon dioxide leads to loss of consciousness or death. Drowning, choking, electric shock, traumatic injury, or the inhalation of toxic gases can induce asphyxia.

ASPIRATIONS

Both freshwater and saltwater aspirations lead to severe hypoxemia due to a ventilation perfusion imbalance and significant pulmonary venous admixture. In victims who do not aspirate, hypoxemia results from apnea. Ninety percent of drowning victims aspirate water into their lungs. Ten percent do not aspirate, and death is secondary to laryngospasms and hypoxia (dry drowning).

DROWNING

Review of Drowning and Near Drowning	
Dry drowning	Dry drowning is asphyxiation caused by decreased oxygen and is a result of laryngotracheal spasm that prevents both water and oxygen from entering the lungs.
Wet drowning	Wet drowning is asphyxiation caused by decreased oxygenation because the lungs filled with water instead of air as the victim takes a breath.
Secondary drowning	Secondary drowning is death caused by respiratory failure commonly from ARDS, pulmonary edema, or aspiration pneumonia that occurs following successful resuscitation. Secondary drowning can occur from hours to several days after the near drowning event.
Seawater drowning	Seawater is a hypertonic solution. Fluid traverses into the alveoli because of osmotic pull across the alveolar capillary membrane and results in pulmonary edema, hemoconcentration, and hypovolemia.
Fresh water drowning	Fresh water is a hypotonic solution. Fluid transverses rapidly out of the alveoli into the blood by diffusion. The water may contain contaminants (chlorine, algae, and mud particles) that break down the surfactant. Fluid seeps into the alveoli and results in pulmonary edema, hemodilution, and hypervolemia.

IRRIGATION OF THE EYE

Review of the Technique for Eye Irrigation

Review of the Technique for Eye Irrigation
Wash the entire area about the eye. Anesthetize the eye. Saline bullets can be used to irrigate the eyes until the equipment can be assembled.
Assemble the equipment: Warmed irrigating solution of normal saline IV tubing IV cannula with the needle removed attached to the tubing
Place the patient on the affected side or on their back for bilateral irrigation. Pad well with towels.
Run a gentle stream of solution over the eye from the inner canthus to the outer.
Ask the patient to occasionally blink, look up, down, and from side-to-side to assure that the irrigating solution reaches all surfaces of the eye.
Evert (turn inside out) the upper eyelid by placing a cotton swab over the eyelid, pulling the eyelashes down and then up over the swab to irrigate under the upper lid.
Use copious amounts of fluids. Four liters is common.

INFECTIONS

Aspiration of contaminated water poses additional risks of infection and obstruction of small bronchioles by particulate substances.

PULMONARY EDEMA

Pulmonary Edema	
Description	Pulmonary edema is an effusion of serous fluids into the air vesicles and into the interstitial tissues of the lungs.
Signs and symptoms	Signs and symptoms may include severe dyspnea, decreased oxygenation, metabolic acidosis, crackles, wheezes, and productive cough of foam or pink-tinged sputum.
Tests	Chest x-ray may show bilateral interstitial and alveolar infiltrates.
Treatment	Treatment may include strict fluid restriction, high flow oxygen, bronchodilators, BiPAP or mechanical ventilation, diuretics, dobutamine, nitroglycerin, and intravenous morphine.
Note	Patients who require mechanical ventilation have a 50% mortality rate. Pulmonary edema can be the result of water aspiration. Both fresh and saltwater drowning present with similar clinical pictures. There is a difference in how the pulmonary edema develops in fresh and saltwater. However, the treatment is the same. Pulmonary edema can develop up to 72 hours after a near drowning event and close observation is essential.

PULSE OXIMETRY SATURATION AND CORRESPONDING pO2

Saturation	Oxygen Levels (pO2)
80% SpO2	40 to 49 pO2
85% SpO2	46 to 56 pO2
87% SpO2	49 to 60 pO2
90% SpO2	55 to 67 pO2
93% SpO2	63 to 78 pO2
95% SpO2	72 to 89 pO2

RESPIRATORY ACIDOSIS

Review of Respiratory Acidosis	
Definition	Respiratory acidosis is CO2 retention due to respiratory failure.
Symptoms	Symptoms may include confusion and a lowered level of consciousness.
Causes	Causes include sedatives, stroke, chronic pulmonary disease, airway obstruction, severe pulmonary edema, and cardiopulmonary arrest.
Management	Management is aimed at improvement of ventilation with pulmonary toilet and reversal of bronchospasm. Intubation may be required.

RESPIRATORY ALKALOSIS

Review of Respiratory Alkalosis	
Definition	Respiratory alkalosis is excessive ventilation causing a primary reduction in CO2 and increase in pH.
Symptoms	Symptoms may include a fast-respiratory rate and a pH > 7.45. Severe alkalosis can cause seizures, tetany, cardiac arrhythmia, and loss of consciousness.
Causes	Pain and psychogenic causes are common. Others causes include pneumonia, pulmonary edema, interstitial lung disease, asthma, fever, hypoxemia, sepsis, delirium tremens, salicylates, hepatic failure, mechanical over ventilation, and central nervous system lesions.
Management	Management is directed towards correcting the underlying disorder. For psychogenic cases, sedation or a rebreathing bag may be used.

STATISTICS

- In 2007, there were 3,443 fatal unintentional drowning victims in the United States, averaging ten deaths per day.
- More than one in five fatal drowning victims are in children 14 and younger.
- A nonfatal drowning can cause brain damage that may result in long term disabilities including memory problems, learning disabilities, and permanent loss of basic functions.

WARMING

Review of ACLS Hypothermia Algorithm	
Mild hypothermia 34° to 36° C 93° to 96.8° F	Institute passive rewarming techniques by moving the patient to a warm environment, wrapping with warmed blankets, giving warmed oxygen, and warm oral liquids high in glucose to provide calories. Passive rewarming raises the temperature 0.5° to 2.0° C/hr (1.4° to 3.3° F/hr). Discontinue when core temperate is > 35° C (95° F) to avoid hyperthermia.
Moderate hypothermia 30° to 34° C 86° to 93° F	Institute passive rewarming techniques by moving the patient to a warm environment, wrapping with warmed blankets, giving warmed oxygen, and warm oral liquids high in glucose to provide calories. Initiate active external rewarming to the truncal areas only with the Bear Hugger, radiant heating lamps, heating pads, and a warming bed.
Severe hypothermia < 30° C < 86° F Death usually occurs below 25.6° C (78° F)	Active internal warming efforts are essential. The heart is resistant to drug therapy and to electro conversion at a core temperature of less than 86 degrees. Active internal rewarming may include warmed intravenous fluids to 43° C (109.4° F), warmed humidified oxygen 42° to 46° (107.6° to 114.8° F), warm fluids for peritoneal lavage, extra corporeal rewarming, hemodialysis, and esophageal rewarming tubes.
Complications	Moderate and severe hypothermia carry a risk of rewarming shock. Shock occurs when the peripheral areas are warmed faster than the core causing a large amount of lactic acid from the extremities to be rapidly shunted to the heart. Fibrillation can occur. Discontinue when core temperate is > 35° C (95° F) to reduce the risk of hyperthermia.

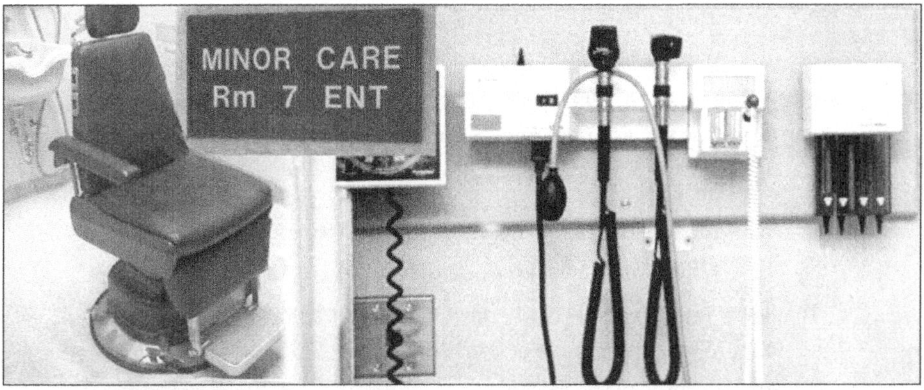

14 EAR, NOSE, THROAT, AND DENTAL EMERGENCY

For details on triage see Chapter 34, Triage in a Nutshell.

PATIENT'S STORY – INTERVIEW QUESTIONS

1. Have you had a recent injury?
2. When did the symptoms begin?
    a. Are the symptoms still present?
    b. If the symptoms are no longer active, how long did they last?
    c. If the symptoms were intermittent, how long did each episode last and what was the frequency?
3. Where is the problem located and are any associated symptoms present?
    a. Is drainage present?
    b. When was the onset of the drainage?
    c. What is the character, color, and amount of the drainage?
    d. Is fever present?
4. Did anything cause the symptoms, e.g., trauma, cleaning the ear or nose, swallowing a specific food?
5. How does the problem affect the patient's normal function, e.g., loss of hearing, inability to swallow, inability to chew?
6. Has any treatment been initiated, and has it helped?
7. Has the patient had similar problems before?
    a. hen was the problem?
    b. What was the diagnosis and treatment?
8. Does the patient have any pertinent past history? For a nosebleed, ask specifically if the patient has a history of anemia.

9. Does the patient take any routine medications?
    a. What is the name, dosage, route, and frequency of each medication?
    b. When was the last dose?
10. Does the patient take any complementary or alternative therapies, herbal products, over-the-counter medications or supplements, or natural therapies?
    a. What is the name, dosage, route and frequency of each therapy?
    b. When was the last dose or therapy?
11. Does the patient have allergies to drugs or foods?
    a. What is the name of the allergen?
    b. What was the reaction?
12. When was the patient's last tetanus immunization?
13. If the patient is female and between the ages of 10 to 50 years, when was the first day of her last menstrual period?

NURSING DOMAIN

Domain 3. Elimination and Exchange. Class 4. Respiratory function.
Domain 11. Safety/Protection. Class 1. Infection.
Domain 2. Nutrition Class 5. Hydration.

ANTICIPATED MEDICAL CARE

Review of the Anticipated Medical Care of Ear, Nose, Throat, and Dental Emergencies	
Exam	Exam of the area involved including chest for ENT complaints that might have systemic involvement
Urine tests	None
Blood tests	CBC, blood cultures if febrile, monospot
ECG	None
X-ray	Soft tissue films of the throat for foreign bodies
Diet	NPO
IV	None
Medications	Analgesics, antibiotics, sore throat gargles, ear analgesic and antibiotic solutions (solutions are contraindicated when the ear drum is ruptured)
Disposition	Home

Review of the Anticipated Medical Care of Ear, Nose, Throat, and Dental Emergencies	
Worst-case scenario	The worst-case scenario is an obstructed airway that requires endotracheal intubation and mechanical ventilation in a minor care setting.

INITIAL CARE PLAN

Alcohol-based hand sanitizers are the preferred method for cleaning your hands in most clinical situations. Wash your hands with soap and water whenever they are visibly dirty, before eating, and after using the restroom.

1. Ask the patient to undress and remove all jewelry that might interfere with the examination. A gown is commonly required for sore throats for ease of auscultating the lungs.
2. Position the patient in a sitting position to enhance breathing and to elevate the injury.
3. Obtain vital signs including pulse oximetry. Place the patient on oxygen if the saturation is < 94%. Severe COPD patients may be unable to maintain saturation >88% to 92%.
4. Perform a focused physical examination by examining the site of injury or complaint.
5. Give initial medications and treatments covered by hospital protocol, e.g., local analgesia and antipyretics.
6. Consider obtaining throat cultures.
7. Order indicated x-rays covered by hospital protocol.
8. Inform the patient not to eat or drink and teach the patient and family the rationale for the NPO status.
9. Elevate the siderails and place the stretcher in the lowest position.
10. Inform the patient, family, and caregivers of the usual plan of care and the anticipated time before disposition.
11. Provide the patient with a device to reach someone for assistance and explain how to use it. Ask the patient to call for help before getting off the stretcher.

ONGOING CARE PLAN

Inform the medical provider of adverse changes noted during ongoing evaluation. Document that the medical provider was notified of the adverse change. Document if orders were or were not received.

1. Monitor vital signs including temperature.
2. Monitor therapy closely for the patient's therapeutic response.

   a. The usual time for a medication effectiveness check is 20 to 30 minutes after giving the drug.
   b. If therapy is not effective, ask the medical provider for a repeat dose or an alternative.
3. Monitor closely for the development of adverse reactions to therapy.
   a. Perform interventions to relieve the adverse reaction.
   b. Ask the medical provider for a remedy.
4. If not NPO, provide the patient with food at mealtimes and fluids during the stay.
5. Keep the patient, family, and caregivers well informed of the plan of care and the remaining time anticipated before disposition.
6. Monitor the patient's laboratory and x-ray results.
7. Notify the medical provider of critical abnormalities.
8. Remedy abnormalities as ordered.
9. Notify the medical provider when all diagnostic results are available for review. Ask for establishment of a diagnosis and disposition.

DISCHARGE INSTRUCTIONS

1. Provide the patient with the name of the nurse and doctor in the emergency room.
2. Inform the patient of their diagnosis or why a definitive diagnosis couldn't be made. Explain what caused the problem if known.
3. Teach the patient how to take the medication as prescribed and how to manage the common side effects. Instruct the patient not to drive or perform any dangerous tasks while taking narcotic pain medications.
4. Instructions for patients with nosebleeds include:
   a. Not to pick, rub, or blow the nose for the next few days.
   b. If bleeding recurs, sit up, avoid the head down position, and pinch the nose firmly and continuously for 15 minutes.
   c. If a pack was placed, expect removal in 1 to 3 days by the follow-up medical provider. If bleeding continues, call the follow-up medical provider or return to the emergency room.
5. Teach the patient how to use the medication prescribed and follow-up as recommended. If any new symptoms or drainage develop or the pain worsens, call the follow-up medical provider. If contact with the follow-up medical provider is not available in a reasonable amount of time, return to the emergency room.
6. For dental emergencies, instruct the patient to see the follow-up dentist within the length of time recommended. If treatment is delayed, serious consequences can develop.

7. Recommend a medical provider or dentist for follow-up care. Provide the name, address, and phone number with a recommendation of when to schedule the care.
8. Instruct the patient to call the follow-up medical provider immediately or return to the emergency room if the problem worsens in any way or any unusual symptoms develop. Encourage the patient NOT to IGNORE WORSENING OR PERSISTENT SYMPTOMS.
9. Ask for verbal confirmation or demonstration of understanding and reinforce teaching as needed.

RELATED CONDITIONS AND INFORMATION

BELL'S PALSY

Review of Bell's Palsy	
Definition	Bell's palsy is an idiopathic unilateral facial paralysis
Cause	The cause of Bell's palsy is unknown.
Symptoms	Symptoms may include rapid onset of ear and facial pain with maximal paralysis over 2 to 5 days. The patient is unable to move the affected side. The patient may experience difficulty eating.
Tests	No tests are commonly done. Diagnosis is made by history and physical examination, but a brain CT Scan may routinely be performed to confirm the absence of other pathology.
Treatment	The most common treatment is an antiviral regimen. Other treatments may include steroids, analgesics, and artificial tears. Protection of the eye during sleep is essential to avoid damage to the eye. Moist heat and passive range of motion exercises to improve comfort may be recommended.
Complications	Complications include corneal abrasions, facial muscle atrophy, and residual weakness.
Note	Bell's palsy is the most common of the facial paralyses and found in 23 of 100,000 people annually. It is most common in patients over 40 years old and occurs with equal incidence in both males and females.

DENTAL CARIES AND ABSCESSES

Dental caries is commonly caused by poor oral hygiene allowing bacteria to grow and break down the teeth. Abscesses are usually confined to the local area, but they but can spread to the head, neck, and throughout the system. The symptoms are pain and swelling. Medical management of dental caries and abscesses may include topical anesthetics, nerve blocks, analgesics, antibiotics, and referral to a dentist for definitive dental care.

FOREIGN BODIES OF THE EAR

Children, between the ages of 9 months and 4 years, present with beads, stones, foods, and other foreign bodies in their ears. The object may not be discovered until infection develops and a purulent drainage is noticed. Insects including roaches can crawl into ears and their scratching and movements cause great distress for the patient. Methods of removing foreign objects include suction, irrigation, or tools under direct visualization. Do not irrigate foreign bodies that will absorb water and increase in size. Roaches are difficult to kill. Filling the ear canal with 2% Lidocaine solution thus drowning the roach and numbing the ear canal is effective. The roach or insect can then be removed under direct visualization or irrigation. Irrigation is contraindicated if the patient has a history of ruptured tympanic membrane or has tubes in place.

FOREIGN BODIES OF THE NOSE

In children, foreign bodies in the nose are not usually found until a purulent drainage is noticed. Medical management includes removal of the foreign object and may include analgesic and antibiotic medication. The nasal septum and mucous membranes are vascular and easily damaged. Extreme care must be taken not to drive the object into the airway and lungs. Conscious sedation may be needed for foreign body removal in children.

FRACTURED, CHIPPED, AND AVULSED TEETH

Avulsed teeth are a dental emergency. Implantation should occur within 30 minutes to maximize chances of success. Transport the tooth in milk, saline, or under the tongue of an alert patient. A commercial tooth transport solution is available. Primary teeth of children 6 months to 6 years are not implanted. If the tooth cannot be found, a chest x-ray is indicated. Chipped and broken teeth are commonly a result of trauma. Management is determined by the patient's age and relationship of the fracture to the pulp. Cosmetic restorations need dental evaluation in 24 to 48 hours. Tooth fractures in children are urgent. Bacteria can pass into the pulp causing infection in approximately 6 hours. Adults can wait up to 24 hours for treatment as the dentin is thicker and protects the pulp more effectively. Warm moist gauze over the tooth minimizes the sensitivity of the exposed nerve. Medical management may include analgesics or nerve block and referral to a dentist for definitive care. Primary (baby) teeth are seldom re-implanted.

IRRIGATION OF THE EAR

Review of Ear Irrigation	
Equipment	Equipment: 1. Tap water warmed to 98.6 degrees Fahrenheit 2. 30- or 60-ml syringe 3. Large bore Angiocath with needle removed 4. Kidney shaped basin to catch irrigating liquid 5. Towels

Review of Ear Irrigation	
Procedure	The integrity of the tympanic membrane must be confirmed prior to irrigation by visualization and documented. Irrigation is only done if the tympanic membrane is intact. Position patient in a sitting position, drape towels over the shoulders, and ask the patient to hold basin against his neck under the ear. Straighten the ear canal (up and back for adults, down and back for children). Direct the irrigating stream superiorly against the ear canal wall to get behind the cerumen and drive it forward and out of the ear.
Post procedure	After the procedure, ask the patient to lie on the affected side to drain excess irrigating fluid.
Note	Commercial otic irrigating devices are available.

LARYNGITIS

Review of Laryngitis	
Definition	Laryngitis is an inflammation of the vocal cords.
Causes	The cause of laryngitis includes overuse of the vocal cords, allergies, irritants, and both viral and bacterial infections.
Symptoms	Symptoms may include partial or total voice loss.
Tests	Tests may include CBC and throat culture.
Management	Medical management may include prescription of topical anesthetic throat lozenges, antibiotics, and instruction to rest the voice, increase fluid intake, and to avoid smoking.
Complications	Complications include vocal cord hemorrhage, airway obstruction, and vocal cord scarring.
Note	Aspirin is contraindicated for pain because of its anticoagulant effects increase the risk of vocal cord hemorrhage.

LUDWIG'S ANGINA

Ludwig's angina is an infection of the submandibular, sublingual, and submental space. Patients may present with pain, fever, drooling, tongue displacement, and dysphagia. Complications include spread of the infection down to the mediastinum with respiratory distress and airway obstruction. CT makes the diagnosis. Medical treatment may include surgical drainage and high dose antibiotics.

NOSEBLEED

Review of Nosebleed	
Definition	A nosebleed is a hemorrhage from the nose.
Causes	The causes of nosebleed include local infections, drying of the nasal membranes, trauma including picking, hypertension, bleeding tendencies, and a complication of anticoagulants.

Review of Nosebleed	
Symptoms	Symptoms include bleeding from the nose. An anterior nosebleed is the most frightening for the patient. Posterior bleeding is evidenced by blood running into the nasal pharyngeal cavity and then swallowed.
Tests	Tests may include CBC, PT, aPTT, and type and screen.
Management	Management includes maintaining the patient in a sitting position and pinching the nostrils against the nasal septum for 5 to 10 minutes while the patient breathes through their mouth. Medical management may include application of topical vasoconstrictors, e.g., 2% or 5% cocaine hydrochloride and Neo-Synephrine, and cauterization with silver nitrate or electrocautery if the bleeding site can be visualized. Direct pressure is accomplished by anterior or posterior nasal packing, e.g., petroleum gauze, nasal sponges, foam, tampons, and balloons. The easiest for the patient is a pack that will dissolve and does not require removal. Coating packing material with antibiotic ointment may prevent infections. Surgical ligation of bleeding vessels is sometimes necessary.
Follow-up management	Anterior packing is left in place for 24 to 72 hours and then removed. Posterior packing and balloons are often left for 2 to 3 days and hospital admission may be necessary. Toxic shock has been reported in patients with nasal packing and is due to *Staphylococcus aureus*.

OTITIS EXTERNA

Review of Otitis externa	
Definition	Otitis externa is an infection of the external ear canal and auricle. Most often seen in the summer and called swimmer's ear. Moisture, warmth, and microorganisms are the three factors involved in otitis externa.
Symptoms	Symptoms may include a painful erythematous external canal with pustular drainage. Chewing worsens the pain.
Management	Medical management may include antibiotic and steroid solution eardrops. Wick placement is needed if the canal is occluded to allow the medication to enter the canal.
Complications	Complications include regional cellulitis, lymph adenopathy, and partial hearing loss.
Note	External otitis resolves in a week and often recurs.

OTITIS MEDIA AND RUPTURED TYMPANIC MEMBRANES

Review of Otitis Media and Ruptured Tympanic Membrane

Review of Otitis Media and Ruptured Tympanic Membrane	
Definition	Otitis media is a bacterial infection of the middle ear occurring more frequently in children and is commonly preceded by a viral upper respiratory infection.
Symptoms	Symptoms may include rapid onset of ear pain, tinnitus, hearing loss, nausea, vomiting, fever, and otorrhea secondary to drum rupture. Children who can't verbalize rub and pull at their ears and sleep restlessly.
Tests	Visualization of the tympanic membrane (ear drum) is essential for diagnosis. Cerumen must be removed if it blocks visualization of the drum.
Management	Medical management may include antibiotics, analgesics, topical otic anesthetic, and antibiotic solutions. Otic solutions are never used if the drum is ruptured.
Complications	Complications include ruptured tympanic membrane, meningitis, mastoiditis, abscesses, and permanent hearing loss.
Note	A ruptured tympanic membrane is often associated with an ear infection. Pain and pressure are often relieved when the drum ruptures. Irrigation is contraindicated. Lateral sinus thrombosis is a serious complication of otitis media caused by the spread of injection to the lateral sinus and mastoid.

PERITONSILLAR ABSCESS

Review of Peritonsillar Abscess	
Definition	The most common deep infection of the head and neck that occurs in adults and is typically formed by a combination of aerobic and anaerobic bacteria. Peritonsillar abscesses form in the area between the palatine tonsil and its capsule. If the abscess progresses, it can involve the surrounding anatomy, including the masseter muscles and the pterygoid muscle. If severe, the infection can also penetrate the carotid sheath.
Symptoms	Presenting symptoms include trismus, progressively worsening sore throat, often localized to one side, fever, dysphagia, otalgia, odynophagia, erythematous, swollen tonsil with contralateral uvular deviation, edema of palatine tonsils, purulent exudate on tonsils, drooling, and a muffled voice with cervical lymphadenopathy.
Tests	Needle aspiration remains the gold standard for diagnosis but ultrasonography and computed tomographic scanning are also useful.

Review of Peritonsillar Abscess	
Management	After performing aspiration, appropriate antibiotic therapy must be initiated. In advanced cases, incision and drainage or immediate tonsillectomy may be required. Analgesics and hydration may also be necessary.
Complications	Complications may include recurrences of tonsillitis or peritonsillar abscess, airway obstruction, aspiration from ruptured abscess resulting in pneumonia or pneumonitis, jugular vein thrombosis, carotid artery rupture, cerebral abscess, mediastinitis, meningitis, sepsis, and death.

PHARYNGITIS

Review of Pharyngitis	
Definition	Pharyngitis is an inflammation or infection of the pharynx.
Symptoms	Symptoms may include bright-red throat, swollen tonsils, exudates on the tonsils and pharynx, a swollen uvula, and tender swollen cervical nodes.
Tests	Tests may include culture with gram stain.
Management	Medical management may include analgesic medications and recommendation for warm saline gargles. Most cases of pharyngitis are viral and do not require antibiotics. Bacterial pharyngitis is treated with antibiotics.
Complications	Complications include retropharyngeal abscess and subacute bacterial endocarditis that can result from streptococcal pharyngitis.

SINUSITIS

Review of Sinusitis	
Definition	Sinusitis is an acute inflammation or infection of the mucous membranes in the sinus cavity.
Symptoms	Symptoms may include fever, dull-achy pain over the affected sinus, and periorbital or forehead pain worsened by bending forward.
Tests	Tests may include CBC, culture, and gram stain, x-ray of the sinus (not conclusive), CT, and sinus endoscopy.
Management	Medical management may include nasal decongestant sprays, warm compresses, analgesics, and antibiotics.
Complications	Complications include chronic sinusitis, cellulitis, abscess, sepsis, brain abscess, meningitis, and osteomyelitis.

SWIMMER'S EAR

External otitis or swimmer's ear is an inflammation or infection that involves moisture, warmth, and microorganisms. The external canal may become painful and erythematous. Pustular drainage is often present. Management may include antibiotic and steroid solutions. Wick placement is needed if the canal is occluded so medications can be delivered to the inside of the ear.

TEMPOROMANDIBULAR JOINT DISLOCATION

Review of Temporomandibular Joint Dislocation	
Definition	TMJ dislocation is an anterior and superior bilateral dislocation of the jaw. Unilateral dislocation seldom occurs.
Cause	The cause of the dislocation is commonly opening the mouth too wide (yawning or laughing) or a dystonic reaction to medication.
Symptoms	The symptoms include an open mouth, pain at the joints, and inability to close the mouth, talk, or swallow.
Tests	Diagnostic workup may include pre and post reduction x-rays.
Management	Medical management may include muscle relaxants, analgesia, and manual relocation of the jaw.
Note	Keep the patient sitting or if unable to tolerate a sitting position, place in the rescue position (lying on the right side) to protect the airway.

TONSILLITIS

Review of Tonsillitis	
Definition	Tonsillitis is an infection of the tonsils.
Symptoms	Symptoms may include sore throat, painful swallowing and breathing, fever, difficulty opening the jaw, and swollen lymph nodes.
Tests	CBC, throat culture, monospot, chest x-ray
Management	Medical management may include analgesia, antibiotics, and ice packs to the neck.
Complications	Complications include peritonsillar abscess, aspiration, airway obstruction, dehydration, and subacute bacterial endocarditis resulting from streptococcal tonsillitis.
Note	The tonsils are lymphatic tissue that filter bacteria and guard against infection entering the respiratory and gastrointestinal tract.

PEDIATRIC CONSIDERATIONS

Review of Pediatric Anatomical Considerations	
Nose and Mouth	Smaller and more easily obstructed than adult
Pharynx	Proportionately larger than adult

Review of Pediatric Anatomical Considerations	
Trachea	Narrower and more easily obstructed especially by swelling
Cricoid Cartilage	Less developed, less rigid, and narrowest part of the airway in children
Diaphragm	Chest wall softer and children more dependent on diaphragmatic breathing

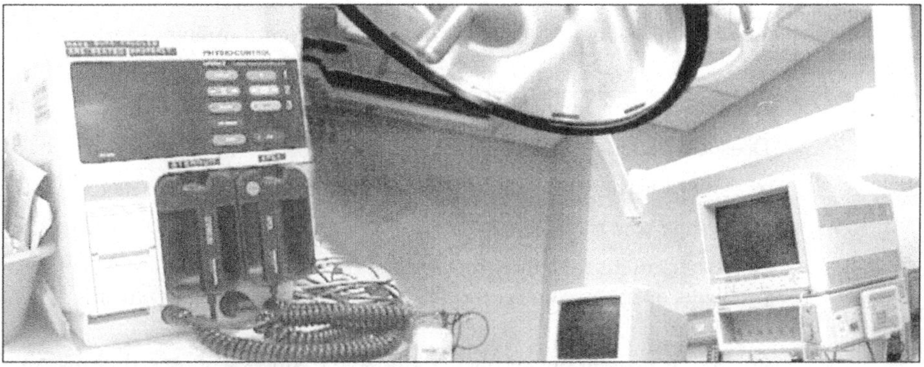

15 ELECTROCUTION

For details on triage see Chapter 34, Triage in a Nutshell.

PATIENT'S STORY – INTERVIEW QUESTIONS

1. When did the injury occur?
2. Are any obvious injuries present?
   a. Where are the injuries located?
   b. Does the patient have any entrance or exit wounds?
   c. Are any associated symptoms present?
3. What caused the electrical shock, e.g., working on home electrical wires, putting up a roof antenna, working on a high voltage power line?
   a. Was the electrical shock from an AC or DC line?
   b. Is the voltage known?
   c. What area of the body was exposed to the electricity?
   d. What was the length of contact with the current?
4. How is the patient's normal function affected?
   a. Did the patient stop breathing?
   b. Was CPR initiated and by whom?
   c. Does the patient have normal neurovascular function distal to all injuries?
   d. Does the patient have normal function of injured areas?
5. Has any treatment been initiated, and has it helped?
6. Is unlawful activity suspected?
   a. Was law enforcement at the scene?
   b. What agency?

Medical personnel are obligated to notify law enforcement if unlawful activity is suspected.

7. Does the patient have any pertinent past history?
8. Does the patient take any routine medications?
    a. What is the name, dosage, route, and frequency of each medication?
    b. When was the last dose?
9. Does the patient take any complementary or alternative therapies, herbal products, over-the-counter medications or supplements, or natural therapies?
    a. What is the name, dosage, route, and frequency of each therapy?
    b. When was the last dose or therapy?
10. Does the patient have allergies to drugs or foods?
    a. What is the name of the allergen?
    b. What was the reaction?
11. When was the patient's last tetanus immunization?
12. If the patient is female and between the ages of 10 to 50 years, when was the first day of her last menstrual period?

NURSING DOMAIN

The nursing domain, nursing diagnosis and plan of care can only be determined after an in-depth interview and consideration of the patient's story.

Domain 12. Comfort. Class 1. Physical comfort.
Domain 4. Safety/Protection. Class 4. Environmental hazards

ANTICIPATED MEDICAL CARE

Review of the Anticipated Medical Care of Electrocutions	
Exam	Full body
Urine tests	Urinalysis or urine dip to look for blood; pregnancy test for women of reproductive age unless they have had a hysterectomy
Blood tests	ABG, electrolytes, renal studies, CBC
ECG	12 lead electrocardiogram
X-ray	Chest, areas of suspected bony damage
Diet	NPO
IV	Normal saline or Ringer's solution
Medications	Analgesics

Review of the Anticipated Medical Care of Electrocutions	
Other	Anticipate the use of sterile linens and sterile dry dressings. If the burn is < 10% of the TBSA (total body surface area), cool moist sterile saline dressings may be used to reduce the burning. For hand burns, a referral is commonly made to a hand specialist. Anticipate nasogastric or orogastric tube for >25% burned TBSA to decompress the stomach and reduce the risk of aspiration.

Burn Classification	**Presence of Pain**	**Clinical Signs**
Superficial-Thickness Burns		
First Degree Epidermis and superficial dermis	Yes	Erythema, minor pain, no blisters
Partial-Thickness Burns		
Second Degree Moderate to deep dermis	Yes	Moderate: Blisters, moderate pain, clear fluid Deep: Whiter appearance, with decreased pain. Difficult to distinguish from full thickness burns
Full-Thickness Burns		
Third degree Through the dermis and into subcutaneous fat and muscle	No	White, brown, or black dry leathery tissue (eschar), severe swelling
Fourth degree Through the subcutaneous fat and into the muscle or bone	No	Eschar, muscle and possible bone exposure

INITIAL CARE PLAN

> Alcohol-based hand sanitizers are the preferred method for cleaning your hands in most clinical situations. Wash your hands with soap and water whenever they are visibly dirty, before eating, and after using the restroom.

1. Ask the patient to undress, remove jewelry that might interfere with the exam, and put on an exam gown. Assist as needed.
2. Remove ALL jewelry near the burns.

3. Cover burns with sterile dressings. Sterile linens are recommended if the burns are moderate or severe.
4. Obtain vital signs including pulse oximetry or test capillary refill. Place on continuous heart monitor, automatic blood pressure cuff, and pulse oximetry monitoring. Document the initial heart monitor strip and document changes of rhythm.
5. Place on oxygen if saturation is < 94% for a minor burn and on 100% oxygen with a non-rebreather mask if the burn is moderate or severe regardless of the saturation level.
6. Assure the patient that pain relief will be a priority.
    a. Obtain an order for morphine and administer 2 to 5 mg IV every 10 to 20 minutes until the patient has relief.
    b. Medication may be used for anxiety.
    c. Morphine can be reversed with Narcan if respiratory function becomes ineffective due to decreased level of consciousness.
    d. Valium and Versed can be reversed with Romazicon.
7. Perform a physical examination.
8. Auscultate lungs.
    a. Examine the site of injury.
    b. Evaluate the level of consciousness based on the mnemonic **AVPU** or **ACDU** level of consciousness score.
    AVPU: **A**lert, **V**erbal, **P**ain, **U**nresponsive.
    ACDU: **A**lert, **C**onfused, **D**rowsy, **U**nresponsive.
    c. Look for entrance and exit wounds.

> Damage is done along the path of the electricity. Consider the potential of damage to the organs in the path of the electrical current.

    d. What is the size and reaction of the pupils?
    e. Does the patient have any head pain or injuries to the head?
    Is the tongue or mouth injured?
    Is any drainage present from the nose or ears?
    f. Is the trachea midline?
    Is jugular venous distention present (unable to detect under fluorescent light)?
    g. Does the chest expand equally?
    Is subcutaneous emphysema present?
    Are the heart tones within normal limits?
    Are the heart tones diminished?
    Are any murmurs present?
    Does the patient complain of chest pain?
    Is the chest tender to palpation?

h. Are the lung sounds clear on the right and left?
Are wheezes or crackles present?
Are the lung sounds decreased or absent in any area of the lungs?

i. Is the abdomen soft, flat, rigid, or distended?
Are bowel sounds normal, hypoactive, hyperactive, or absent?
Does the patient complain of abdominal pain?
Is the patient's abdomen tender to palpation?

j. Is the patient incontinent?
Examination of the genitalia may be deferred if trauma is not suspected.
Do the genitalia appear normal?
Does the patient have bleeding from the urethral meatus or vagina?
Is priapism present?
Does the patient complain of genital pain?
Is the perineal area or genitalia tender to palpation?

k. Does the patient complain of pain when light pressure is applied to the iliac crests?
Is the pelvis stable or unstable?

l. Does the patient have normal motion and sensation in the upper and lower extremities?
Are distal pulses present in the upper and lower extremities?

m. Does the patient have normal movement of his back?
Does the patient complain of back pain?
While keeping the back immobilized, turn the patient.
Inspect the posterior surfaces.
Does the patient have obvious back injuries?
Is the back tender to palpation?

n. Does skin inspection reveal any damage to the skin; e.g., abrasions, lacerations, bruises, needle tracks, or petechiae?

9. Minor burns need a saline lock for medication administration.

10. Moderate and major burns need two large bore intravenous lines with normal saline or Ringer's Solution. Large amounts of intravenous solutions are needed. Infuse intravenous fluids to maintain an hourly urinary output of 75 to 100 cc per hour. Collect laboratory specimens. Draw a variety of tubes and hold for orders.

> In electrical burns, the TBSA is not clinically significant and cannot be used to determine fluid needs.

11. Patients with moderate and major burns have lost some the ability for temperature regulation. Warm the intravenous and irrigation fluids, increase the temperature in the room, and keep the patient covered with warmed blankets.

12. If debris is present, clean and irrigate the burns with sterile water and cover loosely with sterile gauze dressings.

13. Accurate intake and output measurements are essential. All moderate and major burns need an indwelling urinary catheter. Burns in the genitalia can cause swelling that will make voiding and catheterization impossible later.
14. Consider placing a nasogastric or orogastric tube to decompress the stomach and decrease the risk of vomiting and aspiration.
15. Consider drawing ABG analysis for suspected inhalation or respiratory injury.
16. Order diagnostic tests included in hospital protocols.
17. Administer medications covered by hospital protocol, e.g., tetanus toxoid and pain medications.
18. Inform the patient not to eat or drink and teach the patient and family the rationale for the NPO status.
19. Elevate the siderails and place the stretcher in the lowest position.
20. Inform the patient, family, and caregivers of the usual plan of care. Include time involved for each aspect of the stay and anticipated time before disposition. Inform the patient and family if transfer to another facility is a possibility.
21. Provide the patient with a device to reach someone for assistance and explain how to use it. Ask the patient to call for help before getting off the stretcher.

ONGOING CARE PLAN

Inform the medical provider of adverse changes noted during ongoing evaluation. Document that the medical provider was notified of the adverse change. Document if orders were or were not received.

1. Monitor core temperature, heart rate and rhythm, blood pressure, and effectiveness of breathing.
2. Monitor for signs of worsening; e.g., restlessness, difficulty swallowing, dyspnea, and hoarseness.
3. Monitor pain management therapy closely for the patient's therapeutic response.
   a. Burn patients need pain medication frequently.
   b. The usual time for a medication effectiveness check is every 10 to 20 minutes.
   c. Morphine is the drug of choice.
   d. Regional blocks can be used for severe extremity burns.
   e. If therapy is not effective, ask the medical provider for a repeat dose or an alternative.
4. Monitor closely for the development of adverse reactions to therapy.
   a. Perform interventions to relieve the adverse reaction.

   b. Ask the medical provider for a remedy.

5. If not NPO, provide the patient with food at mealtimes and fluids during the stay.
6. Keep the patient, family, and caregivers well informed of the plan of care and the remaining time anticipated before disposition.
7. Monitor the patient's laboratory and x-ray results and notify the medical provider of critical abnormalities. Remedy abnormalities as ordered.
8. Notify the medical provider when all diagnostic results are available for review. Ask for establishment of a diagnosis and disposition.

DISCHARGE INSTRUCTIONS

1. Provide the patient with the name of the nurse and doctor in the emergency room.
2. Inform the patient of their diagnosis or why a definitive diagnosis couldn't be made. Explain what caused the problem if known.
3. Teach the patient how to take the medication as prescribed and how to manage the common side effects. Instruct the patient not to drive or perform any dangerous tasks while taking narcotic pain medications.
4. Instruct the patient in the following:
   a. Any burn is a potential serious injury.
   b. Minor burns are treated with pain medications and elevation of the burned area.
   c. Use soap and water to wash the burned area three times a day and apply the medication as prescribed.
   d. Burns that are more serious require outpatient dressing changes and treatment by a medical professional.
5. Recommend a medical provider for follow-up care. Provide the name, address, and phone number with a recommendation of when to schedule the care.
6. Instruct the patient to notify the follow-up medical provider immediately if fever or pus-like drainage develops. If the medical provider is not available in a reasonable amount of time, return to the emergency room. Encourage the patient NOT to IGNORE WORSENING OR PERSISTENT SYMPTOMS.
7. Ask for verbal confirmation or demonstration of understanding and reinforce teaching as needed.

COMMONLY USED MEDICATIONS

MORPHINE

Morphine sulfate (MSO4)	
Indications	Moderate to severe pain

Morphine sulfate (MSO4)	
Dose	4 to 10 mg IV over 5 min. A large dose is needed for burns. Give repeated doses until the patient has obtained relief.
Pediatric dose	50 to 100 mcg/kg IV, maximum 10 mg/dose
Onset	IV onset rapid, peak 20 minutes, duration 4 to 5 hours
Side effects	Confusion, sedation, hypotension, respiratory depression
Monitor	CNS changes, sedation level, effectiveness of respirations

NARCAN

Narcan (naloxone)	
Indications	Opioid overdose
Dose	0.4 to 2 mg IV every 2 to 3 min. A maximum dose has not been established. However, if the patient does not respond after 10 mg of Narcan, the diagnosis of an opioid overdose must be questioned.
Pediatric dose	0.01 mg/kg IV every 2 to 3 min.
Onset	IV onset 1 min., duration 45 min.
Side effects	High doses may cause nervousness, ventricular tachycardia, and increased systolic blood pressure.
Monitor	Watch for the return of sedation. Duration of Narcan is 45 minutes and the duration of most narcotics is 4 to 5 hours.

RELATED CONDITIONS AND INFORMATION

COMMON CAUSES OF ELECTROCUTION

Review of Common Causes of Electrocution
Extension Cords
Electrical outlets
Electrical appliances
Swimming pools, hot tubs, and spas
Power lines
Lightning

ELECTRICAL BURNS

Electrical burns are caused by electricity as it passes through the body and meets resistance from the body tissue. The heat it causes is proportional to the amperage of the current and the electrical resistance of the body. External burns are usually caused at the entry and exit sites. Nerves, blood vessels, and muscles are less resistant and easily damaged. Organs, such as the brain, heart, and lungs, are damaged quickly. Fat and bone are more resistant. The smaller the body part through which the electricity passes, the more intense the heat; therefore, considerable damage can be caused in the extremities. Electrical current can also cause the heart to fibrillate. AC current can cause tetany that intensifies the patient's grip on the electrical source and increases the time of exposure. The electrical current in homes in the United States is AC 110 volt.

ELECTRICAL SHOCK

Approximately 1000 persons are accidentally electrocuted (killed by electricity) annually and over 4000 are injured. Electrical burn injuries constitute 5% of the admissions to burn centers. The degree of injury varies with the type and strength of the current, the length of contact, and location of the contact. A critical difference between electric burns and thermal burns is the damage done by the electrical current as it passes through the body. Tissue in the current's path may be injured to the point of necrosis. Damage is done to body parts not visible to the eye. Muscle contractions can paralyze the respiratory system and fibrillate the heart. All organs in the path of the electrical current must be evaluated for injury. A small amount of electricity applied directly to the heart may be enough to cease activity. One milliampere of 60-cycle current applied directly to the ventricle can cause fibrillation. Conversely, a relatively large amount of electricity may not be able to penetrate a rubber gloved or calloused hand and not cause any injury. Muscle tissue contracts in response to an applied current of greater than 15 milliamperes alternating current (AC) and 75 milliamperes direct current (DC).

LIGHTNING

Lightning flows electrical current around and through the body capable of causing fractures. People surviving lightning strikes describe temporary paresthesias and paralysis. Most lightening victims behave as if they had electroconvulsive therapy. They are confused and have anterograde amnesia for several days. Generally, lightening victims who do not experience cardiopulmonary arrest at the time of the strike do well with supportive therapy.

CALCULATING SURFACE BURN AREA

The rule of nines is a method for calculating the percentage of total body surface area burned. To determine the total body surface burned calculate the head at 9%, front of trunk at 18%, back of trunk at 18%, arms at 9% each, legs at 18% each, and perineum at 1% and add the percentages together. Another method for calculating the total body surface area burned is to compare the burned area to the size of the patient's hand. The palmer surface of the patient's hand equals one percent of their body surface area.

ELECTRICAL INJURY DURING PREGNANCY

Fetal injury can result to a fetus if it is exposed to electrical current. The common route of electrical current during accidents in the home is the hand to foot. The fetus lives in the path of the current. If the fetus survives, growth development may be retarded. Baseline fetal monitoring and referral for follow-up with an obstetrician is essential.

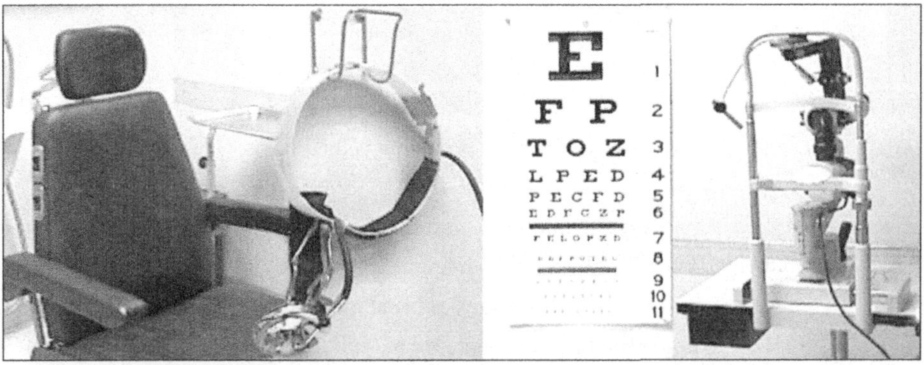

16 EYE EMERGENCY

For details on triage see Chapter 34, Triage in a Nutshell.

PATIENT'S STORY – INTERVIEW QUESTIONS

1. When did the symptom begin?
    a. If the symptoms are no longer active, how long did they last?
    b. If the symptoms were intermittent, how long did each episode last and how frequent were they?
2. Where is the injury located?
    a. Which eye and what part of the eye is injured?
    b. Are the eye symptoms associated with any other symptom; e.g., burning, itching, sensation of something in the eye, nausea, halos, or a visual color disturbance?
    c. Is a headache associated with the eye symptoms?
        i. What part of the head is involved?
        ii. Does the pain radiate?
        iii. What is the severity of the headache?
3. Did any known event cause the symptoms, e.g., a chemical spill, flying foreign body, a penetrating object, or a welding flash?
4. How does the eye injury affect the patient's normal function?
    a. Does the patient normally wear corrective lens or glasses?
    b. Can the patient count fingers and perceive light? Complete visual acuity is performed during the initial assessment. Corrective lens or glasses are used during visual acuity testing.
    c. Is the patient's vision loss monocular (one eye) or binocular (both eyes)?

Binocular changes indicate a neurological problem refer to #30 Stroke, CVA, and TIA.

5. Has any treatment been initiated, and has it helped?
6. Has the patient had similar problems before?
   a. When was the problem?
   b. What was the diagnosis and treatment?
7. Does the patient have any pertinent past history?
   a. Does the patient take any routine medications including eye drops?
   b. What is the name, dosage, route, and frequency of each medication?
   c. When was the last dose?
8. Does the patient take any complementary or alternative therapies, herbal products, over-the-counter medications or supplements, or natural therapies?
   a. What is the name, dosage, route, and frequency of each therapy?
   b. When was the last dose or therapy?
9. Does the patient have allergies to drugs or foods?
   a. What is the name of the allergen?
   b. What was the reaction?
10. When was the patient's last tetanus immunization?
11. If the patient is female and between the ages of 10 to 50 years, when was the first day of her last menstrual period?

NURSING DOMAIN

The nursing domain, nursing diagnosis and plan of care can only be determined after an in-depth interview and consideration of the patient's story.

Domain 12. Comfort. Class 1. Physical comfort.
Domain 11. Safety/Protection. Class 1. Infection. Class 2. Physical Injury.

ANTICIPATED MEDICAL CARE

Review of the Anticipated Medical Care of Eye Emergencies	
Exam	Eye exam
Urine tests	Pregnancy test for women of reproductive age unless they have had a hysterectomy if surgical intervention is required
Blood tests	None
ECG	None

Review of the Anticipated Medical Care of Eye Emergencies	
X-ray	X-rays of the eye if a foreign body is suspected.
Diet	NPO
IV	None
Medications	Topical eye medications may include miotics, mydriatics, cycloplegics, anesthetics, antibiotics, steroids, herpes simplex virus inhibitors, systemic analgesics, and antibiotics.
Disposition	Hospital admission may be required if the eye problem is severe or surgery is necessary.
Worst-case scenario	The worst-case scenario is an unnoticed alkaline or acid erosion of the eye globe. This scenario can be prevented with a good history, pH testing, and immediate irrigation with the proper solution.

INITIAL CARE PLAN

Alcohol-based hand sanitizers are the preferred method for cleaning your hands in most clinical situations. Wash your hands with soap and water whenever they are visibly dirty, before eating, and after using the restroom.

1. Place the patient in an ENT exam room.
2. Consider the appropriateness of contact removal.
   a. Do not remove contacts if the eye is ruptured. The contacts may be supporting the segments of the eye globe. An ophthalmologist should make the decision to remove contacts when the globe is ruptured.
   b. If contacts are removed, mark sterile containers right and left. Place each contact in the appropriate container of normal saline.
3. For chemical or powder burns (including alkaline powder from air bags), test acidity with pH paper before instilling eye drops.
4. When indicated, irrigation is a priority.
   a. 1st pH testing
   b. 2nd Anesthetizing medications
   c. 3rd Irrigation
   d. 4th Visual acuity testing after irrigation
5. Obtain vital signs.
6. Perform a focused examination.
   a. Examine the eyelid and eye globe.
   b. Determine the pupil size and reaction.
   c. Perform a visual acuity with glasses or corrective lens in place.

   d. Test ocular motility.

7. Clean and dress wounds.
   a. Consider collecting wound cultures.
   b. Place a sterile protective covering over the injured eye.
   c. Loosely cover a perforated globe with an eyecup or eye shield. Do not apply any pressure to the globe.
8. Administer medications covered under nurse-initiated hospital protocols, e.g., tetanus toxoid immunization.
9. Initiate diagnostic tests covered by hospital protocol. Consider establishing intravenous access and preoperative blood work if surgery is anticipated.
10. Instruct the patient not to eat or drink and teach the patient and family the rationale for the NPO status.
11. Inform the patient, family, and caregivers of the usual plan of care, the expected overall time before disposition.
12. Provide the patient with a device to reach someone for assistance and explain how to use it.

ONGOING CARE PLAN

Inform the medical provider of adverse changes noted during ongoing evaluation. Document that the medical provider was notified of the adverse change. Document if orders were or were not received.

1. Monitor visual changes and vital signs.
2. Monitor therapy closely for the patient's therapeutic response.
   a. Eye anesthetizing drops act instantly.
   b. The usual time for systemic medication effectiveness check is 20 to 30 minutes after giving the drug.
   c. If therapy is not effective, ask the medical provider for a repeat dose or an alternative.
3. Monitor closely for the development of adverse reactions to therapy.
   a. Perform interventions to relieve the adverse reaction.
   b. Ask the medical provider for a remedy.
4. If not NPO, provide the patient with food at mealtimes and fluids during the stay.
5. Keep the patient, family, and caregivers well informed of the plan of care and the remaining time anticipated before disposition.
6. Monitor the patient's laboratory and x-ray results and notify the medical provider of critical abnormalities. Remedy abnormalities as ordered.

7. Notify the medical provider when all diagnostic results are available for review. Ask for establishment of a diagnosis and disposition.

DISCHARGE INSTRUCTIONS

1. Provide the patient with the name of the nurse and doctor in the emergency room.
2. Inform the patient of their diagnosis or why a definitive diagnosis couldn't be made. Explain what caused the problem if known.
3. Instruct the patient with an eye infection that:
    a. bacterium and viruses are highly contagious;
    b. the patient should avoid rubbing the eye to reduce the risk of spreading the infection;
    c. a good hand washing with soap and water should be performed after touching the eye;
    d. a follow-up visit before the scheduled time may be necessary if swelling of the eyelid, fever, or headache develop.
4. Instruct the patient with an eye inflammation caused from welding, dust, or allergies that healing usually takes place in 24 hours. Encourage them to follow-up with the recommended medical provider if symptoms get worse.
5. Instruct the patient with an eye injury that the eye needs to be rested for 24 to 48 hours.
6. If medication is prescribed, remove the patch, instill the medication, and replace the patch with a clean one.
7. If severe eye pain or pus-like drainage develops, see the follow-up medical provider or return to the emergency room. Otherwise, follow-up with the recommended medical provider at the recommended time.
8. Instruct the patient with blunt eye trauma that:
    a. Resting in bed and wearing an eye patch will rest the eye.
    b. Cold compresses to the eye will help reduce the swelling.
    c. Occasionally problems are not detectable during the ER visit. If vision changes, pain increases, double vision develops, or any other significant problems develop before the follow-up medical provider can arrange an appointment; return to the emergency room.
9. Teach the patient how to take the medication as prescribed and how to manage the common side effects. Instruct the patient not to drive or perform any dangerous tasks while taking narcotic pain medications.
10. Recommend a medical provider for follow-up care. Provide the name, address, and phone number with a recommendation of when to schedule the care.

11. Instruct the patient to call the follow-up medical provider immediately or return to the emergency room if the problem persists for over eight hours, worsens in any way, or if any unusual symptoms develop. Encourage the patient NOT to IGNORE WORSENING OR PERSISTENT SYMPTOMS.
12. Ask for verbal confirmation or demonstration of understanding and reinforce teaching as needed.

COMMONLY USED MEDICATIONS

AAO (AMERICAN ACADEMY OF OPHTHALMOLOGY) OPHTHALMIC MEDICATIONS COLOR CODES

Review of Ophthalmic Medications Color Codes	
Blue	Beta-blockers. Used to treat glaucoma. Blue indicates a lower dosage than yellow.
Gray	Non-steroidal anti-inflammatories (NSAIDs)
Green	Pupil constriction (miotics)
Orange	Carbonic anhydrase inhibitors used to treat glaucoma
Pink	Anti-inflammatories or steroids
Purple	Adrenergic agnostics used to treat glaucoma
Red	Pupil dilation (mydriatics and cycloplegics)
Tan	Anti-invectives or antimicrobials
Turquoise	Prostaglandin analogues used to treat glaucoma
White	Topical anesthesia
Yellow	Beta-blockers. Used to treat glaucoma and reduce intraocular pressure

RELATED CONDITIONS AND INFORMATION

ACTINIC EYE INJURIES

Actinic eye injuries are burns caused by ultraviolet light or sunrays. Dark glasses are recommended when out in the sunshine.

BINOCULAR VISION LOSS

Binocular vision loss causes include bilateral anterior ischemic optic neuropathy, cerebral infarct or hemorrhage, and pituitary apoplexy.

BLEPHARITIS

Blepharitis is an ulcerative or non-ulcerative inflammation of the edges of the eyelids. Symptoms may include red, tender, and swollen eyelids. Treatment may include cleansing with baby shampoo, applying an antibiotic eye ointment to the eyelid margins, and warm compresses.

BLUNT TRAUMA

Review of Injuries Caused by Blunt Trauma

Review of Injuries Caused by Blunt Trauma	
Hyphema	A hyphema is blood in the anterior chamber of the eye in front of the iris. Treatment may include strict resting in bed, sedation, and bilateral eye patches without pressure for several days. Treatment is controversial and many schools of thought are in the current literature.
Iris injury	An iris injury is inflammation to the iris and ciliary bodies from a contusion. Treatment may include cycloplegic and steroidal agents. Complications include vision loss and loss of the eye.
Lens injury	Lens injuries may include total and partial dislocation and opacification. Treatment may include surgery. Repair is not emergent unless the injury is causing acute angle-closure glaucoma.
Sub-conjunctival hemorrhage	A subconjunctival hemorrhage is bleeding beneath the conjunctiva making the white part of the eye bright red. It can be caused by trauma, spontaneous hemorrhage, or by simple sneezing and coughing. This painless benign problem heals spontaneously without treatment.

CENTRAL RETINAL ARTERY OCCLUSION

Occlusion of the central retinal artery is EMERGENT. The occlusion of the central retinal artery stops blood supply to the retina. Retinal circulation must be established within 1 to 1 ½ hours to reduce the risk of permanent vision loss. Symptoms are sudden painless blindness in the affected eye. Treatment may include hospitalization and surgical decompression.

CHEMICAL BURNS TO THE EYE

Chemical burns to the eye are EMERGENT. The alkaline, acid, or chemical irritant denatures the tissue. The denatured cornea appears white. Some chemicals are neutralized on impact. Alkaline such as concrete, lye, and drain cleaners continue to damage until the substance is removed. Initial treatment is immediate copious irrigation with normal saline or water at an eyewash station. Irrigation continues until the pH reaches 7.4. Irrigation is commonly 2 liters over 30 minutes. For severe cases, irrigation can last as long as 2 to 4 hours. When the pH reaches 7.4, a topical antibiotic, cycloplegic, and steroid are instilled, and bilateral eye patches are applied. Systemic analgesia is recommended. An ophthalmology consult is essential.

CONJUNCTIVAL LACERATION

A laceration to the conjunctiva is common. The most common cause is a scratch from a fingernail. Treatment for lacerations <5 mm are antibiotics and patching; lacerations >5 mm require suturing.

CONTACT LENSES

Contact lenses tend to get lost both in the department and in the patient's eye. To reduce the risk of loss in the emergency room, careful placement of the contact lenses in sterile containers filled with normal saline, safe storage, and documentation are essential. To find contacts in the eye, evert the upper lid and remove the lens. If the contact is not found, sweep the cul-de-sac with a moistened swab. If still not found, examine with fluorescein stain for corneal abrasions. The abrasion may feel like the lens is still present in the eye. Lubricating drops are essential before removing a dried lens. A hard lens is removed with a suction cup made for that purpose. Remove soft contacts by grasping them between the thumb and index finger and lifting the lens off the eye.

> Do not remove a contact lens if the eye is ruptured. The contact may be the only support for the ruptured globe. An ophthalmologist should make the decision if removal of the contact is appropriate in the ER.

CORNEAL ABRASION

Corneal abrasions occur when a foreign body denudes the epithelium. Diagnosis is made by fluorescein stain. Treatment may include pressure patching for 24 to 48 hours to reduce the risk of the eyelid scraping against the denuded area.

EMERGENT EYE EMERGENCIES

Emergent eye problems threaten vision and are second only to emergencies that threaten life. Among the true emergent problems are angle-closure glaucoma, retinal artery occlusion, ruptured globe, intraocular foreign bodies, and ocular chemical burns.

ENUCLEATION

Enucleation is removal of the eye globe. This may occur traumatically or may be performed surgically.

EXTERNAL EXAMINATION AND EVALUATION OF EYE MOTILITY

Review of External Exam of the Eye and Evaluation of Eye Motility
Begin the exam away from the eye and gradually move closer.
Inspect for lacerations, bruises, and differences between the eyes.
Inspect the eyelids, eyelashes, and how the eyes lay in their sockets.
Inspect the conjunctiva and sclera for color.
Evaluate the patient's ability to move the eyes through the six positions of gaze by asking the patient to follow a finger moved around the eye. In children, asking them to follow a toy is more apt to be successful.

EXOPHTHALMOS

Exophthalmos is an abnormal protrusion of the eyeball commonly associated with Graves' disease (thyrotoxicosis). It is a chronic process and when seen in the ER, no treatment is necessary.

FLUORESCEIN STAINING OF THE EYE

Review of Fluorescein Staining of the Eye
Moisten the end of a fluorescein strip with sterile normal saline solution.
Pull down the patient's lower eyelid to expose the cul-de-sac.
Touch the strip to the fluid inside the lower eyelid and remove the strip.

Review of Fluorescein Staining of the Eye
Ask the patient to blink several times to distribute the stain over the eye.
Examine the cornea with a cobalt blue light (Wood's lamp). Denuded areas of the cornea will show as a bright yellow spot.

HYPHEMA

Review of Hyphema	
Definition	A hyphema is blood in the anterior chamber of the eye in front of the iris.
Cause	The cause is commonly a blunt force that causes bleeding from depression of the iris and ciliary bodies.
Symptoms	Symptoms may include pain, blurred vision, photophobia, and blood in the anterior chamber in front of the iris.
Tests	No tests are required. Diagnosis is made clinically. A good history and physical exam are essential.
Treatment	Medical treatment of a hyphema may include strict resting in bed, sedation, and bilateral eye patches without pressure for several days. Treatment is controversial and many schools of thought are in the current literature.
Complications	Complications include a second bleed in 2 to 14 days, staining of the cornea, and loss of vision.

INSTILLATION OF EYE MEDICATIONS AND APPLICATION OF PATCHES

Review of Eye Medication Instillation and Application of Patches
Pull the lower eyelid downward and ask the patient to look up.
Instill eye drops or a thin line of ointment into the cul-de-sac of the lower eyelid. Do not place eye drops in the inner canthus. When eye drops are placed in the inner canthus, the solution drains into the lacrimal duct and immediately into the nose. If more than one drug is administered, wait several minutes between drugs.
Ask the patient to blink several times and roll his eyes gently and slowly to expose the entire eye surface to the medications.
After administration, ask the patient to apply pressure for a few minutes to the tear duct near the nose to minimize systemic absorption.
Instruct the patient not to tightly squeeze the eyelids together. Squeezing the eyelids together causes the medication to leak out.
To patch an eye, ask the patient to close both eyes and place a horizontally folded eye patch over the lid. The folded patch fills the indention between the brow and the cheek. Place a second patch unfolded over the first patch and tape obliquely with paper tape.

Review of Eye Medication Instillation and Application of Patches
If the purpose of the patch is to keep the eyelid closed at nighttime to reduce the risk of damage caused by a dry eye, taping the eyelid shut with paper tape is effective. The cotton filled eye patches make applying enough pressure to keep the lid closed difficult to impossible. In Bell's palsy, the lid should be taped shut for sleeping and when the eye is exposed to dust-filled air.

IRRIGATION OF THE EYE

Review of Irrigation of the Eye
Wash the entire area around the eye.
Gather the following equipment: Warmed irrigating solution of normal saline IV tubing IV cannula with the needle removed and attached to the tubing. Use of a nasal cannula attached to the tubing and placed over the bridge of the nose for bilateral irrigation is a questionable practice. The sterility and debris free interior of the tubing cannot be guaranteed.
Place the patient on the affected side or on their back for bilateral irrigation. Pad the patient well with towels.
Run a gentle stream of the solution over the eye from the inner (internal) canthus to the outer (external) canthus of the eye.
Ask the patient to occasionally blink, look up, down, and from side-to-side to assure that the irrigating solution reaches all surfaces of the eye.
Evert (turn inside out) the upper eyelid by placing a cotton swab over the eyelid, pulling the eyelashes down, and then up over the swab to irrigate under the upper lid.

CHALAZION

A chalazion is a small hard tumor like cyst on the eyelid from a distended meibomian gland. Treatment may include surgical excision or incision and drainage.

CONJUNCTIVITIS

Conjunctivitis is inflammation of the conjunctiva. Symptoms include red swollen eyelids with purulent discharge. Causes are foreign bodies, allergies, and bacterial infections. Cleansing of the eyelids is essential. Ivory soap is the most effective cleanser. Treatment is directed towards the cause, e.g., removal of the foreign object, antibiotics for bacterial infections, and antihistamines for allergies. Common bacterial infections include staphylococcal, gonococcal, pneumococcal, and pseudomonal organisms. Treatment of bacterial infection is topical and systemic antibiotics. Instruct the patient and family in good handwashing techniques and methods to prevent the spread of infection.

CORNEAL LACERATION

Small lacerations are treated the same as corneal abrasions. Larger ones require suturing in surgery.

CORNEAL ULCER

A corneal ulcer is often caused by irritation from a contact lens left in the eye too long. The ulcer appears as a white spot on the cornea. Symptoms may include pain, photophobia, vascular congestion, and profuse tearing. Fluorescein stain is used for diagnosis. Treatment may include systemic antibiotics, warm compresses, and an eye patch.

EYELID WOUNDS

Wounds to the eyelids often cause an injury to the eye. Careful examination of the eye is essential. The eyelids are vascular, and edema develops quickly preventing good approximation of wound edges. Cooling the area with an ice pack placed over sterile saline moistened gauze is a priority intervention. Closure by a plastic surgeon is recommended.

FOREIGN BODY

Foreign bodies are anything that will fit into the eye. The most common is a dust particle. Symptoms are pain, hypersensitivity to light, and excessive tearing. Treatment may include local anesthesia to facilitate examination and removal of the foreign object. A needle is not recommended to facilitate removal of an object imbedded in the cornea. Antibiotic ointment and patching are essential. Organic foreign bodies have a high incidence of infection. Metallic objects can cause rust rings if left in the eye for over 12 hours. Ocular burr drills are used to remove rust rings. Topical anesthetics are not for long-term use because the substance retards healing.

GLAUCOMA, ACUTE

Acute glaucoma is EMERGENT. Acute glaucoma occurs when the anterior chamber angle near the root of the iris is blocked. Symptoms may include severe eye pain, a fixed and slightly dilated pupil, a foggy appearing cornea, hard globe, halos, and disturbances of the peripheral vision. Treatment may include decreasing the intraocular pressure by decreasing the volume and increasing the flow. Topical timolol decreases aqueous production and oral glycerol or intravenous Mannitol reduces the volume in the globe. Outflow is enhanced by pilocarpine. When the acute attack is under control, surgery is required.

GLAUCOMA, CONGENITAL

Infantile or juvenile glaucoma is a failure of the anterior chamber to develop normally. Symptoms may include tearing and photophobia. A child protects the eye from light by keeping the eyelid closed. The treatment is surgery.

GLAUCOMA, OPEN ANGLE

Open angle glaucoma is a chronic condition that progresses slowly. Treatment may include miotic eye drops and surgery.

GLAUCOMA, SECONDARY

Secondary glaucoma causes include increased intraocular pressure secondary to surgery, trauma, and tumors. Treatment is directed towards correcting the cause.

GLOBE RUPTURE

Globe rupture is EMERGENT and can be caused by blunt or penetrating trauma. Symptoms may include altered light perception, a deep anterior chamber, hyphema, and occasionally vitreous hemorrhage. AVOID EYE MANIPULATION,

DO NOT REMOVE CONTACTS, and DO NOT USE EYE MEDICATIONS. If the penetrating object is still present, stabilize it, and loosely patch both eyes to decrease eye movement. Treatment is surgical repair or enucleation.

HERPES SIMPLEX

Herpes simplex can infect both the eye and the eyelids. Painful red swollen lesions are present on the lids. The infections of the eyelid can quickly spread to the eye. Corneal ulcers are a complication of eye infections. Treatment may include topical antiviral medication. Steroids make the symptoms worse.

HERPES ZOSTER

Symptoms of herpes zoster infection of the peripheral trigeminal nerve include eruptions of acute inflammatory herpetic vesicles along the peripheral trigeminal nerve distribution. All parts of the eyelid and eye can become infected. Symptoms may include severe pain and herpetic vesicles usually associated with shingle lesions in the scalp and on the face. Good hygiene is essential. Treatment may include analgesia (both topical and systemic) and oral acyclovir to decrease the severity of the lesions.

HORDEOLUM

A hordeolum is an inflammation of a sebaceous gland on the eyelid and is commonly referred to as a sty.

INTRAOCULAR FOREIGN BODIES

Intraocular foreign bodies of the eye are EMERGENT. Small projectiles striking the eye at a high rate of speed can penetrate the eye and come to rest in the anterior chamber. The most common object is a metal fragment from a metal drill. Symptoms may be only minor discomfort. A good history is essential. X-rays of the eye are used to identify the size and position of the fragment if it is metal. CT is used for nonmetal objects. Treatment may include surgical removal of the object, antibiotics, tetanus toxoid, and patching.

IRITIS

Iritis is an inflammation of the iris (the colored contractile membrane suspended between the lens and the cornea). Symptoms may include deep severe achy pain, blurred vision, photophobia, and tearing. The iris may appears swollen, dull and muddy, and the pupil irregularly contracted and sluggish to react. Treatment may include 1% atropine to keep the pupil dilated and systemic and topical steroids.

KERATITIS

Keratitis is an inflammation of the cornea usually caused by a bacteria or fungus. Culture and sensitivity are recommended. Warm compresses are helpful for the pain and swelling. Treatment may include antibiotics or antifungal medications.

MONOCULAR VISION

Monocular vision loss causes include ischemia from vascular occlusion and retinal detachment.

ORBITAL CELLULITIS

Orbital cellulitis is an acute infection of the orbital tissue commonly caused by bacterium. The cause is usually secondary to sinusitis or an orbital injury. Symptoms may include pain, swelling, tenderness, and redness of the periorbital tissues. A CT scan is necessary to rule out orbital and intracranial abscesses.

Treatment may include hospitalization, intravenous antibiotics, evaluation by an ophthalmologist, and an evaluation by a neurologist or neurosurgeon.

PAPILLEDEMA

Review of Papilledema	
Definition	Papilledema is an inflammation and swelling of the optic nerve at the entrance to the eyeball
Cause	The cause of papilledema is an obstruction of venous return from the retina that may develop with intracranial cerebral pressure, retrobulbar neuritis, blood vessel changes from trauma, hemorrhage, infections, and brain tumors.
Note	Papilledema may be the defining factor between hypertension and hypertension crisis.

PH TESTING OF THE EYE

The pH of the eye is tested on all suspected acid or alkaline burns. If the pH is >7.4 or <7.4 the eye is irrigated until the pH returns to 7.4. Testing of the pH must be done before anesthetic eye drops are instilled. The pH of the drops changes the reading temporarily and the actual pH of the eye may be misjudged.

PUPIL EXAMINATION

Review of Pupil Examination	
Shape	The pupil is normally round. An irregular shape can be an acute emergency, from an old injury, or secondary to eye surgery. A good history is essential. Tear shaped pupils are associated with globe ruptures with the tear dropping toward the rupture site.
Size	The size of the pupil changes in response to direct and consensual light (concurrent constriction of one pupil in response to light shined in the other).
Reaction to light	Reaction to light describes a pupil that constricts to light. Documentation for a pupil that constricts from 6 mm to 2 mm in light is 6 → 2.
Accommodation	Accommodation refers to the automatic adjustment in the focal length of the lens of the eye to permit retinal focus of images of objects at varying distances.
OD	Right eye
OS	Left eye
OU	Both eyes
Documentation	PERRLA, pupils are equal, round, regular, and reactive to light and accommodation.

RADIATION AND WELDING BURNS TO THE EYE

Infrared and ultraviolet rays cause radiation burns. The degree of the burn depends on the wavelength and length of exposure. Ultraviolet rays burn welders, winter sport participants, sunbathers, and sun lamp users. Symptoms occur 6 to 10 hours after exposure and may include severe pain, photophobia, vision loss, and corneal irregularity. Treatment may include anesthetics, topical antibiotics, and a patch for 24 hours. The cornea heals fast usually within 24 hours without any residual vision loss. Infrared burns are rare. People working with infrared radiation wear protective eyewear. These types of burns include long exposure to intense heat, e.g., a glassblower watching his work or exposure to an eclipse or x-ray radiation. The burns can cause permanent vision loss. Treatment may include anesthetics, topical antibiotics, and a patch for 24 hours.

RETINAL DETACHMENT

A retinal detachment is a retinal tear that allows the vitreous humor to seep between the retina and the choroids. Loss of blood supply to the retina makes it unable to perceive light. Symptoms may include flashes of light, veil or curtain effects, floaters, or dark spots. Treatment may include hospitalization, resting in bed, bilateral patches, and ophthalmology consultation.

THERMAL BURNS

Thermal burns to the eye are EMERGENT. Eye globe burns are commonly caused by hot metal, steam, or gasoline. Treatment may include analgesia, sedation, eye irrigation, antibiotics, and bilateral eye patches. Ophthalmology consult is essential.

VIRAL KERATO-CONJUNCTIVITIS

Acute conjunctivitis and keratitis are caused by an adenovirus. Symptoms may include redness of the conjunctiva, pain, tearing, photophobia, and swollen eyelids. Warm compresses help decrease the pain and swelling. Treatment may include analgesia. The healer is the passage of time. Meticulous hand washing and equipment sterilization is essential to avoid spread.

OPHTHALMIC TONOMETER

An ophthalmic tonometer is an instrument used for measuring the intraocular pressure of the eye. A tonometer that does not touch the eye measures the alteration in the cornea with a puff of air. The Schiotz tonometer is placed directly on the anesthetized eye globe to obtain an intraocular pressure reading. Normal is 12 mm Hg with a normal increase of 1 mm Hg per decade after age 40. The Schiotz tonometer reads low when the pressure in the eye is high because the plunger of the tonometer cannot indent the cornea as deeply.

VISUAL ACUITY

Visual acuity testing is essential for all eye problems. The test is a measurement of the patient's ability to see normally. In chemical burns, irrigation takes priority over testing the patient's visual acuity. If the patient normally wears corrective lens or glasses, the exam is done with the glasses or corrective lens in place. If glasses or lens are not available, a pinhole can be utilized to measure the visual acuity. Pierce an 18-gauge needle through a card and ask the patient to look through the pinhole. The pinhole can correct an error of up to approximately 20/30. First, test the affected eye by asking the patient to cover the unaffected eye and read the chart. Second, test the unaffected eye by asking the patient to cover the affected eye and read the chart. Last, test both eyes by asking the patient to read the chart with both eyes open. The Snellen chart is the most commonly used. The patient's distance from the Snellen chart must be 20 feet and is inconvenient in an emergency room. The Rosenbaum Pocket Vision Screener is held 14 inches from the nose and is more convenient for ER use.

Documentation for Visual Acuity	
20/20	The patient can read what is expected of a person to normally read at 20 feet.
20/20 2	The patient missed two letters, otherwise, can read what is expected of a person to normally read at 20 feet. Change the last number missed to match the patient's ability.
20/200	At 20 feet, the patient can only read what the normal person can read at 200 feet. This is the level of legal blindness.
10/200	The 10 indicates the number of feet that the patient must stand from the Snellen chart and read what the normal person can read at 200 feet. Change the number of feet to describe the patient's ability.
CF/3 ft	The patient can count fingers at 3 feet. Change the number of feet to match the patient's ability.
HM/4	The patient can see hand motion at 4 feet. Change the number of feet to match the patient's ability.
LP/position	The patient can perceive light and determine the direction the light comes from.
LP/no position	The patient can perceive the light but is unable to determine the direction of the light.
NLP	The patient is unable to perceive light.

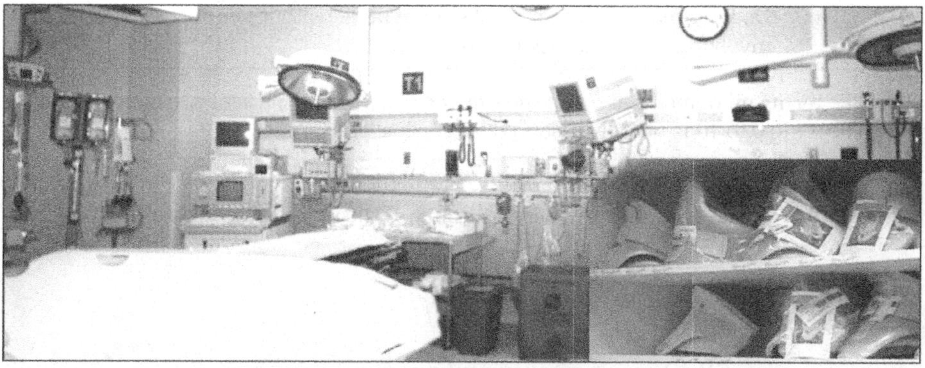

17 FALLS AND SPINAL INJURY

For details on triage see Chapter 34, Triage in a Nutshell.

PATIENT'S STORY – INTERVIEW QUESTIONS

1. When and how was the patient injured?
2. Where are the injuries and are any associated symptoms present?
3. What caused the injury; e.g., a fall from a cliff, roof, or ladder?
   a. If the incident was a fall, what was the height of the fall?

A fall is commonly > 6 feet. If the fall was < 6 feet, a vertical deceleration injury may not be present. Consider using chapter #32 Traumatic Injury.

   b. What brought about the fall; e.g., stumbling or tripping over a mechanical obstacle, losing a grip on a mechanical support, or a medical problem (e.g., dizziness, lightheadedness, vertigo, or faintness)?
   c. For a slip and fall, consider chapter #32 Traumatic Injury.
   d. For fainting, consider chapter #33 Syncope and Near Syncope.
   e. For electrocution, consider chapter #15 Electrocution.
4. How does the injury affect normal function and how severe is the injury?
   a. What is the appearance of the injured area?
   b. Is neurovascular function normal distal to the injury?
   c. Does the patient have normal use of the injured area?
   d. Has the injury affected normal body functions, e.g., incontinence, grips, sensations?
5. Does the patient have pain not directly associated with an obvious injury?
   a. Where is the pain located and is radiation present?
   b. What is the severity of the pain?

6. Does the patient complain of skin hypersensitivity or burning sensations involving localized or generalized areas?

The terms mild, moderate, or severe or the words of the patient are appropriate. The scale 0 to 10 is usually reserved for cardiac pain.

7. Has any treatment been initiated, and has it helped?
8. Has the patient had serious injury to the same areas before?
   a. What was the diagnosis?
   b. What was the treatment?
9. Is unlawful activity suspected?
   a. Was law enforcement at the scene?
   b. What agency?

Medical personnel are obligated to notify law enforcement if unlawful activity is suspected.

10. Does the patient have any pertinent past history?
11. Does the patient take any routine medications?
    a. What is the name, dosage, route, and frequency of each medication?
    b. When was the last dose?
12. Does the patient take any complementary or alternative therapies, herbal products, over-the-counter medications or supplements, or natural therapies?
    a. What is the name, dosage, route, and frequency of each therapy?
    b. When was the last dose or therapy?
13. Does the patient have allergies to drugs or foods?
    a. What is the name of the allergen?
    b. What was the reaction?
14. When was the patient's last tetanus immunization?
15. If the patient is female and between the ages of 10 to 50 years, when was the first day of her last menstrual period?

NURSING DOMAIN

The nursing domain, nursing diagnosis and plan of care can only be determined after an in-depth interview and consideration of the patient's story.

Domain 12. Comfort. Class 1. Physical comfort.
Domain 11. Safety/Protection. Class 2. Physical Injury.

Domain 4. Activity/Rest Class 5. Self-care.
Domain 5. Perception/Cognition Class 3. Sensation/perception.

ANTICIPATED MEDICAL CARE

Review of the Anticipated Medical Care of Falls and Traumatic Spinal Injuries	
Exam	Full body
Urine	Urine dip for blood; pregnancy test for women of reproductive age unless they have had a hysterectomy
Blood	Hemogram, electrolytes, renal studies, type and screen
ECG	ECG for females and males over 35 years, and for all ages with a cardiac history
X-ray	X-rays of areas with suspected bony injury, CT scan and/or MRI may also be considered if a spinal cord injury is suspected and to rule out any occult injuries.
Diet	NPO
IV	Normal saline or Ringer's solution 200 cc bolus for symptoms of shock, intravenous fluid rate titrated to maintain a urinary output of > 30 cc/hr
Medications	Pain medications, nonsteroidal anti-inflammatories, and muscle relaxants. Intravenous steroids (Decadron or Depo-Medrol) may be considered for spinal cord involvement though the effectiveness is currently being studied.
Other	Nasogastric tube, indwelling Foley catheter
Disposition	Hospitalization may be required for moderate or severe body damage. For acute spinal cord injury, anticipate a transfer to a facility specializing in spinal cord injury.
Worst-case scenario	Worst-case scenario is the patient presents with vague complaints which could be consistent with a possible SCI, leaves without a proper diagnosis later resulting in death of the patient.

INITIAL CARE PLAN

> Alcohol-based hand sanitizers are the preferred method for cleaning your hands in most clinical situations. Wash your hands with soap and water whenever they are visibly dirty, before eating, and after using the restroom.

1. Ask the patient to undress, remove all jewelry that might interfere with the examination, and put on an exam gown. Assist as needed.

2. For the patient in C-Spine immobilization, remove shoes, socks, necklaces and earrings. After the C-spine immobilization equipment is removed, expose the full body.
3. Obtain vital signs. Vital signs on trauma patients include temperature, respiratory rate and rhythm, heart rate and rhythm, blood pressure, and pulse oximetry.
4. Place on oxygen if saturation < 94%.
5. Assure the patient that all efforts will be taken to keep him comfortable and safe during the diagnostic work-up and treatment.
6. Evaluate the level of consciousness based on the mnemonic **AVPU** or **ACDU** level of consciousness score.
   AVPU: **A**lert, **V**erbal, **P**ain, **U**nresponsive.
   ACDU: Alert, **C**onfused, **D**rowsy, **U**nresponsive.
7. Perform a head-to-toe physical examination.

> If two nurses are at the bedside, one can ask the following questions and document the answers of the other who performs the exam. Document positive and negative findings.

   a. What is the size and reaction of the pupils?
   b. Does the patient have any head pain or injuries to the head?
      Is the tongue or mouth injured?
      Is any drainage present from the nose or ears?
   c. Is the trachea midline?
      Is jugular venous distention present (unable to detect under fluorescent light)?
   d. Does the chest expand equally?
      Is subcutaneous emphysema present?
      Are the heart tones within normal limits?
      Are the heart tones diminished?
      Are any murmurs present?
      Does the patient complain of chest pain?
      Is the chest tender to palpation?
   e. Are the lung sounds clear on the right and left?
      Are wheezes or crackles present?
      Are the lung sounds decreased or absent in any area of the lungs?
   f. Is the abdomen soft, flat, rigid, or distended?
      Are bowel sounds normal, hypoactive, hyperactive, or absent?
      Does the patient complain of abdominal pain?
      Is the patient's abdomen tender to palpation?

g. Is the patient incontinent?
   Examination of the genitalia may be deferred if trauma is not suspected.
   Do the genitalia appear normal?
   Does the patient have bleeding from the urethral meatus or vagina?
   Is priapism present?
   Does the patient complain of genital pain?
   Is the perineal area or genitalia tender to palpation?

h. Does the patient complain of pain when light pressure is applied to the iliac crests?
   Is the pelvis stable or unstable?

i. Does the patient have normal motion and sensation in the upper and lower extremities?
   Are distal pulses present in the upper and lower extremities?

j. Does the patient have normal movement of his back?
   Does the patient complain of back pain?
   While keeping the back immobilized, turn the patient.
   Inspect the posterior surfaces.
   Does the patient have obvious back injuries?
   Is the back tender to palpation?

k. Does skin inspection reveal any damage to the skin; e.g., abrasions, lacerations, bruises, needle tracks, or petechiae?

8. Establish intravenous access and draw laboratory blood specimens. Draw a variety of tubes that will allow the lab to perform hematology, chemistry, and coagulation studies. Patients on anticoagulants and cirrhotic patients need a PT and a PTT. Consider drawing other labs; e.g., type and screen, blood cultures.

9. Keep the patient warm with heated blankets. Shawl a warmed blanket around the head, neck, and shoulders. Place another blanket over the body and tightly tuck it around the patient.

10. Administer medications covered by protocols, e.g., tetanus toxoid.

11. Clean and dress wounds. Consider collecting wound cultures.

12. Consider placing drains.

    a. Nasogastric tube to decrease the risk of vomiting and aspiration

    b. Indwelling Foley catheter to monitor urinary output.

13. Initiate orders for x-rays of areas with suspected bony damage if covered by hospital protocol.

14. Instruct the patient not to eat or drink and teach the patient and family the rationale for the NPO status.

15. Elevate the bed siderails and place the stretcher in the lowest position.

16. Inform the patient, family, and caregivers of the usual plan of care and the expected overall time in the ER.

17. Inform the patient, family, and caregivers of the necessity to cooperate with any immobilization procedures.
18. Provide for protection of the patient's extremities when sensory deficits are apparent.
19. Provide the patient with a device to reach someone for assistance and explain how to use it. Ask the patient to call for help before getting off the stretcher.

ONGOING CARE PLAN

Inform the medical provider of adverse changes noted during ongoing evaluation. Document that the medical provider was notified of the adverse change. Document if orders were or were not received.

1. Monitor temperature, heart rate and rhythm, respiratory rate and rhythm, blood pressure, and effectiveness of breathing.
2. Monitor therapy closely for the patient's therapeutic response.
    a. The usual time for a medication effectiveness check is 20 to 30 minutes after giving the drug.
    b. If therapy is not effective, ask the medical provider for a repeat dose or an alternative.
3. Monitor extremity movements by asking the patient to wiggle toes and fingers and gently lift arms and legs. Compare with the baseline.
4. Monitor extremity sensation with a gentle touch on all extremities and compare with the baseline.
5. Monitor closely for the development of adverse reactions to therapy.
    a. Perform interventions to relieve the adverse reaction.
    b. Ask the medical provider for a remedy.
6. Keep the patient, family, and caregivers well informed of the plan of care and the remaining time anticipated before disposition.
7. Monitor the patient's laboratory and x-ray results and notify the medical provider of critical abnormalities. Remedy abnormalities as ordered.
8. Notify the medical provider when all diagnostic results are available for review. Ask for establishment of a diagnosis and disposition.

DISCHARGE INSTRUCTIONS

1. Provide the patient with the name of the nurse and doctor in the emergency room.
2. Inform the patient of their diagnosis or why a definitive diagnosis couldn't be made. Explain what caused the problem if known.
3. Teach the patient how to take the medication as prescribed and how to manage the common side effects. Instruct the patient not to drive or perform any dangerous tasks while taking narcotic pain medications.

4. Instruct the patient with minor neck injuries that:
   a. Symptoms often worsen over one to three days and then improve.
   b. Rest is essential.
   c. A soft cervical collar allows the neck muscles to rest and should be removed only for bathing.
   d. Use an ice pack to cool the area for the first 24 hours to decrease the inflammation and swelling. Then, use warm moist heat to increase the blood circulation and aid healing.
   e. When the symptoms are gone, gradually increase activity.
   f. Do not go back to full activities until released by the follow-up medical provider. Follow-up is very important.
5. Instruct the patient with minor back injuries that:
   a. Symptoms often get worse over the first three days after the injury.
   b. Rest is essential.
   c. Use an ice pack to cool the area for the first 24 hours to decrease the inflammation and swelling. Then, use warm moist heat to increase the blood circulation and aid healing.
   d. Since the back contains the most muscles in the body, injuries do not get better quickly.
   e. When the symptoms are gone, gradually increase activity.
   f. Do not go back to full activity until released by the follow-up medical provider. Follow-up is very important.
6. Recommend a medical provider for follow-up care. Provide the name, address, and phone number with a recommendation of when to schedule the care.
7. Instruct the patient to call the follow-up medical provider immediately or return to the emergency room if the pain worsens or any problems develop with movement or sensation of the arms or legs or bowel/bladder retention or incontinence occurs. Encourage the patient NOT to IGNORE WORSENING OR PERSISTENT SYMPTOMS.
8. Ask for verbal confirmation or demonstration of understanding and reinforce teaching as needed.

COMMONLY USED MEDICATIONS

DILAUDID

Dilaudid (hydromorphone)	
Indications	Moderate to severe pain
Dose	Typical dose 1 to 5 mg IV. Titrate to response. No maximum dose.
Onset	IV onset rapid, peak 15 to 30 minutes, duration 3 to 4 hours

Dilaudid (hydromorphone)	
Side effects	Drowsiness, dizziness, confusion, sedation, increased intracranial pressure, nausea, vomiting, urinary retention, respiratory depression
Monitor	CNS changes, respiratory effectiveness, allergic rash
Note	Dilaudid 5 mg equivalent to Morphine 10 mg IM. Dilute to 4 or 5 ml with NS or sterile water for injection and administer slowly over at least 2 to 3 minutes Antidote is naloxone.

PHENERGAN

Phenergan (promethazine)	
Indications	Nausea, vomiting
Adult Dose	12.5 to 25 mg IV every 4 to 6 hours. When used intravenously, promethazine injection should be given in concentration no greater than 25 mg/ml at a rate not to exceed 25 mg/min. Preferably inject through a medication port in IV tubing that is known to be functioning satisfactorily. 25 mg IM every 4 to 6 hours
Pediatric dose	More than 2 years IM or IV 0.25 to 0.5 mg/kg every 4 to 6 hours
Onset	IM onset 20 min., duration 4 to 6 hours IV onset 3 to 5 min., duration 4 to 6 hours
Side effects	Drowsiness, sedation, hypotension, palpitations, tachycardia
Monitor	Vital signs, respiratory effectiveness

VERSED

Versed (midazolam hydrochloride)	
Indications	Conscious sedation
Adult dose	1 to 2.5 mg IV over 2 min., every 2 min. (a total dose of over 5 mg is not usually necessary) If patients have narcotic medications before the Versed, use approximately 30% less Versed.
Pediatric dose	Pediatric patients age 12 to 16 years should be dosed as adults. Pediatric dose is weight based. IV initial loading dose is 0.05 to 0.2 mg/kg given over 2 to 3 min. (Usually not used in pediatric patients that are not intubated.)
Onset	IV onset 3 to 5 min.
Compatibility	Use normal saline in IV line before and after giving the dose.

Versed (midazolam hydrochloride)	
Side effects	Serious life threatening decreased respiratory tidal volume and respiratory rate
Monitor	Heart rate and rhythm, blood pressure, and oxygenation
Note	Versed is a potent sedative that requires slow administration and individualization of dosage. Versed is 3 to 4 times as potent as Valium. The reversing agent for Versed is Romazicon.

ROMAZICON

Romazicon (flumazenil)	
Indications	Valium or Versed (benzodiazepine) overdose
Adult dose	First dose 0.2 mg IV over 15 sec Second dose 0.3 mg IV over 15 seconds Third dose 0.5 mg IV over 30 seconds If no response, may repeat every minute until response is adequate or the maximum of 3 mg are given. If more than 3 mg are required, the diagnosis of a benzodiazepine overdose must be questioned.
Onset	IV onset 1 minute, peak 10 min., duration unknown
Side effects	Nausea, vomiting, seizures, dizziness, agitation, pain at injection site
Note	Effects of flumazenil may wear off before the benzodiazepine. Repeat dose to the maximum levels.
Monitor	Respiratory effectiveness

VALIUM FOR BACK PAIN

Valium (diazepam)	
Indications	Muscle spasm
Dose	IM 5 to 20 mg single dose, IV 5 to 10 mg single dose
Onset	IV onset 5 min., peak 15 minutes IM onset 15 min., peak ½ to 1 ½ hours, duration 1 to 1 ½ hours
Side effects	Dizziness, drowsiness, orthostatic hypotension, blurred vision, tachycardia
Monitor	Level of consciousness, respiratory effectiveness

RELATED CONDITIONS AND INFORMATION

AUTONOMIC DYSREFLEXIA

Autonomic dysreflexia is a syndrome of massive imbalanced reflex sympathetic discharge occurring in patients with spinal cord injury. Symptoms include elevated blood pressure, profuse sweating above the cord injury level, especially in the face, neck, and shoulders and cool pale skin below the cord injury level. The most common cause is a distended bladder and fecal impaction. One of the first interventions in the ER is an insertion of an indwelling Foley catheter. First recognized in 1890, this syndrome may occur in about 60% of all individuals injured at T6 or above. Morbidity is association with hypertension and can cause retinal and cerebral hemorrhage, myocardial infarction, or seizures. Mortality is rare.

CRUTCHFIELD TONGS

Crutchfield tongs is a skeletal traction device used to stabilize cervical fractures. It is inserted into holes drilled into the skull and attached to weights that provide traction to the cervical spine.

CORD FUNCTION LEVELS

Level of Injury Related to Level of Function	
C1 to C3	Usually fatal, requires immediate and continuous respiratory support
C4	Respiratory difficulty, no function in all extremities, head and neck control, shoulder shrug
C5	Shoulder control and shrug, elbow flexion, wrist rotation
C6	Shoulder control, elbow flexion, wrist rotation and extension
C7	Shoulder control, elbow flexion and extension, wrist rotation and extension
C8 to T1	Neck weakness, limited or natural hand function
T2 to T6	Normal upper extremity function, increased control of trunk muscles
T7 to T12	Normal upper extremity function, increased abdominal muscle control
L1 to L5	Movement of hips and knees
S1 to S5	Increasing return of bladder, bowel and sexual functions

DECELERATION INJURIES

Both rapid deceleration and acceleration forces can cause the spine to move beyond the tolerance of the vertebral column. Vertical deceleration is the type of force that results from a fall. Axial loading is the vertical compression force that is applied to the vertebral column on landing. Different patterns of injuries result from different types of falls. Since the head is the largest part of a child, children often land on their heads. Adults landing on their feet often suffer bilateral calcaneus fractures, bilateral ankle fractures, hip fractures or dislocations, and vertebral compression fractures. Adults who land on their outstretched hands suffer wrist, elbow, and shoulder injuries. In diving accidents, the driving force and impact is downward on the head and cervical vertebral column causing neck fractures from the axial loading forces. When the vertebral bodies are compressed, the wedging of the vertebra may cause compression of the cord or fragments of the bone may sever or damage the spinal cord.

FRACTURES

Fractures Associated with Falls	
Closed	A closed fracture means the skin over the fracture site is intact.
Comminuted	A comminuted fracture means the bone is splintered into fragments.
Complete	A complete fracture means the bony continuity is interrupted.
Compression	A compression fracture is seen in the spinal column, usually the lumbar region, and is the collapse of the bone tissue of the vertebral body. It may be caused by osteoporosis, tumor, or trauma.
Displaced	A displaced fracture means the proximal and distal segments of bone are not aligned.
Greenstick	A greenstick fracture means the bone is bent.
Impacted	An impacted facture means the distal and proximal fracture sites are wedged together.
Open	An open fracture means the skin over the site or near the site is not intact.

FRACTURE MANAGEMENT

Management of Fractures	
Expose the area	Remove all clothing and jewelry near the suspected fracture.
Perform a physical assessment	Inspect for color, position, and obvious differences as compared to the uninjured side, look for a break in the skin, assess for bleeding and deformity. Assess the extremity for pain, pallor, pulses, paresthesia, and paralysis (five Ps).
Determine the need for immobilization	Splint for deformity, pain, bony crepitus, edema, ecchymosis, vascular compromise, open wounds, paralysis, and paresthesia

Management of Fractures	
Immobilize	Splint with the appropriate splint to immobilize the joints below and above the injury Avoid manipulations of the bone Rigid splints such as plastic and metal splints are used for lower extremity fractures. Soft splints such as pillows and slings are used for upper extremity fractures. Traction splints are used for femur and proximal tibial fractures. A thumb spica splint is applied as if the hand was holding a soda can.
PRICE	Protect, rest, ice, compress, and elevate the area. Ice and elevation have a high priority and are essential ER procedures. If necessary, use heated blankets on the rest of the body to maintain a normal core body temperature.
Medications	Administer analgesics. Open fractures are often treated with prophylactic intravenous antibiotics.
Diagnostic Testing	X-ray the area of suspected bony injury to include the joints above and below the injury in the film.
On-going monitors	Frequently reassess the five Ps (pain, pallor, pulses, paresthesia, and paralysis).
Anticipate	Anticipate definitive stabilization, traction, internal or external fixation, and hospitalization for closed or open reduction.

NEUROGENIC SHOCK

Neurogenic shock is associated with a sympathetic blockade due to spinal cord injury and managed with interventions to increase vascular tone such as Dopamine. Symptoms may include bradycardia, vasodilation, and hypotension. The skin is warm and dry due to the vasodilation compared to the cool and clammy skin characteristic of hypovolemic shock. Bradycardia, not tachycardia, occurs in neurogenic shock due to the sympathetic blockade.

STATISTICS OF SPINAL CORD INJURY

Over ten thousand people in the United States suffer spinal cord injuries each year. Sixty percent are men between the ages of 16 and 30 years. The largest number of spinal cord injuries is caused by motor vehicle crashes (many alcohol related) and falls. In the older population, over 60 years, falls are the most common cause of spinal injuries. The remainder of the vertebral column and spinal cord injuries is related to gunshot wounds, stabbings, assaults, and sports-related injuries including diving injuries.

TYPES OF SPINAL CORD INJURIES

Types of Spinal Cord Injuries

Types of Spinal Cord Injuries	
Complete spinal cord injury	Complete spinal cord injury is a complete decrease or loss of movement and/or sensation below the injury site. Tetraplegia (a.k.a. quadriplegia) is usually defined as an injury from C1 to T1 and can result in varying degrees of loss of sensation and movement to the head, neck, chest, torso, and extremities. Paraplegia is usually defined as an injury from T2 to S5 and can result in varying degrees of loss of sensation and movement to the chest, abdomen, and lower extremities.
Incomplete spinal cord injuries	Anterior cord syndrome is damage to the anterior portion of the cord and results in loss or impaired sensation of pain, temperature and touch below the injury level. Posterior cord syndrome is damage to the posterior portion of the spinal cord and results in difficulty in coordinating movement below the injury level. Central cord syndrome is damage to the center of the cord and results in loss of function to the upper extremities with lower extremity involvement to a lesser degree. Brown-Sequard syndrome is damage to one side of the spinal cord and results in impaired or loss of movement to the extremities on the injured side of the cord and impaired sensation of pain, temperature, and touch to the opposite side. Conus medullaris syndrome is damage to the sacral cord and lumbar nerve roots and results in loss of reflexes to the bladder, bowel, and lower extremities. Caudal equina lesion is damage to the lumbosacral nerve root extending from the spinal cord at L1 to L2 and results in loss of sensation and movement below the injury.

VERTEBRAL FRACTURES AND DISLOCATIONS

Vertebral Fractures and Dislocations	
Burst	A vertebral burst fracture is a comminuted fracture of the vertebral body. The mechanism of injury is axial loading. Compression of the cord may or may not be present.
Compression	A vertebral compression fracture is a fracture of the vertebral body. The mechanism of injury is compression, hyperflexion, and anterior or lateral flexion. The spinal column is compressed and can be wedged. Compression of the cord may or may not be present.

Vertebral Fractures and Dislocations	
Simple	A simple vertebral fracture is a linear fracture of the transverse process or pedicles. The mechanism of injury is acceleration or deceleration. The spinal column maintains alignment. Spinal cord injury is rare.
Teardrop	A teardrop vertebral fracture is a small fracture of the anterior edge of the vertebra. The mechanism of injury is hyperflexion. Fragmentation of the bone may impinge the cord and may be associated with damage to the posterior cord.

VERTEBRAL FRACTURE STABILITY CLASSIFICATION

Frequently vertebral fractures are classified as stable or unstable. Stable means no potential for progressive injury to the spinal cord, for displacement of the vertebra, and no displacement or angulation is expected during healing. Unstable means that a potential for progressive injury to the spinal cord, displacement of the vertebra, or for displacement or angulation is expected during healing.

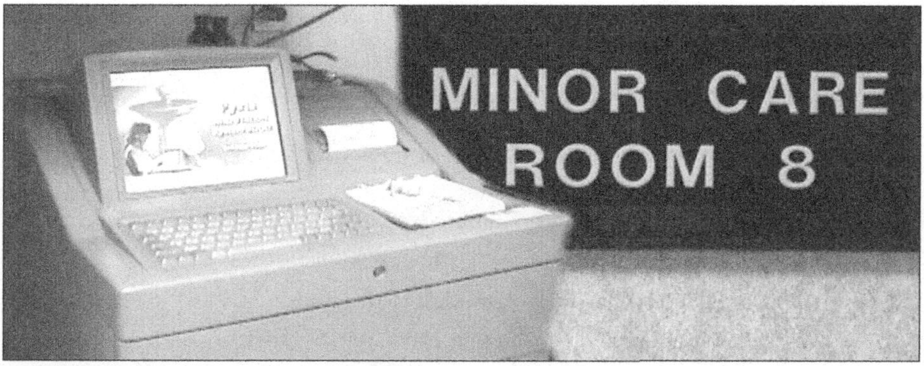

18 HEADACHE

For details on triage see Chapter 34, Triage in a Nutshell.

PATIENT'S STORY – INTERVIEW QUESTIONS

1. When did the headache begin?
2. Is the headache present now?
    a. If the headache is no longer active, how long did it last?
    b. If the symptoms were intermittent, how long did each episode last and what were the frequency of the episodes?
3. Where is the headache located and are any associated symptoms present?
    a. Is the headache associated with nausea, vomiting, or dizziness?
    b. Is the headache associated with any visual changes, e.g., loss of vision, changes in light perception, blurring, halos around lights?
4. Does the patient know why the headache is present?
    a. Is there a recent history of injury, blow to the head, or emotional stress?
    b. For recent head trauma, consider chapter #32 Traumatic Injury and Head Injury.
5. How does the headache affect normal function and how severe is the headache?
    a. Is the patient able to sleep or rest?
    b. How does the patient describe the severity of the pain, e.g., mild, moderate, or severe?

The terms mild, moderate, or severe or the words of the patient are appropriate. The scale of 0 to 10 is commonly used for cardiac patients.

6. Is this headache the patient's first headache or does the patient have a headache history?
    a. If the patient has a history of headaches, is this headache similar to the patient's usual headaches?
    b. If the patient has a history of similar headaches, what was the diagnosis and treatment?
7. Has any treatment been initiated, and has it helped?
8. Does the patient have any pertinent past history?
9. Does the patient take any routine medications?
    a. What is the name, dosage, route, and frequency of each medication?
    b. When was the last dose?
10. Does the patient take any complementary or alternative therapies, herbal products, over-the-counter medications or supplements, or natural therapies?
    a. What is the name, dosage, route and frequency of each therapy?
    b. When was the last dose or therapy?
11. Does the patient have allergies to drugs or foods?
    a. What is the name of the allergen?
    b. What was the reaction?
12. If the patient is female and between the ages of 10 to 50 years, when was the first day of her last menstrual period?

NURSING DOMAIN

The nursing domain, nursing diagnosis and plan of care can only be determined after an in-depth interview and consideration of the patient's story.

Domain 12. Comfort. Class 1. Physical comfort.

ANTICIPATED MEDICAL CARE

Review of the Anticipated Medical Care for Headaches	
Exam	Full body
Urine tests	Patients with a history of headaches and with the same symptoms as their usual headaches commonly do not need any urine tests.
Blood tests	CBC, electrolytes, renal study function studies (Patients with a history of headaches and with the same symptoms as their usual headaches commonly do not have any blood work.)
ECG studies	None

Review of the Anticipated Medical Care for Headaches	
Radiographic studies	Brain CT before spinal tap (CT is done first to rule out masses and situations where lumbar puncture would risk herniation of the brain.)
Diet	NPO
IV	Normal saline or Ringer's solution if patient is dehydrated from vomiting.
Medications	Antipyretics, analgesics, antiemetics
Other	ANTICIPATE INTRAVENOUS ANTIBIOTICS STAT IN THE ER FOR BACTERIAL MENINGITIS
Disposition	Hospital admission may be required if the cause of the headache represents a serious problem.
Worst-case scenario	Worst-case scenario is when a surgically correctable lesion progresses undetected to cause the brain stem to infarct. Result is often death or severe neurological deficit.

INITIAL CARE PLAN

Alcohol-based hand sanitizers are the preferred method for cleaning your hands in most clinical situations. Wash your hands with soap and water whenever they are visibly dirty, before eating, and after using the restroom.

1. Ask the patient to undress, remove all jewelry that might interfere with the examination, and put on an exam gown. Assist as needed.
2. Obtain vital signs including pulse oximetry or test capillary refill.
3. Assure the patient and advise that prompt administration of pain medications may be considered an unsafe practice. Drugs mask important signs and symptoms. They may not be ordered until the medical provider determines the cause of the pain. It is appropriate to give antiemetics and anti-inflammatory medications promptly.
4. If the patient has fever or appears unstable, establish intravenous access and draw laboratory blood specimens.
    a. Draw a variety of tubes that will allow the lab to perform hematology, chemistry, and coagulation studies. Cirrhotic patients and those on anticoagulants need a PT and aPTT.
    b. Consider drawing other labs, e.g., type and screen, blood cultures.
5. Perform a focused physical examination
    a. Evaluate the level of consciousness based on the mnemonic **AVPU** or **ACDU** level of consciousness score.
    AVPU: **A**lert, **V**erbal, **P**ain, **U**nresponsive.
    ACDU: **A**lert, **C**onfused, **D**rowsy, **U**nresponsive.
    b. Test pupil size and reaction of each pupil.

Review of Pupil Examination	
Shape	The pupil is normally round. An irregular shape can be an acute emergency, from an old injury, or secondary to eye surgery. A good history is essential. Tear shaped pupils are associated with globe ruptures with the tear dropping toward the rupture site.
Size	The size of the pupil changes in response to direct and consensual light (concurrent constriction of one pupil in response to light shined in the other).
Reaction to light	Reaction to light describes a pupil that constricts to light. Documentation for a pupil that constricts from 6 mm to 2 mm in light is 6 → 2.
Accommodation	Accommodation refers to the automatic adjustment in the focal length of the lens of the eye to permit retinal focus of images of objects at varying distances.
OD	Right eye
OS	Left eye
OU	Both eyes
Documentation	PERRLA, pupils are equal, round, regular, and reactive to light and accommodation.

6. Perform a cursory assessment for stroke symptoms.
   a. Evaluate for facial droop by asking the patient to smile. Normally both sides move equally well. The smile is abnormal when one side of the face does not move as well as the other side.
   b. Evaluate arm weakness by asking the patient to hold his arms outstretched with his eyes closed. Normally both arms move equally well. The arms are considered abnormal when one arm does not move as well as the other or one arm drifts down compared with the other.
   c. Evaluate the speech by asking the patient to say, "You can't teach an old dog new tricks." Normally the patient uses correct words with no slurring. The speech is abnormal if the patient slurs words, uses inappropriate words, or is unable to speak.
7. Keep the patient warm.
8. Give initial medications covered by hospital protocol, e.g., antipyretics, acetaminophen.
9. Instruct the patient not to eat or drink and teach the patient and family the rationale for the NPO status.
10. Elevate the siderails and place the stretcher in the lowest position.

11. Inform the patient, family, and caregivers of the usual plan of care, the anticipated overall time in the ER.
12. Provide the patient with a device to reach someone for assistance and explain how to use it. Ask the patient to call for help before getting off the stretcher.

ONGOING CARE PLAN

Inform the medical provider of adverse changes noted during ongoing evaluation. Document that the medical provider was notified of the adverse change. Document if orders were or were not received.

1. Monitor temperature, heart rate and rhythm, blood pressure, and effectiveness of breathing.
2. Monitor level of consciousness and compare to the AVPU or ACDU baseline.
3. Monitor pupil size and reaction. Compare to the baseline.
4. Monitor smile, arm movement, and speech. Compare to the established baseline. Instruct the patient and family to inform the staff of any noticeable changes in movement, behavior, speech, or sensation.
5. Monitor therapy closely for the patient's therapeutic response to medications.
   a. The usual time for a medication effectiveness check is 20 to 30 minutes after giving the drug.
   b. If therapy is not effective, ask the medical provider for a repeat dose or an alternative.
6. Monitor closely for the development of adverse reactions to therapy.
   a. Perform interventions to relieve the adverse reaction.
   b. Ask the medical provider for a remedy.
7. If not NPO, provide the patient with food at mealtimes and fluids during the stay.
8. Keep the patient, family, and caregivers well informed of the plan of care and the remaining time anticipated before disposition.
9. Monitor the patient's laboratory and x-ray results and notify the medical provider of critical abnormalities. Remedy abnormalities as ordered.
10. Notify the medical provider when all diagnostic results are available for review. Ask for establishment of a diagnosis and disposition.

DISCHARGE INSTRUCTIONS

1. Provide the patient with the name of the nurse and doctor in the emergency room.
2. Inform the patient of their diagnosis or why a definitive diagnosis couldn't be made. Explain what caused the problem if known.

3. Instruct the patient to rest in a cool, dim, quiet room and use cold compresses to help relieve the headache.
4. Teach the patient how to take the medication as prescribed and how to manage the common side effects. Instruct the patient not to drive or perform any dangerous tasks while taking narcotic pain medications.
5. Instruct the patient to avoid MSG and nitrates, e.g., bologna and salami, chocolate, caffeine, cheese, fermented food, and alcoholic beverages. These food products are thought to contribute to vascular or migraine headaches.
6. Recommend a medical provider for follow-up care. Provide the name, address, and phone number with a recommendation of when to schedule the care.
7. Instruct the patient to call the follow-up medical provider if the problem persists for over eight hours, worsens in any way, or any unusual symptoms develop. ENCOURAGE THE PATIENT NOT TO IGNORE WORSENING OR PERSISTENT SYMPTOMS.
8. Ask for verbal confirmation or demonstration of understanding and reinforce teaching as needed.

COMMONLY ORDERED MEDICATIONS

DILAUDID

Dilaudid (hydromorphone)	
Indications	Moderate to severe pain
Dose	Typical dose 1 to 5 mg IV. Titrate to response. No maximum dose.
Onset	IV onset rapid, peak 15 to 30 minutes, duration 3 to 4 hours
Side effects	Drowsiness, dizziness, confusion, sedation, increased intracranial pressure, nausea, vomiting, urinary retention, respiratory depression
Monitor	CNS changes, respiratory effectiveness, allergic rash
Note	Dilaudid 5 mg equivalent to Morphine 10 mg IM. Dilute to 4 or 5 ml with NS or sterile water for injection and administer slowly over at least 2 to 3 minutes Antidote is naloxone.

PHENERGAN

Phenergan (promethazine)	
Indications	Nausea, vomiting

Phenergan (promethazine)	
Dose	12.5 to 25 mg IV or IM and repeat 12.5 to 25 mg IV or IM every 4 to 6 hours When used intravenously, promethazine injection should be given in concentration no greater than 25 mg/ml at a rate not to exceed 25 mg/min. Preferably inject through a medication port in IV tubing that is known to be functioning satisfactorily.
Pediatric dose	More than 2 years IM or IV 0.25 to 0.5 mg/kg every 4 to 6 hours
Onset	IM onset 20 min., duration 4 to 6 hours IV onset 3 to 5 min., duration 4 to 6 hours
Side effects	Drowsiness, sedation, hypotension, palpitations, tachycardia
Monitor	Vital signs, sedation, respiratory effectiveness
Note	Must to be diluted when given IV to reduce the risk of a chemical burn to the vein. Painful infusion means the drug is causing a chemical burn to the interior of the vein.

RELATED CONDITIONS AND INFORMATION

ALTERED LEVEL OF CONSCIOUSNESS TREATMENT

Treatment for Altered Level of Consciousness
• Dextrose • Oxygen • Narcan • Thiamine

DECREASING LEVEL OF CONSCIOUSNESS

The noticeable effects of decreasing level of consciousness are the same as the behavior noticed when a person takes one alcoholic drink after another until the drink has to be poured down his throat and death occurs. Sequence of noticeable behavior changes is as follows:

Review of Behavior Associated with Decreasing Level of Consciousness
Inappropriateness
Clumsiness
Sleepiness
When stimulated, can wake up
When stimulated, can't wake up
When pinched, hand moves to pain with purpose of movement
When pinched, patient moves with no purposeful movement

Review of Behavior Associated with Decreasing Level of Consciousness
When pinched, no movement occurs

HEADACHES

Headaches	
Coital headaches	Coital headaches are benign but must be distinguished from subarachnoid hemorrhage.
Exertion	Exertion headaches are an acute headache of short duration after strenuous physical activity. They are usually benign and resolve spontaneously shortly after stopping the activity.
Hypertension	Hypertension rarely causes headaches.
Increased ICP	Increased intracranial pressure can produce severe headache with nausea and vomiting. Treatment may include reduction of the intracranial pressure.
Infection of the CNS	Headaches associated with CNS infection are usually accompanied by fever and stiff neck. Diagnostic workup may include CT first and then LP for gram stain and culture with sensitivity. Management may include STAT intravenous antibiotics and arrangements for hospitalization.
Post lumbar puncture	Post lumbar puncture (LP) headaches are caused by decreased intracranial pressure. Symptoms are history of a recent LP and a headache that is relieved by lying down. The cause is a leak of spinal fluid through the needle puncture site in the dura. Of patients having lumbar punctures, 10 to 40% will develop headache. Treatment may include injection of 10 ml of the patient's blood in the epidural space at the site of the LP. The blood may provide a patch for the hole in the dura. An anesthesiologist commonly does the procedure. Untreated, the headache usually subsides in 5 to 7 days.
Subarachnoid hemorrhage headaches The worst headache of my life	Subarachnoid hemorrhage (SAH) begins with a rapid loss of consciousness in 45% of the cases. In another 45% the initial symptom is an excruciating headache, often described as the "worst headache of my life." Vomiting in combination with severe headache suggest SAH. Treatment may include surgical correction. Surgery may be within the first 48 hours but can be delayed for 10 to 14 days after the SAH to stabilize the patient and minimize vasospasm in the postoperative period.

Headaches	
Temporal arteritis	Temporal arteritis is a unilateral or bilateral headache accompanied by visual loss, tender swollen temporal arteries, and an elevated ESR. It is usually seen in the elderly. Early diagnosis and treatment preserves vision that is comprised by the ischemia to the optic nerve. ER treatment includes steroids and analgesia.
Tension	Tension headache is associated with chronic contraction of the muscles of the scalp and often is associated with chronic emotional stress. ER treatment includes analgesia.

MIGRAINE HEADACHES

Migraine Headaches	
Classic migraine	Classic migraines are precipitated by an aura and severe pain, usually unilateral and lasting from minutes to days. Migraine headaches are thought to be caused by arterial spasms. Basilar artery migraines are located near the occipital area of the brain and affect vision, sensation, balance, and thought processes. Commonly associated symptoms are nausea, vomiting, and photophobia. Straining, walking, sudden position changes, and increased stress worsens the pain. Treatment may include opioid analgesia, ergotamines, and the triptan class medications. New medications are frequently introduced for migraines.
Cluster migraine	Cluster migraines involve clusters of attacks over several weeks and then remission for months or years. They are more common in men. Symptoms include excruciating unilateral pain that can wake a patient from sleep. ER treatment may include oxygen, ergotamines, subcutaneous sumatriptan, and steroids.
Common migraine	The symptoms of the common migraine are irritability, depression, yawning, and generalized edema. ER treatment may include dihydroergotamine (DHE) and the triptan class medications.
Hemiplegic migraine	Hemiplegic migraines include sensation defects in the mouth and extremities and occasionally unilateral extremity weakness or paralysis.
Migraine equivalent	A migraine equivalent headache includes all the features of the migraine without the head pain.

Migraine Headaches	
Ophthalmoplegic migraine	Ophthalmoplegic migraine symptoms may include headache and paralysis of the third cranial nerve. They begin in infancy or early childhood. If untreated, they can lead to visual defects and blindness.

PEDIATRIC CONSIDERATIONS

NEUROLOGICAL DISORDERS IN CHILDREN

Disorder	Symptoms
Brain Tumors	Headache, vomiting in relation to the child getting out of bed, diplopia, strabismus, nystagmus, papilledema, ataxia, personality changes
Guillain-Barre Syndrome	Symptoms usually develop 1 to 3 weeks after an upper respiratory or GI infection. It is demyelination as an immune response to a viral illness, surgery, immunizations or HIV. Onset is a rapid progressive symmetrical weakness traveling upward, muscle pain, ascending loss of deep tendon reflexes, flaccid paralysis
Reye's Syndrome	May be linked to the use of aspirin for flu-like symptoms or fever. Symptoms may include intractable vomiting, rapidly changing mental status, increased vital signs, hyperactive reflexes, irritability, severe agitation, delirium

MENINGITIS SIGNS AND SYMPTOMS BY AGE

Meningitis Signs and Symptoms by Age		
< 2 months old	3 months to 2 years old	> 2 years old
Altered LOC	Altered LOC	Altered LOC
Apnea	Ataxia	Fever
Bulging fontanel	Bulging fontanel	Headache
Cyanosis	Fever	Irritability
Fever	High-pitched cry	Petechiae/purpura
Irritability	Irritability	Positive Brudzinski sign
Petechiae/purpura	Petechiae/purpura	Positive Kernig's sign
Poor feeding	Seizures	Seizures
Seizures	Stiff neck	Stiff neck

SIGNS AND SYMPTOMS OF HYDROCEPHALUS

Hydrocephalus Signs and Symptoms	
Infant	Child

Hydrocephalus Signs and Symptoms	
Increased head circumference	Nausea
Setting sun eyes	Headache
Widening sutures	Altered LOC
Dilated scalp veins	Papilledema
Irritability	Diplopia
High pitched cry	Seizures
Seizures	

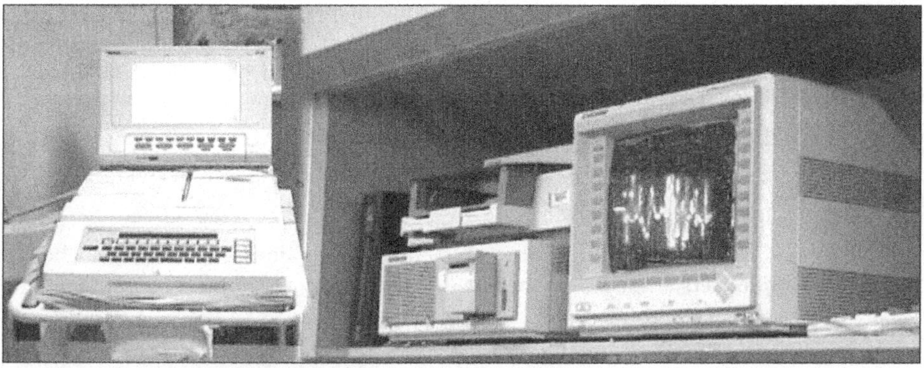

19 HEART EMERGENCY

For details on triage see Chapter 34, Triage in a Nutshell.

PATIENT'S STORY – INTERVIEW QUESTIONS

1. When did the symptoms begin?
2. Are the symptoms still present?
   a. If the symptoms are no longer active, how long did they last?
   b. If the symptoms were intermittent, how long did each episode last and what were the frequency of the episodes?
3. Does the patient feel the symptoms?
   a. Where does the patient locate the heart symptoms?
   b. Are any associated symptoms present; e.g., nausea, lightheadedness, or sweating?
4. Does the patient know why the problem started?
   a. Did the patient sustain an injury?
   b. What was the patient activity at the onset; e.g., exercising, straining to have a bowel movement, at rest, or asleep?
5. Has any treatment been initiated, and has it helped?
6. Has the patient had similar problems before?
   a. When was the problem?
   b. What was the diagnosis and treatment?
7. Is there a history of heart problems?
8. Does the patient have a pacemaker implant?
   a. When was it implanted?
   b. What is the type?
9. Does the patient have an internal cardiac defibrillator implant?

a. Has it fired today?

b. When and how many times did it fire?

10. Does the patient have any pertinent past history?

11. Does the patient take any routine medications?

a. What is the name, dosage, route, and frequency of the medication?

b. When was the last dose?

12. Does the patient take any complementary or alternative therapies, herbal products, over-the-counter medications or supplements, or natural therapies?

a. What is the name, dosage, route, and frequency of the therapy?

b. When was the last dose or therapy?

13. Does the patient have allergies to drugs or foods?

a. What is the name of the allergen?

b. What was the reaction?

14. If the patient is female and between the ages of 12 to 50 years, when was the first day of her last menstrual period?

NURSING DOMAIN

The nursing domain, nursing diagnosis and plan of care can only be determined after an in-depth interview and consideration of the patient's story.

Domain 12. Comfort. Class 1. Physical comfort.
Domain 3. Activity/Rest Class 4. Cardio/pulmonary responses

ANTICIPATED MEDICAL CARE

Review of the Anticipated Medical Care of Heart Emergencies	
Medical provider Exam	Anticipate a full body examination. If the patient is unstable, the initial exam can be limited to the chest and inspection of feet and ankles for peripheral edema. When stability is reached, the full body exam can be done.
Urine tests	None
Blood tests	Hemogram, electrolytes, cardiac markers, serum levels of digitalis, quinidine, PT and aPTT if on anticoagulants or cirrhotic; TSH for new onset atrial fibrillation.
ECG	12 lead electrocardiogram
X-ray	Chest
Other	Echocardiogram, electrocardiogram with magnet for pacemakers

Review of the Anticipated Medical Care of Heart Emergencies	
Diet	NPO
IV	Normal saline TKO
Medications	Oxygen at 4 liters per nasal cannula Treatment of arrhythmia by ACLS protocols Cardiac anti-arrhythmia drugs
Disposition	Hospital admission is required for a serious condition or one not responsive to treatment.
Worst-case scenario	The worst-case scenario is a lethal arrhythmia refractory to ACLS protocols resulting in death.

INITIAL CARE PLAN

> Alcohol-based hand sanitizers are the preferred method for cleaning your hands in most clinical situations. Wash your hands with soap and water whenever they are visibly dirty, before eating, and after using the restroom.

1. Ask the patient to undress, remove all jewelry that might interfere with the examination, and put on an exam gown. Assist as needed.
2. Obtain vital signs including pulse oximetry or test capillary refill.
   a. Institute continuous heart monitoring, pulse oximetry, and non-invasive blood pressure monitoring.
   b. Document the initial heart monitor strip and document changes of rhythm.
3. Place on oxygen at 4 liters by nasal cannula.
4. Assure the patient that he is safe.
5. Perform a focused physical examination
   a. Auscultate the lungs.
   b. Listen to heart tones.
   c. Inspect for peripheral edema.
   d. Evaluate the level of consciousness based on the mnemonic **AVPU** or **ACDU** level of consciousness score.
   AVPU: **A**lert, **V**erbal, **P**ain, **U**nresponsive.
   ACDU: **A**lert, **C**onfused, **D**rowsy, **U**nresponsive.
6. Establish intravenous access, hang normal saline at a TKO rate and draw laboratory blood specimens.
   a. Draw a variety of tubes that will allow the lab to perform hematology, chemistry, and coagulation studies. Cirrhotic patients and those on anticoagulants need a PT and aPTT.
   b. Draw other tests to establish drug levels associated with the current drugs the patient is taking, e.g., digoxin and quinidine.

> Any patient taking digoxin is considered toxic until proven otherwise. A method of remembering to check toxicity is the name. Digoxin is dig(italis) + (t)oxin.

   c. Draw blood cultures if the patient is febrile.

7. Initiate any medications covered under nurse or paramedic-initiated hospital protocols, e.g., ACLS drugs.
8. Initiate any diagnostic tests covered by hospital protocol, e.g., electrocardiogram, laboratory studies, and chest x-ray.
9. Instruct the patient not to eat or drink and teach the patient and family the rationale for the NPO status.
10. Elevate the siderails and place the stretcher in the lowest position.
11. Inform the patient, family, and caregivers of the usual plan of care and the probable overall time before disposition.
12. Provide the patient with a device to reach someone for assistance and explain how to use it. Ask the patient to call for help before getting off the stretcher.

ONGOING CARE PLAN

> Inform the medical provider of adverse changes noted during ongoing evaluation. Document that the medical provider was notified of the adverse change Document if orders were or were not received.

1. Monitor temperature, heart rate and rhythm, blood pressure, and effectiveness of breathing.
2. Monitor therapy closely for the patient's therapeutic response.
   a. The usual time for a medication effectiveness check is 20 to 30 minutes after giving the drug.
   b. If therapy is not effective, ask the medical provider for a repeat dose or an alternative.
3. Monitor closely for the development of adverse reactions to therapy.
   a. Perform interventions to relieve the adverse reaction.
   b. Ask the medical provider for a remedy.
4. Keep the patient, family, and caregivers well informed of the plan of care and the remaining time anticipated before disposition.
5. Monitor the patient's laboratory and x-ray results and notify the medical provider of critical abnormalities. Remedy abnormalities as ordered.
6. Notify the medical provider when all diagnostic results are available for review. Ask for establishment of a diagnosis and disposition.

DISCHARGE INSTRUCTIONS

1. Provide the patient with the name of the nurse and doctor in the emergency room.

2. Inform the patient of their diagnosis or why a definitive diagnosis couldn't be made. Explain what caused the problem, if known.
3. Teach the patient how to take the medication as prescribed and how to manage the common side effects. Instruct the patient not to drive or perform any dangerous tasks while taking narcotic pain medications.
4. Inform the patient that the medical provider has determined there is no serious problem. Avoid smoking, excessive caffeine, stress, and stimulant medications.
5. Recommend a medical provider for follow-up care. Provide the name, address, and phone number with a recommendation of when to schedule the care.
6. Instruct the patient to call the follow-up medical provider immediately or return to the emergency room if the problem worsens in any way or any unusual symptoms develop. Encourage the patient NOT to IGNORE WORSENING OR PERSISTENT SYMPTOMS.
7. Ask for verbal confirmation or demonstration of understanding and reinforce teaching as needed.

COMMONLY ORDERED MEDICATIONS

ADENOCARD IV

Adenocard IV (adenosine)	
Indications	Narrow complex paroxysmal supraventricular tachycardia
Adult dose	Initially 6 mg IV rapid bolus over 1 to 3 sec.. If tachycardia is not eliminated in 1 to 2 minutes, give 12 mg IV and repeat one time. Do not dilute. Push rapidly over 1 to 3 seconds and follow with 20 ml NS to push the medication through the IV tubing. A syringe of NS and one of adenosine can be placed in the same IV port. Push adenosine and then immediately push the NS. The goal is to get ALL the medication in rapidly.
Pediatric dose	0.1 to 0.2 mg/kg IV maximum first dose 6 mg. May give 0.2 mg/kg for second dose; maximum second dose: 12 mg; flush immediately with >5 mL NS
Onset	IV onset rapid, duration 1 to 2 minutes
Side effects	Brief heart block, asystole, transient chest pain, back pain, flushing, heaviness in the arms
Monitor	Heart rate and rhythm, blood pressure, oxygenation

AMIODARONE

Cordarone (amiodarone)	
Indications	Life-threatening, recurrent ventricular arrhythmias; recurrent ventricular fibrillation

Cordarone (amiodarone)	
Adult dose	Pulseless VT or VF: 300 mg IV push Recurrent VT or VF: 150 mg IV push up to a maximum dose of 2.2g IV/24 hours
Pediatric dose	5 mg/kg rapid IV push; may repeat up to a maximum of 15 mg/kg (300 mg)
Onset	IV onset rapid; half-life 40 to 55 days
Compatibility	Y site compatible: Dopamine, Dobutamine, isoproterenol, lidocaine, potassium chloride.
Side effects	Hypotension, bradycardia, impaired memory, nausea, vomiting, hypothyroidism
Note	Do not use with other medications that prolong QT interval (e.g. procainamide). Multiple complex drug interactions.
Monitor	Heart rate and rhythm, blood pressure

ATROPINE

Atropine	
Indications	Symptomatic bradycardic or pulseless electrical asystole (PEA)
Adult dose	0.5 mg IV, every 3 to 5 min., maximum 0.03 to 0.04 mg/kg (70 kg patient maximum is 2 mg) PEA: 1 mg IV, every 3 to 5 minutes to a maximum of 3 doses (3 mg) ET tube dose is 2 to 3 mg diluted with 10 ml of NS.
Pediatric dose	0.02 mg/kg IV, minimum dose 0.1 mg IV, maximum single dose 0.5 mg IV for a child, maximum total child dose: 1 mg; 1.0 mg IV for an adolescent; maximum total adolescent dose: 2 mg
Onset	IV onset 2 to 4 min., duration 4 to 6 hours
Compatibility	Compatible at Y-site with potassium chloride, Tagamet, dobutamine, epinephrine, Heparin, and Pronestyl
Side effects	Tachycardia
Note	Use atropine with caution in patients with myocardial ischemia. Doses less than 0.5 mg can lead to paradoxical tachycardia.

BRETYLIUM

Bretylol (bretylium)	
Indications	May be used in cardiac arrest from ventricular fibrillation, ventricular tachycardia, resistant ventricular arrhythmias; not a first line agent.

Bretylol (bretylium)	
Adult dose	5 mg/kg IV If the heart is not converted to an effective rhythm, give 10 mg/kg IV in five minutes after the first dose. Repeat at 15 to 30 min. intervals up to a total dose of 30 to 35 mg/kg. If conversion is successful, follow with a maintenance infusion of 1 to 2 mg/min. IV.
Pediatric dose	5 mg/kg IV may increase to 10 mg/kg IV Maximum dose 30 mg/kg.
Onset	IV onset 5 min., duration is 6 to 24 hours IM onset ½ to 2 hours, duration 6 to 24 hours
Compatibility	Compatible at Y-site with Aminophylline, Dopamine, Inocor, Lidocaine, Nitroglycerin, diltiazem, and Pronestyl. NOT Compatible at Y-site with Dilantin (phenytoin and Propofol.
Side effects	Syncope, hypotension, nausea, vomiting, respiratory depression
Note	Monitor blood pressure every 15 minutes until stable for four readings.

CARDIZEM

Cardizem (diltiazem)	
Indications	Atrial fibrillation, atrial flutter, paroxysmal supraventricular tachycardia, hypertension
Adult dose	First bolus is 0.25 mg/kg IV over 2 min. (average 20 mg). If no response in 15 min., administer a second bolus of 0.35 mg/kg IV over 2 min. Bolus may be followed with an IV infusion of 10 to 15 mg/ IV for up to 24 hours with titration to heart rate.
Onset	IV onset unknown, PO onset ½ hour, duration 6 to 8 hours
Compatibility	NOT compatible at Y-site with Lasix, diazepam, phenytoin, sodium bicarbonate.
Side effects	Cardiac conduction prolongation at the AV node, 1st and 2nd degree block, headache, nausea, CHF, hypotension, syncope, peripheral edema, acute hepatic injury, premature ventricular contractions
Note	Do not use calcium channel blockers (Cardizem) for wide QRS complexes of unknown origin.
Monitor	Heart rate and rhythm, blood pressure

DIGOXIN

Digoxin	
Indications	Digoxin is used for atrial fibrillation and flutter with a fast-ventricular response. May be alternative drug for reentry supraventricular tachycardia.
Adult dose	IV loading, 10 to 15 mcg/kg IV lean body weight, give over > 5 min. Maximum dose is affected by renal function. Maintenance dose in end stage renal disease is 0.125 mg PO every other day.
Pediatric dose	Child >2 years., IV LOADING dose 0.015 to 0.035 mg/kg IV given over >5 min.
Onset	IV onset 5 to 30 minutes, peak 1 to 5 hours, duration 6 to 8 days
Compatibility	Compatible at Y-site with potassium chloride, morphine sulfate and midazolam.
Side effects	Arrhythmias, hypotension, AV block
Note	Digoxin is 70% excreted by the kidneys. It takes 5 to 7 days to be excreted from the system. Rule of Three: A creatinine of 3 equals a dig level of 3 after 3 days of normal dosing. Avoid electrical cardioversion if patient is receiving digoxin unless rhythm is life threatening and then use lower current settings (10 to 20j). Toxic effects are common and associated with serious arrhythmias. The drug of choice in some textbooks for non-life-threatening ventricular arrhythmias from digitalis toxicity is Dilantin. However, the first drug of choice at the bedside for life threatening ventricular arrhythmias is epinephrine.
Toxic effects	Toxic effects may include visual color defects, mostly yellows and greens with halos, severe fatigue unrelieved with rest, and psychosis. Nausea and vomiting are the least common effect of toxicity.
Monitor	Heart rate, rhythm, blood pressure

DOBUTREX

Dobutrex (dobutamine)	
Indications	Cardiac decompensation from ineffective heart pumping action (CHF, pulmonary congestion)
Adult dose	2.5 to 15 mcg/kg/min. IV up to 40 mcg/kg/min. IV. Start at 2.5 mcg/kg/min IV and increase by approximately 2 to 3 mcg/kg/min. IV to the desired response.

Dobutrex (dobutamine)	
Pediatric dose	2 to 20 mcg/kg per min. and titration to the desired effect
Compatibility	Compatible at Y-site with Dopamine, epinephrine, Inocor, Isuprel, Lidocaine, Neo-Synephrine, Nitroglycerin, Levophed, Pronestyl, morphine, potassium chloride and propofol. NOT compatible with phytonadione, acyclovir, alteplase, aminophylline., sodium bicarbonate.
Note	A Swan Ganz cardiac catheter is recommended to monitor cardiac output and wedge pressures. Do not mix Dobutrex in alkaline solutions. Use with extreme caution post myocardial infarction. Correct volume depletion before use.
Monitor	Hemodynamic status; heart rate, rhythm, blood pressure.

DOPAMINE

Dopamine	
Indications	Dopamine is used for hypotension with signs of shock and as a second line drug for symptomatic bradycardia.
Adult dose	IV Titration Low dose: 1 to 5 mcg/kg/min. Intermediate dose: 5 to 15 mcg/kg/min. High dose: >15 mcg/kg/min. Maximum effective dose is 20 mcg/kg/min.
Pediatric dose	IV titration 2 to 20 mcg/kg
Onset	IV onset 5 minutes, half-life 2 minutes, duration less than 10 minutes
Side effects	Tachycardia, arrhythmias
Note	Increase and decrease by 1 to 2 mcg/kg/min. Swan Ganz catheter or central line is recommended. For extravasations, use Regitine. Do not mix with alkaline solutions.

EPINEPHRINE IV INFUSION

Epinephrine IV Infusion	
Indications	Profound shock
Adult dose	1 to 4 mcg/min. or 0.04 to 0.08 mcg/kg/min.
Pediatric dose	Initially 0.1 mcg/kg and titration to desired effect
Onset	IV onset immediate
Side effects	Hypertension, tachycardia, arrhythmias, cerebral hemorrhage and pulmonary edema

HEPARIN

Heparin	
Indications	Adjunctive therapy in acute myocardial infarction, venous thrombosis, and pulmonary embolus to reduce the risk of further clotting and in atrial fibrillation to reduce the risk of formation of an embolus.
Adult dose	Generic protocol Initial IV bolus of 80 IU/kg Continue IV at 18 IU/kg per hour (rounded to nearest 50 IU) Adjust rate every 6 hours to maintain aPTT 1 ½ to 2 times normal
Onset	IV onset 5 min., peak 10 min., duration 2 to 6 hours
Compatibility	Compatible at Y-site with potassium chloride, Aminophylline, Dopamine, Isuprel, Lidocaine, Neo-Synephrine, Lasix, Atropine, and Levophed
Side effects	Bleeding
Note	Check aPTT per hospital protocol.

IBUTILIDE

Ibutilide	
Indications	A-fib, A-flutter when duration ≤ 48 hr
Adult dose	≥60 kg: 1 mg in 50 mL NS infused over 10 min ≤60 kg: 0.01 mg/kg in 50 mL NS. Over 10 min.
Onset	IV onset 30 minutes; half-life 2 to 12 hr
Side effects	Prolonged QT, torsade de pointes
Monitor	Continuous rhythm monitoring for 4 hours after infusion; blood pressure, EKG after each dose to monitor prolonged QT Magnesium is given either prophylactically before the ibutilide or after the event for torsade de pointes that occurs in approximately 10% of the patients.

ISUPREL IV INFUSION

Isuprel IV Infusion (isoproterenol)	
Indications	Bradycardia unresponsive to atropine and refractory Torsade de pointes
Adult dose	2 to 10 mcg/min. until the pulse reaches 60. When used for Torsade de pointes, it is given until the ventricular tachycardia is suppressed.
Onset	IV onset rapid, duration 10 min.
Compatibility	Compatible at Y-site with potassium chloride, dobutamine, Heparin, Inocor, amiodarone, and Lidocaine.

Isuprel IV Infusion (isoproterenol)	
Side effects	Tachycardia
Note	Contraindicated in cardiac arrest. For bradycardia unresponsive to atropine, use pacing first and use Isuprel only if a pacemaker is not available.

LIDOCAINE BOLUS

Lidocaine Bolus	
Indications	Ventricular arrhythmias
Adult dose	1 mg/kg If arrhythmia continues, administer 0.5 mg/kg every 8 minutes until arrhythmia stops or a maximum dose of 3 mg/kg is reached. ET tube dose: 2 to 4 mg/kg.
Pediatric dose	1 mg/kg
Onset	IV onset immediate
Compatibility	Compatible at Y-site with Aminophylline, Bretylium, dobutamine, Dopamine, epinephrine, Heparin, Inocor, Isuprel, Neo-Synephrine, Nitroglycerin, and Pronestyl
Side effects	Nausea, vomiting, confusion
Note	If arrhythmia is resolved, follow with IV infusion.

LOPRESSOR

Lopressor (metoprolol)	
Indications	PSVT, hypertension, acute MI
Affect	Decreases myocardial oxygen consumption
Adult dose	Administer 5 mg slow IV at 5 minutes intervals until desired effect is achieved or a total of 15 mg is given.
Onset	IV onset immediate, peak 20 minutes, duration 5 to 8 hours
Side effects	Bronchospasm, bradycardia
Note	Hold for bradycardia <40, heart block > 1 degree, and systolic blood pressure <90. Second-line agent after adenosine, Diltiazem, and digoxin. Monitor hemodynamic status.

MORPHINE

Morphine sulfate (MSO4)	
Indications	Moderate to severe chest pain
Dose	2 to 4 mg IV over 1 to 5 min., every 5 to 30 min.
Pediatric dose	50 to 100 mcg/kg IV, maximum 10 mg
Onset	IV onset rapid, peak 20 minutes, duration 4 to 5 hours

Morphine sulfate (MSO4)	
Side effects	Confusion, sedation, hypotension, respiratory depression
Note	Reversing agent is Narcan 0.4 to 2 mg IV.
Monitor	Effectiveness of respirations

NITROGLYCERIN OINTMENT

Nitroglycerin Ointment	
Indications	Chest pain, suspected cardiac ischemia
Adult dose	½ inch to 2 inches applied to the anterior chest
Onset	Topical onset ½ to 1 hour, duration 2 to 12 hours
Side effects	Headache, flushing, dizziness, postural hypotension
Note	Ointment is applied to the anterior chest. Avoid areas of potential cardiac monitoring lead placement. DO NOT apply to extremities to decrease the side effects; the therapeutic action is also decreased.
Monitor	Blood pressure, heart rate, heart rhythm

NITROGLYCERIN

Nitroglycerin IV infusion	
Indications	Chest pain, acute myocardial infarction, left ventricular failure, hypertension
Adult dose	Start at 3 to 5 mcg/min. and increase by 5 mcg/min. every five minutes. No maximum dose is established. Doses of >200 mcg/min. are acceptable. The dose is regulated by the body's hemodynamic response and is commonly limited by a systolic blood pressure of < 90.
Onset	IV onset immediate, duration variable
Compatibility	Compatible at Y-site with Aminophylline, Bretylium, dobutamine, Dopamine, Dobutamine, morphine, heparin, Inocor, Lidocaine, potassium chloride
Side effects	Headache, hypotension
Note	Use a glass bottle or non-latex bag and special non-latex tubing. Some hospital protocols allow the nurse to increase the NTG to relief of pain, but not to decease unless order to wean is received from the medical provider. Some protocols require the nurse to check with the medical provider if over 200 mcg/min. is required.

PRONESTYL

Pronestyl (procainamide)	
Indications	Ventricular arrhythmias uncontrolled by Lidocaine

Pronestyl (procainamide)	
Adult dose	The dose for cardiac arrest is 20 mg/min. IV The dose for refractory arrhythmias is 100 mg IV every five minutes until: (1) the QRS widens by 50%; (2) hypotension develops; (3) the arrhythmia is suppressed; or, (4) a maximum dose of 17 mg/kg is given. Watch for PR interval lengthening, hypotension, heart block, and AV node disturbances. Maintenance 1 to 4 mg/min. IV.
Onset	IV onset rapid, peak ½ to 1 hour, duration 3 to 4 hours. Therapeutic serum concentrations are reached in about 15 minutes.
Compatibility	Compatible at Y-site with Lidocaine, dobutamine, amiodarone, heparin, and potassium chloride
Side effects	Headache, heart block, cardiovascular collapse
Note	Monitor plasma levels for continuous infusion > 3 mg/min. or if infusion is continued for more than 24 hours.

TENECTEPLASE (TNKASE)

<table>
<tr><td colspan="2">Tenecteplase (TNKase)</td></tr>
<tr><td>Indications</td><td>Acute myocardial infarction, acute ischemic stroke</td></tr>
<tr><td>Adult dose</td><td>Single bolus over 5 sec.: 30 to 50 mg IV, weight adjusted.
<table>
<tr><td>Patient weight in Kg</td><td>TNKase in mg</td><td>Milliliters of reconstituted TNKase</td></tr>
<tr><td><60 kg
(132 lb)</td><td>30</td><td>6</td></tr>
<tr><td>60 to <70
(132 to 154 lb)</td><td>35</td><td>7</td></tr>
<tr><td>70 to <80
(154 to 176 lb)</td><td>45</td><td>8</td></tr>
<tr><td>80 to <90
(176 to 198 lb)</td><td>45</td><td>9</td></tr>
<tr><td>90
(198 lb)</td><td>50</td><td>10</td></tr>
</table>
</td></tr>
<tr><td>Onset</td><td>IV onset 3 to 5 minutes, half-life 90 to 130 minutes</td></tr>
<tr><td>Side effects</td><td>Bleeding, hematoma at site.</td></tr>
<tr><td>Monitor</td><td>Heart rate and rhythm, blood pressure, CBC, aPTT, signs and symptoms of bleeding</td></tr>
</table>

Tenecteplase (TNKase)	
Note	Precautions and exclusion criteria: Active internal bleeding; history of CVA within 3 months, major surgery or recent trauma within 14 days; aortic dissection, severe, uncontrolled hypertension, known bleeding disorders, lumbar puncture within 7 days, recent arterial puncture at noncompressible site.

VALIUM

Valium (diazepam)	
Indications	Conscious sedation, status epilepticus
Dose	IV 5 to 10 mg, single dose IM 5 to 20 mg, single dose Status epilepticus: IV: 5 to 10 mg every 10 to 20 min., up to 30 mg in 8 hr.
Onset	IV onset 5 min., peak 15 minutes IM onset 15 min., peak ½ to 1 ½ hours
Side effects	Dizziness, drowsiness, orthostatic hypotension, blurred vision, hypoxia, tachycardia, urinary retention.
Monitor	Level of consciousness, respiratory effectiveness
Note	When used intravenously, care is essential to reduce the risk of venous thrombosis, phlebitis, local irritation, and vascular impairment. Administer slowly over at least 1 min. for each 5 mg. Do not use small veins such as on the dorsum of the hand or wrist. Do not mix Valium with other solutions or drugs.

VASOPRESSIN

Pitressin(vasopressin)	
Indications	Alternative for epinephrine in shock-refractory VF, asystole, PEA
Dose	One-time dose: 40U IV Endotracheal: 2 to 2 ½ times the IV dose mixed with 10 mL of NS
Onset	Immediate; half-life 10 to 20 min.
Side effects	Arrhythmia, asystole, chest pain, tremors
Monitor	Heart rate and rhythm, blood pressure
Note	Use extreme caution to avoid extravasation because of risk of tissue necrosis and gangrene.

VERAPAMIL

Verapamil	
Indications	Tachyarrhythmias, such as atrial fibrillation, atrial flutter, or atrial tachycardia
Adult dose	2.5 to 5 mg IV, over 1 to 2 min., every 15 min., maximum 30 mg
Onset	IV onset 1 to 5 min., peak 3 to 5 min., duration 2 hours
Compatibility	Compatible at Y-site with dobutamine, dopamine
Side effects	Headache, drowsiness, nausea, dizziness, facial flushing

VERSED

Versed (midazolam hydrochloride)	
Indications	Conscious sedation.
Adult dose	1 to 2.5 mg IV slowly over at least 2 min., wait for 2 minutes to fully evaluate effect before giving another dose. A total dose of over 5 mg is not usually necessary. If the patient was medicated with narcotic medications before the Versed, use approximately 30% less Versed.
Pediatric dose	Pediatric patients 12 to 16 years old should be dosed as adults. Pediatric dose is weight based. IV initial loading dose is 0.05 to 0.2 mg/kg IV administered over 2 to 3 min. Versed should only be used for intubated pediatric patients.
Onset	IV onset 3 to 5 minutes
Compatibility	Compatible at Y site with amiodarone, diltiazem, dopamine, epinephrine, fentanyl, lorazepam, morphine. Flush IV line with normal saline before and after using Versed.
Side effects	Serious life-threatening decreased respiratory rate and decreased tidal volume and hypotension.
Monitor	Heart rate and rhythm, blood pressure, oxygenation, respiratory rate.
Note	Versed is a potent sedative that requires slow administration and individualization of dose. Versed is 3 to 4 times more potent than Valium. The reversing agent is Romazicon (flumazenil).

RELATED CONDITIONS AND INFORMATION

ASYSTOLE

When asystole is seen on the monitor, look at the rhythm in another lead before beginning resuscitation attempts. The reason for the straight line may be a disconnected lead. The patient may not be in asystole.

AUSCULTATION OF HEART SOUNDS

Review of Heart Sounds	
Rationale	Listening to the heart sounds provides vital information about the integrity of the heart muscles, heart valves, and the conduction system.
Location for auscultation	The point of maximum impulse is heard at the left fifth intercostal at the midclavicular line. The tricuspid valve is heard at the left fourth intercostal space, The aortic valve is heard at the right second intercostal space. The pulmonary valve is heard at the left second intercostal space. The mitral valve is heard at the left fifth intercostal space, mid-clavicular line.
1st heart sound S1	The left ventricle fills through the mitral valve from the left atrium and the right ventricle fills through the tricuspid valve from the right atrium. Closure of both the mitral and tricuspid valves produce the first heart sound.
2nd heart sound S2	The left ventricle contracts and blood flows through the aortic valve into the aorta. The right ventricle contracts and blood flows through the pulmonic valve into the lungs. As the ventricles empty, the aortic and pulmonic valves close producing the second heart sound.
3rd heart sound S3	The mitral valve reopens for rapid ventricular filling creating the third sound heard in children and young adults.
4th heart sound S4	The atrium contracts to enhance ventricular filling, producing the fourth heart sound that is not normally heard in adults.

BETA-BLOCKERS

In the early stages of an acute myocardial infarction, beta blockers reduce myocardial workload and can be useful in decreasing the myocardial oxygen consumption.

BRADYCARDIA WITH SYMPTOMS OF SHOCK

Management of Bradycardia with Symptoms of Shock
Initially: Maintain patent airway; oxygen, monitor ECG, blood pressure, pulse oximetry, and establish IV access.
Administer atropine 0.5 to 1 mg IV and repeat every 3 to 5 min. Maximum dose is 0.03 to 0.04 mg/kg (approximately 2.5 mg for a 71 kg patient). Go directly to pacing if IV access is not available. Heart transplants do not respond to atropine.

Management of Bradycardia with Symptoms of Shock
Initiate pacing.
Administer dopamine 5 to 20 mcg/kg/min. IV.
Administer epinephrine 2 to 10 mcg/kg/min. IV.
Administer isoproterenol 2 mcg to 10 mcg/min. IV until pulse reaches 60. To be used with extreme caution. In low doses, it is a Class IIb (possibly helpful) and in high doses Class III (not useful or effective).
Observe heart rate and rhythm, blood pressure, changes in level of consciousness, and for complaints of chest pain.

CARDIAC MARKERS

CK/MB levels usually remain elevated for up to 72 hours.

Troponin levels remain elevated for up to 7 days

Myoglobin usually normalized 8 hours after an injury.

CARDIOGENIC SHOCK

Cardiogenic shock is defined as persistent hypotension (SBP <80mm Hg) for more than 30 minutes in the absence of hypovolemia. Patients in cardiogenic shock have an elevated central venous pressure due to increased preload and afterload that is associated with pump failure. A narrowing pulse pressure (the difference between the systolic and diastolic blood pressure) is a sign of deterioration. A narrow pulse pressure indicates a low stroke volume (decreasing systolic pressure) or a high peripheral resistance (increasing diastolic pressure). Causes of cardiogenic shock include left ventricular infarct (80% of shock patients), right ventricular infarct (10% of shock patients), and mechanical complications such as valvular dysfunction, ventricular septal rupture, open-heart surgery, cardiac arrest, cardiomyopathies, and arrhythmias. Cardiogenic shock is associated with a 40% loss of myocardial function. Primary percutaneous transluminal coronary angioplasty is the treatment of choice for cardiogenic shock.

CONGESTIVE HEART FAILURE

Review of Congestive Heart Failure	
Definition	Heart failure is a progressive condition in which the heart's muscle becomes weakened after it is injured. The weakened heart gradually losses its ability to pump enough blood to supply the body's needs.

Review of Congestive Heart Failure	
Causes	Congestive heart failure is a fluid overload in the body caused by the heart not pumping effectively. Forward failure causes fluid to accumulate in the lungs and backward failure causes fluid to accumulate in the body (peripheral edema, ascites, hepatosplenomegaly). The most common cause of right ventricular failure is a failure of the left ventricle. As the pulmonary venous and arterial pressures increase, the preload of the right ventricle is increased, and fluid accumulates in the body. Other causes of right ventricular failure are lung disease, valvular disease, and right myocardial ventricular infarction.
Forward failure	Failure of the left ventricle causes activity intolerance, tachypnea, orthopnea, shortness of breath, tachycardia, and production of pink frothy sputum, indicative of pulmonary edema.
Backward failure	Failure of the right ventricle causes peripheral edema and hepatosplenomegaly (with and without tenderness) from systemic vascular engorgement.
Diagnostic findings	ABG analysis reveals findings of hypoxia and respiratory acidosis. Electrocardiogram shows left ventricular enlargement. Chest x-ray reveals findings of infiltrates (pulmonary fluid overload) and an enlarged heart.
ER goal	The goal is to maintain sufficient oxygenation to body tissues by increasing oxygenation, decreasing preload, decreasing afterload, and increasing the contractility of the heart.
Management	Medical management may include: • oxygen therapy to keep oxygen saturation >94%; • fluid restriction; • diuretics (Lasix, Bumex) to reduce the fluid preload; • inotropic medications (digoxin, dobutamine) to increase the pumping action of the heart; • morphine to decrease anxiety and the workload placed on the heart; • blood pressure reducing medications (nitroglycerin, nitroprusside) to decrease afterload.
Discharge Instructions	Maintain a daily sodium intake of 2 grams a day or less and weigh daily. Report weight gain to the follow-up medical provider. Take beta blocker and ace inhibitor daily as prescribed.

ARRHYTHMIA

Review of Arrhythmias in Lead II

Review of Arrhythmias in Lead II	
Atrial fibrillation	Rate: Atrial rate 350 to 600 beats per min. with a ventricular rate of 60 to 160 per min. Rhythm: Irregularly irregular P waves: None QRS: Irregular, narrow P QRS relationship: P waves not present PR interval: No P waves.
Atrial flutter	Rate: Atrial rate 240 to 360 beats per min., most commonly 300 with a 2:1 block resulting in a ventricular rate of 150 Rhythm: Regular, occasional irregular P waves: None, atrial waves are saw-tooth flutter waves QRS: Narrow P QRS relationship: No P waves, relationship between QRS and the flutter waves may be regular, e.g., 4:1, 2:1 PR interval: No P waves
First degree AV block	Rate: 60 to 100 beats a min. Rhythm: Regular P waves: Present with normal configuration QRS: Regular, narrow P QRS relationship: P wave before each QRS PR interval: >0.20 sec (5 small boxes equals 1 large box or 0.20 sec)
Second degree AV block Mobitz I, Wenckebach	Rate: Normal Rhythm: Regularly irregular P waves: One before each QRS except during regularly dropped ventricular conduction occurring at regular intervals QRS: Missed conductions at cyclic intervals P QRS relationship: One P wave before each QRS except during the regular dropped ventricular beat PR interval: Lengthens with each beat until a QRS is dropped and the cycle is repeated
Second degree Mobitz II	Rate: Atrial rate 60 to 100, ventricular rate slower Rhythm: Regularly irregular P waves: Two or more for each QRS QRS: Narrow P QRS relationship: One or more P waves are not followed by a QRS PR interval: Normal and regular

Review of Arrhythmias in Lead II	
Sinus bradycardia	Rate: < 60 Rhythm: Regular P Waves: Present QRS: Present, narrow P QRS relationship: P wave before each QRS PR interval: Normal < 0.20 (5 small boxes equals 1 large box or 0.20 sec)
Sinus tachycardia	Rate: >100, seldom >160 Rhythm: Regular P waves: Normal QRS: Present with normal duration P QRS relationship: P wave before each QRS PR interval: Normal, <0.20 (5 small boxes equals 1 large box or 0.20 sec)
Supra-ventricular tachycardia	Rate: 140 to 220 beats per min. Rhythm: Regular P waves: Appear abnormal, buried in T wave, difficult to identify, or not seen QRS: Normal or prolonged. P QRS relationship and PR interval: Difficult to determine because of unidentifiable P waves
Third degree AV block, complete heart block	Rate: Atrial rate 60 to 100 beats per min. with a ventricular rate of < 60 Rhythm: Regular when atrial and ventricular rhythm are examined separately. P Waves: Normal QRS: Wide > 0.10 seconds (from 2 to 3 small boxes) P QRS Relationship: No relationship to each other PR Interval: No constant interval

ENDOCARDITIS

Review of Endocarditis	
Definition	Endocarditis is an infection of the endocardium.
Cause	The cause is infection by a microorganism.
Symptoms	Endocarditis can be suspected in any patient with a new cardiac murmur associated with a low-grade fever for more than one week or in any IV drug user. Complaints of malaise and arthralgias are common.
Diagnostic findings	Blood cultures are essential. CBC shows normochromic normocytic anemia. The ESR is elevated. Urine shows proteinuria and hematuria. Echocardiogram demonstrates vegetations. A transesophageal echocardiogram can demonstrate intracardiac abscesses.

Management	Medical management includes IV antibiotics and hospitalization for a detailed cardiac workup.

FUNCTION OF THE HEART BY THE NUMBERS

The Work of the Normal Heart	
Rate	72 beats a minute 104,000 beats a day 38,000,000 beats a year
Pumping volume	82 ml of blood a pump stroke 8,193 liters of blood a day
Work force	Equivalent to raising one ton to a height of 41 feet every day

MAGNET ELECTROCARDIOGRAM

A magnet electrocardiogram is performed with a magnet placed over the patient's pacemaker. A myth exists that the magnet stops the pacemaker. Some pacemakers have a magnet activated automatic threshold determination. Activation of the magnet rate is used to evaluate the pacing function of the generator that has been suppressed by the patient's intrinsic rhythm and to evaluate battery depletion. The magnet rate is frequently different from the automatic rate. In some programmable pacemakers, end of life is indicated only by a decrease of the magnet rate making the magnet testing mandatory. The magnet rate results when a magnet is placed over the generator deactivating the sensing mechanism and converting the pacemaker to a fixed rate unit.

MURMURS

Review of Heart Murmurs	
Definition	A heart murmur is an abnormal sound heard by auscultation over the heart that results from disruptions of the normal blood flow, e.g., obstructions, valve irregularities, vegetation, or roughening of the heart surfaces. Murmurs produced by aneurysms (weakened bulges of a blood vessel wall) are called bruits.
Auscultation locations for valvular murmurs	The point of maximum impulse is heard over the left fifth intercostal space at the midclavicular line. An aortic murmur is heard over the right second intercostal space. A pulmonary murmur is heard over the left second intercostal space. A tricuspid murmur is heard over the left fourth intercostal space. A mitral murmur is heard over the left fifth intercostals space, mid-clavicular line.

Review of Heart Murmurs	
Grading	Grade I is barely audible. Grade II is audible immediately, but faint. Grade III is loud without thrust or thrill. Grade IV is loud with thrust or thrill. Grade V is very loud with thrust or thrill and heard with a stethoscope when applied lightly to the chest wall. Grade VI is louder and may be heard without stethoscope. The quality is described as blowing, musical, harsh, or rumbling.

DILATED CARDIOMYOPATHY

Review of Dilated Cardiomyopathy	
Definition	Dilated cardiomyopathy is a dilated left ventricle with poor contractions. The right ventricle may also be involved. Commonly described as a large floppy heart.
Cause	Ischemic cardiomyopathy is the most common cause, followed by myocarditis. Other causes are connective tissue disorders, muscular dystrophies, and peripartum complications.
Symptoms	Symptoms may include congestive heart failure, advanced arrhythmias, and peripheral emboli from left ventricular mural thrombus.
Physical findings	Physical findings may include jugular venous distention (JVD), lung crackles, S3 heart sound, and peripheral edema. Mitral and tricuspid regurgitation murmurs are common.
Tests	The electrocardiogram shows LBBB with left ventricle and right ventricle enlargement and ST T wave abnormalities. Chest x-ray shows cardiomegaly, pulmonary vascular redistribution, and effusions.
Management	Medical management may include diuretics for fluid overload, nitroglycerin, morphine, anticoagulants, and anti-arrhythmic drugs and hospitalization for a detailed cardiac workup. Heart transplant is the only cure.

RESTRICTIVE CARDIOMYOPATHY

Review of Restrictive Cardiomyopathy	
Definition	Restrictive cardiomyopathy is characterized by non-dilated ventricles with a stiffness of the myocardium that impairs ventricular filling.
Cause	Causes include infiltrative disease, e.g., eosinophilic disorders, amyloidosis, hemochromatosis and myocardial fibrosis.
Physical findings	Physical findings may include right heart failure, jugular venous distention, hepatomegaly, peripheral edema, and tricuspid regurgitation murmur.

Review of Restrictive Cardiomyopathy	
Diagnostic findings	Electrocardiogram findings reveal low limb lead voltage, sinus tachycardia, and ST and T wave abnormalities. Chest x-ray shows mild left ventricular enlargement. Echocardiogram shows bilateral atrial enlargement and increased ventricular thickness. Ejection fraction may be normal or mildly deceased.
Management	Medical management may include diuretics for pulmonary congestion, anticoagulants to reduce the risk of emboli, and hospital admission for a detailed cardiac workup.

HYPERTROPHIC OBSTRUCTIVE CARDIOMYOPATHY

Review of Hypertrophic Obstructive Cardiomyopathy	
Definition	Hypertrophic obstructive cardiomyopathy is a marked left ventricular enlargement without an underlying cause.
Cause	Thought to be a genetic disorder characterized by disproportionate hypertrophy of the left ventricle.
Physical findings	Physical findings may include S4 heart sound, a harsh systolic murmur along the left sternal border, and a blowing mitral murmur at the apex.
Tests	Electrocardiogram reveals LV hypertrophy and prominent Q waves in Leads I, aVL, V5, and V6.
Management	Medical management may include beta-blockers, Verapamil, and hospitalization for workup. Digoxin, inotropic drugs, and diuretics are contraindicated. Surgical myectomy is necessary for patients who are refractory to medical therapy.

MYOCARDITIS

Review of Myocarditis	
Definition	Myocarditis is an inflammation of the myocardium.
Cause	Myocarditis is usually secondary to an acute viral infection. The acute disease process can progress to chronic dilated cardiomyopathy and may develop in patients with HIV infections.
Physical findings	Physical findings may include fever, congestive heart failure, fatigue, palpitations, tachycardia, and soft s1 and s3 heart tones.
Diagnostic findings	Electrocardiogram reveals transient ST T wave abnormalities. Chest x-ray shows cardiomegaly. Echocardiogram shows decreased left ventricular function and pericardial effusions if pericarditis is present.
Management	Medical management may include treatment of congestive heart failure and fever and hospitalization for a detailed cardiac work-up.

PAROXYSMAL SUPRAVENTRICULAR TACHYCARDIA

Management of Paroxysmal Supraventricular Tachycardia
Vagal maneuvers are the first course of action for paroxysmal supraventricular tachycardia. Vagal maneuvers are described as any maneuver that increases the parasympathetic tone and slows the conduction through the AV node. The maneuvers include breath holding, facial immersion in ice water, coughing, nasogastric tube placement, gag reflex stimulation, squatting, carotid sinus massage, and a circumferential digital sweep of the anus. Eyeball pressure should never be performed as it may result in retinal detachment. Avoid carotid sinus massage in the elderly or late middle age because of potentially undiagnosed carotid atherosclerosis.
Administer Adenosine IV initial rapid bolus of 6 mg over 1 to 3 seconds. Do not dilute. Push rapidly over 1 to 3 seconds and follow with 20 ml NS to push the medicine through the IV tubing. A syringe of NS and adenosine can be placed in the same IV port. Push adenosine and then immediately push the NS.
If the tachycardia is not eliminated in 1to 2 minutes, give a second Adenosine IV dose of 12 mg and repeat one time. Do not dilute. Push rapidly over 1 to 3 seconds and follow with 20 ml NS to push the medicine through IV tubing. A syringe of NS and adenosine can be placed in the same IV port. Push adenosine and then immediately push the NS.
For narrow complex supraventricular tachycardia, administer Diltiazem 15 to 20 mg IV over 2 minutes; may give another IV dose in 15 minutes give 20 to 25 mg. May also use beta-blockers (Metoprolol) but with caution in patients with CHF and pulmonary diseases.
For wide complex supraventricular tachycardia, administer Amiodarone 150 mg. IV over 15 min or Lidocaine 1 mg/kg. If not resolved, perform synchronized cardioversion.

PERICARDITIS

Review of Pericarditis	
Definition	Pericarditis is an infection of the pericardium.
Cause	The cause is a microorganism infection secondary to a viral infection, acute myocardial infarction, metastatic neoplasm, radiation therapy (up to 20 years earlier), chronic renal failure (CRF), rheumatoid arthritis, and post open-heart surgery (up to several months earlier).
Symptoms	Symptoms may include intense chest pain, characteristically sharp, pleuritic, and positional (relieved by leaning forward), fever, and palpitations. Pericarditis can imitate an acute myocardial infarction.

Review of Pericarditis	
Tests	Electrocardiogram shows diffuse ST elevation, concave upward, usually in all leads except aVR and V1. Chest x-ray shows increased heart size; a large pericardial effusion may present with a water bottle configuration. Echocardiogram is the most specific test for pericardial effusion.
Management	Medical management may include aspirin and pain control. Anticoagulants are generally contraindicated because of the risk of pericardial hemorrhage.
Disposition	Hospitalization may be required for detailed cardiac workup and possible pericardiectomy.
Comment	Pericarditis is most readily identified by auscultation of a pericardial friction rub best heard along the left sternal border. Cardiac tamponade is the most life-threatening complication of pericarditis leading to ventricular fibrillation.

POTASSIUM

High potassium levels show tall peaked T waves, depressed ST segments on an electrocardiogram. Low potassium levels show prominent U waves associated with decreased P waves and T wave flattening on electrocardiogram.

SINUS TACHYCARDIA

Sinus tachycardia may be caused by fever, shock, congestive heart failure, exercise, or anxiety. Before treating the arrhythmia, assess vital signs and determine what symptoms could have provoked the sinus tachycardia and treat the underlying cause.

SYNCHRONIZED ELECTRICAL CARDIOVERSION

Review of Synchronized Electrical Cardioversion Procedure
THE SYNCHRONIZED MODE MUST BE RESET AFTER EACH SHOCK. MOST DEFIBRILLATORS DEFAULT BACK TO UNSYNCHRONIZED MODE TO ALLOW AN IMMEDIATE DEFIBRILLATION IN THE EVENT OF VENTRICULAR FIBRILLATION.
Consider using conscious sedation with Valium or Versed.
Turn on defibrillator and attach monitor leads to the patient.
Press the sync control button and confirm by observing the markers on the R waves.
Select appropriate energy level. Start with 100 joules. PSVT and atrial flutter may respond to a lower energy level. Start with 50 joules.
Position pads or apply gel to paddles and position on the patient's chest.
Announce charging to team members and press the charge button.

Review of Synchronized Electrical Cardioversion Procedure
When paddles are charged, announce, "I am going to shock on three. One I'm clear." Make sure you are clear of the patient, stretcher, and equipment. "Two you are clear." Make sure all team members are clear. "Three everybody is clear." Make sure you are clear one more time, apply 25 pounds pressure on both paddles, and press the discharge buttons simultaneously.
If tachycardia is not resolved, increase the joules to 200, reset the synchronized mode, make sure the markers are still present on the R waves, and repeat.
If tachycardia is not resolved, increase the joules to 300, reset the synchronized mode, make sure the markers are still present on the R waves, and repeat.
If tachycardia is not resolved, increase the joules to 360, reset the synchronized mode, make sure the markers are still present on the R waves, and repeat.

TAMPONADE

Review of Cardiac Tamponade	
Definition	EMERGENT Cardiac tamponade is an accumulation of pericardial fluid under pressure that impairs the filling of the heart and decreases cardiac output.
Cause	The causes of cardiac tamponade include cardiac trauma, myocardial perforation at cardiac catheterization or during pacemaker placement, and previous pericarditis. Penetrating chest trauma is the most common cause. Blunt trauma is the second most common cause. As little as 100 ml of blood in the pericardial sac can cause a severe decrease in cardiac output. Chronic fluid accumulation can result from various medical disorders and the pericardium can accommodate up to 1,500 ml of fluid over time.
Symptoms	Symptoms of tamponade may include chest pain, restlessness, hypotension, hypoxia, pulsus paradoxus (inspiratory fall in systolic blood pressure > 10 mmHg), jugular venous distention, and distant heart sounds, narrow pulse pressure, low voltage on EKG.
Tests	Tests include electrocardiogram, chest x-ray, and heart catheterization to confirm the diagnosis.
Management	Intravenous fluid resuscitation will temporarily increase cardiac output until measures to relieve the pressure can be carried out. Pericardiocentesis is an attempt to temporarily reduce the pressure. An electrocardiogram electrode is attached to the intracardiac needle to monitor as the needle encounters the myocardium. If the needle encounters the myocardium, there is an ST segment elevation. Removing as little as 20 ml of blood can save the patient's life.

Review of Cardiac Tamponade	
Disposition	Hospital admission may be required for cardiac catheterization and open-heart surgery.

3RD DEGREE HEART BLOCK

Management of 3rd Degree Heart Block
Prepare for transvenous pacer placement.
Use external pacer until transvenous is placed.

VENTRICULAR TACHYCARDIA

Management of Ventricular Tachycardia
Amiodarone 150 mg. IV over 10 min. or Lidocaine 0.5 to 0.75 mg/kg IV, if symptoms continue give 0.5 mg/kg IV every 8 min., maximum dose 3 mg/kg.
If not resolved, perform synchronized cardioversion.

PEDIATRIC CONSIDERATIONS

CARDIOVASCULAR DISORDERS

Disorder	Symptoms
Endocarditis	Malaise, night sweats, chills, arthralgia, valvular insufficiency, intermittent fever, splenomegaly, petechiae commonly on the upper anterior trunk
Heart failure	Tachycardia, diaphoresis, failure to thrive, peripheral edema, nasal flaring, retractions, ascites, hepatomegaly, pulmonary edema, acute renal failure
Kawasaki disease	An acute systemic vasculitis causing acquired heart disease. Symptoms include fever, cervical lymphadenopathy, erythema to oral cavity strawberry tongue, myocarditis, transient arthritis, and intermittent signs of heart failure.
Rheumatic heart disease	Complications include pancarditis, heart failure, damage to aortic and mitral valves

CONGENITAL HEART DEFECTS

Defect	Related Information
Atrial septal defect (ASD)	Usually benign in infancy Complications may include atrial arrhythmias, frequent respiratory infections, and heart failure.
Patent ductus arteriosus (PDA)	Usually detected by 3 months of age Complications may include heart failure, recurrent pneumonia, and infective endocarditis.

Defect	Related Information
Ventricular septal Defect (VSD)	Usually identified between 4 to 8 weeks of age Complications may include pulmonary hypertension, pneumonia, heart failure, and infective endocarditis.
Coarctation of the aorta	Symptoms develop and worsen by 1 year old Complications may include heart failure, severe hypertension, pulmonary edema, cerebral aneurysm, aortic aneurysm, and infective endocarditis.
Aortic stenosis	Complications may include infective endocarditis, pulmonary edema, heart failure, and sudden death due to myocardial ischemia.
Pulmonary stenosis	Complications may include heart failure and infective endocarditis.
Hypoplastic left heart syndrome	Complications may include heart failure and death.
Transposition of the great vessels	Obvious at birth Complications may include infective endocarditis and death.
Tetralogy of Fallot	Complications may include right ventricular dysfunction, infective endocarditis, polycythemia, and death.
Tricuspid atresia	Complications may include infective endocarditis, brain abscess, and stroke.

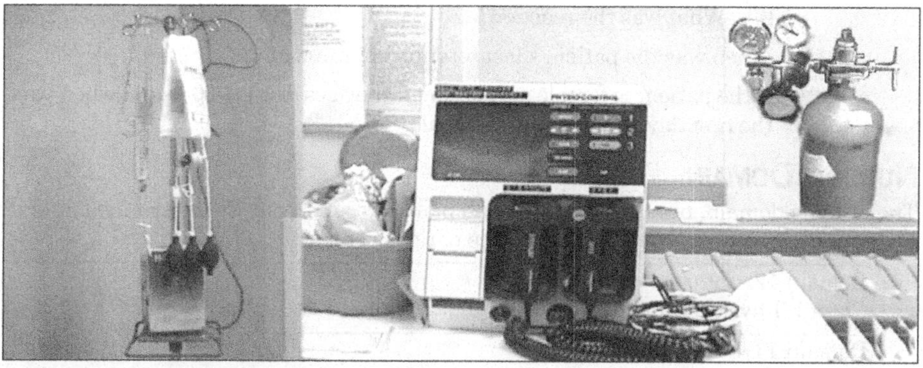

20 HEAT AND COLD EXPOSURE

For details on triage see Chapter 34, Triage in a Nutshell.

PATIENT'S STORY – INTERVIEW QUESTIONS

1. Have you had a recent injury?
2. When did the symptoms begin?
3. Where are the injuries located and are any associated symptoms present?
4. What was the patient doing that might have caused the problem, e.g., slept outside, fell through the ice and climbed out, walked on the desert, stayed in a house without air conditioning or a fan?
5. How do the symptoms affect the patient's normal function?
   a. Is neurovascular function normal distal to the injuries?
   b. Does the patient have normal function of the injured areas?
   c. Is pain present and what is the severity?
6. Has any treatment been initiated, and has it helped?
7. Does the patient have any pertinent past history?
8. Does the patient take any routine medications?
   a. What is the name, dosage, route, and frequency of each medication?
   b. When was the last dose?
9. Does the patient take any complementary or alternative therapies, herbal products, over-the-counter medications or supplements, or natural therapies?
   a. What is the name, dosage, route and frequency of each therapy?
   b. When was the last dose or therapy?
10. Does the patient have allergies to drugs or foods?
    a. What is the name of the allergen?

b. What was the reaction?

11. When was the patient's last tetanus immunization?
12. If the patient is female and between the ages of 10 to 50 years, when was the first day of her last menstrual period?

NURSING DOMAIN

The nursing domain, nursing diagnosis and plan of care can only be determined after an in-depth interview and consideration of the patient's story.

Domain 12. Comfort. Class 1. Physical comfort.
Domain 11. Safety/Protection Class 6. Thermoregulation

ANTICIPATED MEDICAL CARE

Review of the Anticipated Medical Care of Heat and Cold Exposures	
Exam	Full body
Urine tests	Test for proteinuria and hematuria; pregnancy test for women of reproductive age unless they have had a hysterectomy.
Blood tests	CBC, electrolytes, and renal functions studies
ECG	ECG for females and males over 35 years
X-ray	Chest, areas of suspected bony damage
Diet	NPO
IV	Normal saline or Ringer's solution warmed for hypothermia and chilled or room temperature for hyperthermia
Medications	Thorazine for shivering
Other	Gradual warming or cooling
Disposition	Hospital admission may be required for serious problems.
Worst-case scenario	The worst-case scenario is malignant hyperthermia as seen in young males post neuroleptics (Haldol). Reactions can occur up to five days post medication. Treatment may include Dantrolene 1 mg/kg rapidly until symptoms stop or maximum single dose of 10 mg/kg is reached.

INITIAL CARE PLAN

> Alcohol-based hand sanitizers are the preferred method for cleaning your hands in most clinical situations. Wash your hands with soap and water whenever they are visibly dirty, before eating, and after using the restroom.

1. Ask the patient to undress, remove all jewelry that might interfere with the examination, and put on an exam gown. Assist as needed.

   a. For hyperthermia, leave as much exposed skin as the patient will accept.
   b. For hypothermia, protect against heat loss. Place a warmed blanket like a shawl around the head, neck, and shoulders. Place another blanket over the body and tightly tuck it around the patient. Use warm blankets until more active warming begins.
2. Place the patient supine.
3. Obtain vital signs including pulse oximetry or test capillary refill.
   a. Institute continuous heart, pulse oximetry, and non-invasive blood pressure monitoring. Document the initial heart monitor strip and document changes of rhythm.
   b. Obtain a core temperature. A rectal temperature is acceptable if other means is not available. An oral temperature is unacceptable.
4. Administer oxygen at 4 liters by nasal cannula to enrich the environment.
5. Establish intravenous access; draw laboratory blood specimens, and saline lock the cannula.
   a. Draw a variety of tubes that will allow the lab to perform hematology, chemistry, and coagulation studies. Patients that have cirrhosis or are on anticoagulants need a PT and aPTT.
   b. Consider drawing other labs, e.g., type and screen, blood cultures.
6. Perform a focused physical examination.
   a. Auscultate the lungs.
   b. Inspect the skin for pallor or cyanosis of extremities and trunk. Inspect for peripheral edema.
   c. Evaluate the level of consciousness based on the mnemonic **AVPU** or **ACDU** level of consciousness score.
      AVPU: Alert, **V**erbal, **P**ain, **U**nresponsive.
      ACDU: Alert, **C**onfused, **D**rowsy, **U**nresponsive.
7. Assure the patient that all efforts will be made to keep him safe and pain free.
8. Clean and dress wounds with sterile dressings. Consider collecting wound cultures.
9. Inform the patient if he can drink liquids. Provide the alert cold patient with warmed high-carbohydrate drinks. Provide the alert hot patient with cooled high-carbohydrate drinks.
10. Elevate the siderails and place the stretcher in the lowest position.
11. Inform the patient, family, and caregivers of the plan of care and the anticipated time until disposition.
12. Provide the patient with a device to reach someone for assistance and explain how to use it. Ask the patient to call for help before getting off the stretcher.

ONGOING CARE PLAN

Inform the medical provider of adverse changes noted during ongoing evaluation. Document that the medical provider was notified of the adverse change. Document if orders were or were not received.

1. Monitor core temperature, heart rate and rhythm, blood pressure, and effectiveness of breathing.
2. Monitor level of consciousness and compare to AVPU or ACDU baseline.
3. Monitor for changes in skin color and swelling of the injured body parts.
4. Monitor therapy closely for the patient's therapeutic response.
    a. The usual time for a medication effectiveness check is 20 to 30 minutes after giving the drug.
    b. If therapy is not effective, ask the medical provider for a repeat dose or an alternative.
5. Monitor closely for the development of adverse reactions to therapy.
    a. Perform interventions to relieve the adverse reaction.
    b. Ask the medical provider for a remedy.
6. If not NPO, provide the patient with food at mealtimes and fluids during the stay.
7. Keep the patient, family, and caregivers well informed of the plan of care and the remaining time anticipated before disposition.
8. Monitor the patient's laboratory and x-ray results and notify the medical provider of critical abnormalities. Remedy abnormalities as ordered.
9. Notify the medical provider when all diagnostic results are available for review. Ask for establishment of a diagnosis and disposition.

DISCHARGE INSTRUCTIONS

1. Provide the patient with the name of the nurse and doctor in the emergency room.
2. Inform the patient of their diagnosis or why a definitive diagnosis couldn't be made. Explain what caused the problem if known.
3. Teach the patient how to take the medication as prescribed and how to manage the common side effects. Instruct the patient not to drive or perform any dangerous tasks while taking narcotic pain medications.
4. Recommend a medical provider for follow-up care. Provide the name, address, and phone number with a recommendation of when to schedule the care.
5. Instruct the patient to call the follow-up medical provider immediately or return to the emergency room if the problem persists for over eight hours, worsens in any way, or any unusual symptoms develop. Encourage the patient NOT to IGNORE WORSENING OR PERSISTENT SYMPTOMS.

6. Ask for verbal confirmation or demonstration of understanding and reinforce teaching as needed.

COMMONLY ORDERED MEDICATIONS

CHLORPROMAZINE (THORAZINE)

Chlorpromazine (Thorazine)	
Indications	Shivering
Adult dose	25 to 50 mg IV 50 to 100 mg IM not to exceed 400 mg a day by any route
Pediatric dose	0.55 mg/kg IV 0.25 mg/lb IM not to exceed 40 mg/lb per day by any route
Onset	IM onset unknown, duration 4 to 8 hours IV onset rapid, duration unknown
Side effects	Neuroleptic malignant syndrome, extrapyramidal syndromes, dystonia, orthostatic hypotension, laryngospasms
Note	Monitor mental status, blood pressure

RELATED CONDITIONS AND INFORMATION

COLD-EXPOSURES EMERGENCIES

Emergencies Caused by Exposure to Cold Temperatures	
Chilblain (pernio)	Chilblain or pernio is a localized area of itching, redness and edema and commonly seen on the ears, nose, fingers and toes. Treatment is to rewarm by moving to a warm environment. DO NOT RUB the injured tissue and avoid direct heat application. Inform the patient to watch for signs of tissue damage and secondary infection.

Emergencies Caused by Exposure to Cold Temperatures	
Frostbite	Frostbite is freezing of body tissue. Ice crystals form in the body's intracellular spaces. Tissue damage is irreversible. Superficial frostbite involves the skin and subcutaneous tissue. Symptoms may include tingling, numbness, and a burning sensation. When the tissue thaws, the patient commonly has a hot stinging sensation. Tissue appears mottled with blisters. Medical management may include warm soaks, elevation, and hospitalization for observation and prevention of complications. Deep frostbite involves the freezing of muscles, bones, and tendons. Tissue appears white or yellow white. Blisters appear 1 to 7 days after the injury. Edema occurs and may persist for months. Eventually, the tissue appears gray-black and gangrene develops. Medical management may include evaluation, immersing the affected area in warm water, 40o to 43o C (104o to 110o F), analgesia, tetanus toxoid, and avoiding friction and pressure to the injured area. Hospitalization is required for treatment and possible escharotomy. The depth of the injury cannot be assessed for several weeks. Amputation is not considered until the depth of the injury is known.
Trench foot (immersion foot)	Trench foot is damage to the tissue of the toes and feet caused by cold temperatures and a wet foot or by cold temperatures and a dry foot in a boot that does not allow for normal evaporation. Management is gradual rewarming by exposing to air or soaking in warm water. Damage is reversible. Hospitalization is recommended for observation and prevention of complications.

FROSTBITE

Warming is effective when the skin becomes pink and warm indicating the blood flow is increased to near normal levels.

HYPERTHERMIA

Management of Hyperthermia	
Cardinal signs and symptoms	Cardinal signs and symptoms of hyperthermia are skin hot and dry with no sweating, core temperature of > 40.6° C (> 105° F), prostration, rapid pulse, rapid respirations, and a low blood pressure.
Common victims	Common victims are the elderly, persons with chronic disease, persons taking diuretics, military recruits, and users of street drugs.

Management of Hyperthermia	
Diagnostic findings	Diagnostic findings may include an elevated WBC and BUN, protein in the urine, respiratory alkalosis or metabolic acidosis, an abnormal electrocardiogram, and abnormal clotting studies that may culminate to DIC.
Management	Medial management may include placing in a cool environment, removing all clothing, putting into a cool shower on a gurney, and directing fans on the patient. Use chilled normal saline for intravenous fluids; however, these patients are not volume depleted and 1 to 2 liters over the first 4 hours is usually adequate. Lactated Ringer's is not recommended, as the liver may be unable to metabolize lactate. Chlorpromazine (Thorazine) is used to reduce shivering. Continue cooling until the core temperature reaches 39° C (102° F).
Cooling methods	Cooling methods include cooling blankets, spraying with tepid water, placing in direct contact with air directed by a fan, and placing well-padded ice packs in the groin, axilla, and on the neck. DO NOT rub down with isopropyl alcohol because this may cause a toxic exposure if a significant amount of alcohol is absorbed through the skin.

HYPOTHERMIA

Management of Hypothermia	
Mild Hypothermia 34°to 36° C 93.2° to 96.8° F	Warming methods in mild hypothermia include passive rewarming by moving the patient to a warm environment, wrapping with warmed blankets, giving warmed oxygen, and warm oral liquids high in glucose to provide calories. Discontinue when core temperate is > 35° C (95° F) to reduce the risk of hyperthermia.
Moderate Hypothermia 30° to 34° C 86° to 93.2° F	Warming methods in moderate hypothermia include passive rewarming by moving the patient to a warm environment, wrapping with warmed blankets, administering warmed oxygen, and warm oral liquids high in glucose to provide calories. Perform active rewarming (only at 0.5° C/hr (0.9° F/hr)) with the Bear Hugger, radiant heating lamps, heating pads, or a warming bed. Discontinue when core temperate is > 35° C (95° F) to reduce the risk of hyperthermia.

Management of Hypothermia	
Severe Hypothermia Less than 30° C Less than 86° F Death usually occurs below 25.6° C (78° F)	In severe hypothermia, warming efforts are essential. The heart is resistant to drug therapy and electro conversion at a core temperature of less than 86 degrees F. Active internal rewarming includes warm intravenous fluids at 43° C (109.4° F), warm, humid oxygen 42° to 46° (107.6° to 114.8° F), peritoneal lavage, extra corporeal rewarming, hemodialysis, and esophageal rewarming tubes. Discontinue when core temperate is > 35° C (95° F) to reduce the risk of hyperthermia.

HEAT EXPOSURE EMERGENCIES

Emergencies Caused by Exposure to Hot Temperatures	
Heat cramps	Heat cramps are severe cramps of the muscles. Commonly seen in the shoulders, abdominal wall, and thighs. They are often associated with pallor, weakness, nausea, tachycardia, profuse sweating, and cool moist skin and usually occur while resting after exertion in a hot environment. Salt depletion is secondary to sweating and increasing water intake further dilutes the serum sodium worsening the problem. Management includes a cool environment and electrolyte replacement with cool oral electrolyte fluids.
Heat edema	Heat edema is swelling of the feet and ankles. It occurs in non-acclimated people during periods of prolonged sitting and standing. The edema is self-limiting. Treatment includes rest, elevation of the feet and legs, and support hose.
Heat exhaustion	Heat exhaustion is caused by exposure to a hot environment for hours or days. Symptoms may include syncope, extreme thirst, muscle cramping, vomiting, and tachycardia. Management includes a cool environment and electrolyte replacement with cool oral electrolyte fluids or intravenous fluids of normal saline if the patient is vomiting. Hypotension can be corrected with intravenous NS bolus of 200 to 500 ml. The patient who does not respond over several hours may require hospital admission.

GERIATRIC CONSIDERATIONS

THERMOREGULATION

As a person ages, their thirst mechanism and ability to sweat decreases.

PEDIATRIC CONSIDERATIONS

THERMOREGULATION

The thermo-regulating mechanisms are immature in neonates and young infants. They mature toward the end of first year of life. Sweat glands develop and start functioning by six to eight months of age.

The circadian rhythm is established by the age of two and tends to be more pronounced in early childhood. Body temperature in children tends to be higher than in adults. A decrease toward adult levels begins at 1 year and slowly declines to normal body temperature through puberty and stabilizes at 13 to 14 years of age in girls and 17 to 18 years of age in boys.

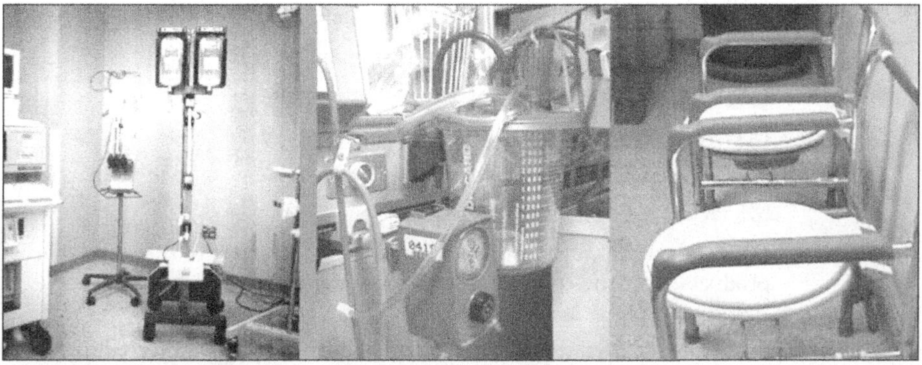

21 HEMORRHAGE

For details on triage see Chapter 34, Triage in a Nutshell.

PATIENT'S STORY – INTERVIEW QUESTIONS

1. When did the bleeding begin?
    a. If the symptoms are no longer active, how long did they last?
    b. If the symptoms were intermittent, how long did each episode last and how frequent were the episodes?
2. Where is the bleeding, e.g., gastrointestinal, vaginal, AV shunt, left leg stump, surgical site on abdomen?
    a. Is the patient with vaginal bleeding pregnant? If yes, considering chapter #26 Pregnancy and Delivery Emergency.
    b. Are any other symptoms associated with the chief complaint, e.g., nausea, vomiting, diarrhea, or lightheadedness?
3. Did anything cause the symptoms, e.g., an injury, taking an enema, having a bowel movement, vomiting?
4. How does the problem affect normal function?
    a. Is the patient able to perform normal duties?
    b. Is lightheadedness present?
    c. Has the patient fainted?
    d. Is any pain or discomfort associated with the bleeding?
        i. Where is the pain located and is any radiation present?
        ii. How severe is the pain?
5. Has any treatment been initiated, and has it helped?
6. Has the patient had similar problems before?
    a. When was the problem?

   b. What was the diagnosis and treatment?

7. Does the patient have any history of anemia?
8. Does the patient have any pertinent past history?
9. Does the patient take any routine medications?
   a. What is the name, dosage, route, and frequency of each medication?
   b. When was the last dose?
10. Does the patient take any complementary or alternative therapies, herbal products, over-the-counter medications or supplements, or natural therapies?
    a. What is the name, dosage, route and frequency of each therapy?
    b. When was the last dose or therapy?
11. Does the patient have allergies to drugs or foods?
    a. What is the name of the allergen?
    b. What was the reaction?
12. When was the patient's last tetanus immunization?
13. If the patient is female and between the ages of 10 to 50 years, when was the first day of her last menstrual period?

> Internal bleeding stops spontaneously in 80% of hospitalized patients without treatment.

NURSING DOMAIN

The nursing domain, nursing diagnosis and plan of care can only be determined after an in-depth interview and consideration of the patient's story.

> Domain 4. Class 4 Cardiovascular/Pulmonary responses

ANTICIPATED MEDICAL CARE

Review of the Anticipated Medical Care of Hemorrhages	
Exam	Full body
Urine tests	Urinalysis, clean catch specimen or a catheterized specimen if vaginal bleeding is present; pregnancy test for women of reproductive age unless they have had a hysterectomy
Blood	Hemogram, type and screen, serum pregnancy test if patient is able to conceive
X-ray	Chest
Other	Guaiac stools and emesis
Diet	NPO
IV	Normal saline or Ringer's solution

Review of the Anticipated Medical Care of Hemorrhages	
Medications	For upper gastrointestinal bleeds, Pepcid or other medications to suppress gastric sections
Other	Anticipate a nasogastric tube, endoscopy at bedside, and a method to monitor blood loss such as a bedside commode, bedpan, or a padded bed.
Disposition	Hospital admission may be required for hemorrhage associated with a significant drop in hemoglobin and for hemorrhages requiring surgery.
Worst-case scenario	The worst-case scenario is circulatory collapse from uncontrollable internal bleeding. Treatment may include STAT blood replacement and surgery to stop the bleeding.

INITIAL CARE PLAN

Alcohol-based hand sanitizers are the preferred method for cleaning your hands in most clinical situations. Wash your hands with soap and water whenever they are visibly dirty, before eating, and after using the restroom.

1. Ask the patient to undress, remove all jewelry that might interfere with the exam, and put on an exam gown. Assist as needed.
2. Obtain vital signs and place on continuous heart and automatic blood pressure monitoring.
3. Establish intravenous access with two large bore cannulas and draw laboratory blood specimens.
    a. Draw a variety of tubes that will allow the lab to perform hematology, chemistry, and coagulation studies. Patients that are cirrhotic or on anticoagulants need a PT and aPTT.
    b. Consider drawing other labs, e.g., type and screen, blood cultures.
4. Assure the patient that he is safe.
5. Perform a focused physical examination.
    a. Auscultate the lungs.
    b. Assess for signs of pallor. Anemia is best assessed by noting the color of the conjunctiva in conjunction with the nail beds and capillary refill in the palm of the hand.
    c. Evaluate the level of consciousness based on the mnemonic **AVPU** or **ACDU** level of consciousness score.
    AVPU: **A**lert, **V**erbal, **P**ain, **U**nresponsive.
    ACDU: **A**lert, **C**onfused, **D**rowsy, **U**nresponsive.
6. For the patient with gastrointestinal bleeding:
    a. Inspect the abdomen for injury and scars of past surgeries.
    b. Look for Gray Turner's sign (bruising of the flank).

   c. Look for Cullen's sign (periumbilical bruising) and distention.
   d. Auscultate abdominal bowel sounds.
   e. Percuss the abdomen.
   f. Palpate the abdomen for tenderness.
7. For the patient with vaginal bleeding:
   a. Inspect the perineum and look for bleeding lacerations.
   b. Estimate vaginal blood flow.
8. Consider placing drains, e.g., nasogastric tube to reduce the risk of vomiting and aspiration, indwelling urinary catheter to monitor urinary output.

> A decreased hourly urinary output is the best indicator of impending shock.

9. Instruct the patient not to eat or drink and teach the patient and family the rationale for the NPO status.
10. Elevate the bedside rails and place the stretcher in the lowest position.
11. Inform the patient, family, and caregivers of the usual plan of care and the expected overall time in the ER.
12. Provide the patient with a device to reach someone for assistance and explain how to use it. Ask the patient to call for help before getting off the stretcher.

ONGOING CARE PLAN

> Inform the medical provider of adverse changes noted during ongoing evaluation. Document that the medical provider was notified of the adverse change. Document if orders were or were not received.

1. Monitor blood loss.
   a. Look under the patient with a vaginal or lower gastrointestinal bleed for blood hidden from view.
   b. The amount of blood in a saturated peri-pad is approximately 30 ml.
   c. Approximately 600 ml is 15% of circulating volume and can cause significant orthostatic hypotension.
2. Monitor temperature, heart rate, blood pressure, and effectiveness of breathing.
3. Monitor level of consciousness and compare to the baseline using the mnemonic AVPU or ACDU.
4. Monitor therapy closely for the patient's therapeutic response.
   a. The usual time for a medication effectiveness check is 20 to 30 minutes after giving the drug.
   b. If therapy is not effective, ask the medical provider for a repeat dose or an alternative.

5. Monitor closely for the development of adverse reactions to therapy.
    a. Perform interventions to relieve the adverse reaction.
    b. Ask the medical provider for a remedy.
6. Keep the patient, family, and caregivers well informed of the plan of care and the remaining time anticipated before disposition.
7. Monitor the patient's laboratory and x-ray results and notify the medical provider of critical abnormalities. Remedy abnormalities as ordered.
8. Notify the medical provider when all diagnostic results are available for review. Ask for establishment of a diagnosis and disposition.

DISCHARGE INSTRUCTIONS

1. Provide the patient with the name of the nurse and doctor in the emergency room.
2. Inform the patient of their diagnosis or why a definitive diagnosis couldn't be made. Explain what caused the problem if known.
3. Teach the patient how to take the medication as prescribed and how to manage the common side effects. Instruct the patient not to drive or perform any dangerous tasks while taking narcotic pain medications.
4. Instruct the patient with gastrointestinal bleeding that:
    a. The bleeding was minor and tests to determine the source of the bleeding are done as an outpatient.
    b. Minor bleeding can often be treated with medications and without further testing.
    c. Endoscopic tests to determine the exact source of the bleeding will be scheduled by the follow-up medical provider.
    d. If the bleeding increases or if dizziness or fainting develops, return to the emergency room. If the bleeding stops, follow-up with the recommended medical provider.
5. Recommend a medical provider for follow-up care. Provide the name, address, and phone number with a recommendation of when to schedule the care.
6. Instruct the patient to call the follow-up medical provider immediately or return to the emergency room if the problem persists for over eight hours, worsens in any way, or any unusual symptoms develop. Encourage the patient NOT to IGNORE WORSENING OR PERSISTENT SYMPTOMS
7. Ask for verbal confirmation or demonstration of understanding and reinforce teaching as needed.

COMMONLY ORDERED MEDICATIONS

AQUAMEPHYTON

AquaMEPHYTON (vitamin K)

AquaMEPHYTON (vitamin K)	
Indications	Indications for vitamin K are hypoprothrombinemia caused by oral anticoagulants.
Adult dose	2.5 to 10 mg PO, SC or IM. The amount is based on the prothrombin level.
Pediatric dose	Neonate dose is 0.5 to 1 mg SC or IM
Onset	PO onset 6 to 12 hours, SC or IM onset 1 to 2 hours, peak 6 hours, duration 14 hours
Side effects	Side effects may include hemolytic anemia, hemoglobinuria, hyperbilirubinemia, and brain damage in large doses.
Note	May give IV after diluting with D5NS 10 ml or more if other routes are not possible (deaths have occurred).

PEPCID

Pepcid (famotidine)	
Indications	Symptoms of duodenal or gastric ulcers
Adult dose	20 mg IV every 12 hours
Onset	IV onset immediate, peak 1 to 3 hours, duration 6 to 12 hours
Compatibility	Y-site compatible with Dopamine, dobutamine, epinephrine, nitroglycerin, potassium chloride, sodium nitroprusside, theophylline, thiamine
Side effects	Seizure, bronchospasm

PITRESSIN

Pitressin (vasopressin)	
Indications	Bleeding and diabetes insipidus
Adult dose	5 to 10 units IM or SC, 0.2 to 0.9 units/min. IV, maximum 0.9 u/min.
Pediatric dose	2.5 to 10 units IM or SC
Onset	IV onset unknown, duration 3 to 8 hours
Side effects	Hypertension, bradycardia, heart block, peripheral vascular collapse
Note	Not recommended for IV use but occasionally given in extreme cases.

RELATED CONDITIONS AND INFORMATION

BLOOD TRANSFUSIONS

Massive blood transfusions require 1 to 2 units of fresh frozen plasma for every five units of blood transfused to treat dilutional coagulation.

CLASSIFICATION OF HEMORRHAGE

	Class I	Class II	Class III	Class IV
Blood loss	Up to 750 cc	750 to 1500 cc	1500 to 2000 cc	> 2000
HR	< 100	> 100	> 120	> 140
BP	Normal	Normal	Decreased	Decreased
RR	14 to 20	20 to 30	30 to 35	> 35
Cap refill	Normal	Slight delay	from 2 to 3 seconds	No filling
Skin	Pink and cool	Pale and cold	Pale, cold, moist	Mottled
Urine	> 30 cc/hr	20 to 30 cc/hr	5 to 15 cc/hr	< 5 cc/hr
Behavior	Slight anxiety	Mild anxiety	Anxious, confused	Lethargic, confused
Fluid	Crystalloid	Crystalloid	Crystalloid and blood	Crystalloid and blood

CONTROL OF EXTERNAL HEMORRHAGE

For hemorrhage of the extremities, elevate the extremity as high as possible above the heart level and compress the area. With the elevation of the extremity maintained, a compression bandage will control the bleeding.

GASTROINTESTINAL HEMORRHAGE

Review of the Causes of Gastrointestinal Hemorrhage by Site	
Esophagus	Esophageal hemorrhage may be caused by aortic aneurysm, eroding esophagus, esophagitis, hiatal hernia, tumors, peptic ulcers, and esophageal varices that are usually caused from portal hypertension (increased pressure in the portal vein from obstruction of the blood flow through the liver).
Liver	Hemorrhage of the liver can be caused by cirrhosis.
Duodenum	Hemorrhage at the duodenum is often caused by peptic ulcer, diverticulum, tumor, or duodenitis.
Dividing point between upper and lower GI bleeds	The ligament of Treitz at the junction of the duodenum and jejunum is the dividing point between upper and lower gastrointestinal bleeding.
Jejunum and ileum	Intussusception, tumors, peptic ulcers, enteritis, Meckel's diverticulum, and tuberculosis can cause hemorrhage at the jejunum and the ileum.
Mouth and Pharynx	Mouth and pharyngeal hemorrhages can be caused by malignant tumors and hemangiomas.

Review of the Causes of Gastrointestinal Hemorrhage by Site	
Stomach	Stomach hemorrhage is commonly caused by tumors, carcinoma, diverticulum, gastritis with erosion, peptic ulcers, and varices.
Pancreas	Hemorrhage of the pancreas can be caused by an eroding carcinoma and pancreatitis.
Colon and Rectum	A malignant tumor, diverticulitis and diverticulosis, fissure, foreign body, hemorrhoids, polyps, and ulcerative colitis can cause colon and rectal hemorrhage.

GENERIC MANAGEMENT OF INTERNAL HEMORRHAGE

Review of the Generic Management of Hemorrhage
Venous access with two large bore (18 to 14 gauge) cannulas or a central venous catheter.
Continuous monitoring of the heart, blood pressure, pulse oximetry, and hourly urine output.
Fluid resuscitation with isotonic intravenous solution (normal saline), albumin, fresh frozen plasma in patients with coagulopathy, and PRBC to maintain a hematocrit of 25 to 30.
Administer vitamin K 10 mg SC or IM for patients with a coagulopathy.
Administration of drug therapy specific to the problem.
Exploratory emergency surgery for uncontrolled or prolonged bleeding.

GLOSSARY

Review of Terms Associated with Hemorrhages	
Breakthrough	Breakthrough bleeding is intermenstrual bleeding that occurs with progestational agents, e.g., birth control or postmenopausal hormones.
Hematemesis	Hematemesis is vomiting of blood or altered blood (coffee-ground) indicating bleeding proximal to the ligament of Treitz. Blood may be mixed with food. Often associated with nausea and stomach pain and a history of gastric problems.
Hematochezia	Hematochezia is bright red or maroon rectal bleeding not tarry stools. Bleeding is usually beyond the ligament of Treitz but can be due to rapid (> 1000 ml of blood) upper gastrointestinal bleeding.
Hemoptysis	Hemoptysis is expectoration of blood arising from the oral cavity, pharynx, larynx, trachea, bronchus, or lungs. Blood is coughed up, frothy, bright red, and may be mixed with sputum. Symptoms may include dyspnea, pain, and a tickling sensation. There is often a history of tuberculosis.

Review of Terms Associated with Hemorrhages	
Melena	Melena is altered blood (black and tarry) from the rectum. Approximately 100 ml or more blood is required for one melenic stool. Melena indicates bleeding proximal to the ligament of Treitz but can be as far distal as the ascending colon. Iron, licorice, beets, blueberries, Pepto-Bismol, and charcoal cause black stools. Melena is common in the newborn.
Occult	Occult hemorrhage means unapparent bleeding. A common site is the intestines and detectable by a chemical test done on the feces.

HEMORRHAGE TYPES

Review of Hemorrhages Types	
Antepartum	Antepartum hemorrhage is a hemorrhage in a pregnant female before the onset of labor.
Arterial	Arterial hemorrhage is bleeding from an artery commonly in spurts of bright red blood.
Post-menopausal	Postmenopausal hemorrhage is uterine bleeding after surgical or natural menopause and is a sign of malignancy.
Postpartum	Postpartum hemorrhage is abnormal bleeding from the uterus following childbirth.
Uterine	Uterine hemorrhage is bleeding from the uterus.
Venous	Venous hemorrhage is bleeding from a vein often a continuous flow of dark red blood.
GI bleeding	Gastrointestinal bleeding (GI) most commonly is related to peptic ulcers and acute mucosal lesions. A common cause of acute mucosal lesions is the regular ingestion of aspirin for arthritis complaints by the elderly. Cancer, bleeding disorders, or vascular abnormalities are seldom related to gastrointestinal bleeding.

HEMORRHAGIC SHOCK

Review of Hemorrhagic Shock	
Definition	Hemorrhagic shock is present when bleeding decreases the circulating blood volume to a point that it is no longer effective for organ and tissue perfusion.
Signs	Signs of hemorrhagic shock may include decreasing arterial pressure, tachycardia, cold and clammy skin, pallor, altered mental status, and decreased kidney function.

Review of Hemorrhagic Shock	
Ongoing Monitoring	Hemorrhagic or hypovolemic shock is best evaluated by hourly urine output. Normal urinary output in a child is 1 to 2 ml/kg per hour and normal adult urinary output is > 30 ml/hr. A mean arterial pressure 80 to 100 is needed to perfuse organs. As the shock develops, the urinary output decreases.
Management	Medical management includes fluid resuscitation with intravenous isotonic fluids and blood replacement. Determining the source of the bleeding and an initial attempt to control the bleeding with endoscopy in the ER is a priority. Hospital admission is required for further fluid resuscitation and treatment of the underlying cause.
Note	Irreversible (refractory) shock is the final stage of shock in which no treatment can reverse the process.

HEMOPHILIA

Even minor trauma can cause major bleeding in the patient with hemophilia. Hemorrhage can occur anywhere in the body. The partial thromboplastin time (PTT) is prolonged. Bleeding into a joint is extremely painful and leads to severe disability. The patients and family are knowledgeable about the disease. Therapy is FFP for hemophilia A and von Willebrand's disease and factor VII for hemophilia B. Patients often have factor VIII at home but are unable to give it because of difficult intravenous access from repeated transfusions.

In the past, the concentrate was made from fractionated freeze-dried antihemophilic factor and contained 250 to 1500 UV of factor VIII:C in a reconstituted volume. Factor VIII is also produced by recombinant DVA techniques and is considered to be the replacement of choice. Cryoprecipitate derived from fresh frozen plasma was once the mainstay of hemophilia A and may be used when noninfectious factor VIII concentrates are not available.

Most hemophiliac patients require large doses of narcotic analgesia because they have built a tolerance from frequent use. Most patients know the amount of medication necessary to relieve their pain. Patients are often under-treated by medical providers for fear of contributing to an addiction.

A hemophilia patient should not be given an IM injection unless factor replacement was given within the past several days.

Intraosseous infusion of intravenous fluids and blood products can be administered into the sternum on adults and the anterior tibia on children.

June 11, 1975, the Governing Body of Jehovah's Witnesses adjusted its previous position and agreed it was acceptable for hemophiliacs to accept repeated treatment. Prior to this date, the hemophiliacs were only allowed treatment once as medicine.

The Jehovah's Witness (JW) doctrine does not believe in accepting homologous or autologous blood transfusions, and acute normovolemic hemodilution. The following procedures may also be refused but are at the discretion of each individual's interpretation of the JW doctrine: autologous blood salvage or cell-saver scavenging, closed-circuit acute normovolemic hemodilution, epidural blood patch, heart-lung machine, hemodialysis, labeling or tagging, platelet gel, and plasmapheresis.

LOWER GASTROINTESTINAL BLEEDS

Review of Lower Gastrointestinal Bleeds	
Definition	A lower gastrointestinal bleed refers to blood loss between the duodenum and the anus.
Common Causes	The most common cause is hemorrhoids. Other causes include anal lesions, fissures, rectal trauma, colitis, polyps, carcinoma, and diverticulosis.
Symptoms	Symptoms may include tachycardia, pallor, weakness, and lethargy. Pain and nausea are not always present.
Tests	Tests may include CBC, type and crossmatch, electrolytes, renal function studies, liver function, coagulation studies, chest x-ray, and electrocardiogram.
Management	Medical management may include fluid replacement followed by blood replacement; continuous monitoring of heart, blood pressure, and pulse oximetry, and hourly urine output. Bedside anoscopy, proctoscopy, or colonoscopy may be necessary for diagnosis and treatment with cautery. Hospital admission is commonly required for further work up; e.g., arteriography and radioisotopic scans, observation, and treatment. Surgical exploration is a last resort.
Complications	Complications include hypovolemic shock and circulatory collapse.

O-NEGATIVE BLOOD

O-negative blood can be administered in an emergency until typed and cross-matched blood is available. O-negative is considered the universal donor.

ORTHOSTATIC VITAL SIGNS

Review of Orthostatic Vital Signs	
Definition	Orthostatic vital signs are lying, sitting and/or standing blood pressure and pulse with less than 1 minute between readings. Commonly, the patient lays flat for 10 minutes prior to taking the vital signs.
Rationale	A patient with a clinically significant circulatory volume loss will have objective findings of a decrease in blood pressure >20 mmHg and an increase in pulse > 20 beats/min. Subjective findings include lightheadedness, nausea, and sweating.

PRESSURE POINTS

Pressure Points to Stop Arterial Hemorrhage

Pressure Points to Stop Arterial Hemorrhage	
Axillary	To control an axillary artery hemorrhage, apply pressure to the head of the humerus. Press high in the axilla against the upper part of the humerus.
Brachial	To control a brachial artery hemorrhage, apply pressure to the shaft of the humerus. Press against the humerus by pulling aside the biceps and pressing deep against the bone.
Carotid	To control a carotid artery hemorrhage, apply pressure against the cervical vertebra. Press one inch to the side of the prominence of the windpipe. Hold pressing deeply towards the back.
Facial	To control a facial artery hemorrhage, apply pressure against the lower part of the jaw. Press an inch in front of the angle of the jaw.
Femoral	To control a femoral artery hemorrhage, apply pressure to the rim of the pelvis or to the shaft of the femur. Press against the pelvis midway between the iliac spine and symphysis pubis or press high on the inner thigh about 3 inches below the rim of the pelvis.
Posterior tibial	To control a posterior tibial hemorrhage, apply pressure against the inner side of the tibia towards the ankle. Press against the tibia above the hemorrhage. For hemorrhage of the foot, press behind the inner ankle.
Subclavian	To control a subclavian artery hemorrhage, apply pressure against the first rib behind the clavicle. Press deep down and backward over the center of the clavicle after depressing the shoulder.
Temporal	To control a temporal artery hemorrhage, apply pressure against the temporal bone. Press against the bony prominence in front of the ear or temple.

LABORATORY TESTS

Laboratory Tests Associated with Hemorrhage	
Bleeding time (BT)	A bleeding time is the time required for blood to stop flowing through a pinprick in the skin.
Prothrombin time (PT)	A prothrombin time is the time for a clot to occur after thromboplastin and calcium are added to decalcified plasma. It is used to determine the effect of Coumadin.
aPTT	PTT is used to determine the effect of Heparin.

Laboratory Tests Associated with Hemorrhage	
Hemoglobin	Hemoglobin measures the amount of iron containing pigment in red blood cells. Hemoglobin is a conjugated protein of heme (iron containing pigment) and globulin (a simple protein). Hemoglobin combines with oxygen to make oxyhemoglobin. The function of hemoglobin is to carry oxygen from the lungs to the tissues. Hemoglobin is measured on a color spectrograph. Normal venous hemoglobin is 12 to 18 g/dl. Decreased means hemorrhage, hemodilution, or lyses of red blood cells (bypass pump). Significant change in the hemoglobin level may take four hours. Increased hemoglobin can mean dehydration. A high WBC or lipemia can elevate the hemoglobin. When the prime objective is maintenance of adequate oxygen transport, monitor the hemoglobin. Typical criteria for red blood cell transfusion is < to 8 gm/dl and < 9 gm/dl in a chronic transfusion patient.
Hematocrit	Hematocrit measures the volume of RBC (mature erythrocytes) packed by centrifugation in a given volume of blood. Results are expressed as a percent of the total. Normal is 37% to 54%. Decreased levels can mean hemodilution. Normal or increased hematocrit can mean hemoconcentration from blood loss.

UPPER GASTROINTESTINAL BLEED

Review of Upper Gastrointestinal Bleed	
Definition	An upper gastrointestinal bleed refers to blood loss between the esophagus and the duodenum.
Common Cause	Common causes of an upper gastrointestinal bleed are peptic ulcer, gastritis (commonly alcohol, aspirin, NSAIDs, or stress induced), esophagitis, and esophageal varices.
Symptoms	Symptoms may include tachycardia, pallor, weakness, and lethargy. Pain, nausea, vomiting and bloody stools are not always present.
Tests	Tests may include CBC, type and crossmatch, electrolytes, renal and liver function studies, coagulation studies, chest x-ray, and electrocardiogram.

Review of Upper Gastrointestinal Bleed	
Management	Medical management may include fluid replacement, intravenous medications to suppress gastric secretions, such as Pepcid, and blood replacement. Continuous monitoring of pulse, blood pressure, pulse oximetry, and hourly urine output is essential. Gastric lavage with saline to remove blood clots, bedside endoscopy for diagnosis, and treatment with cautery may be ordered. Hospital admission is required for further workup, e.g., arteriography and radioisotopic scans, observation, and treatment. Surgical exploration is a last resort.
Complications	Complications include aspiration, hypovolemic shock, and circulatory collapse.

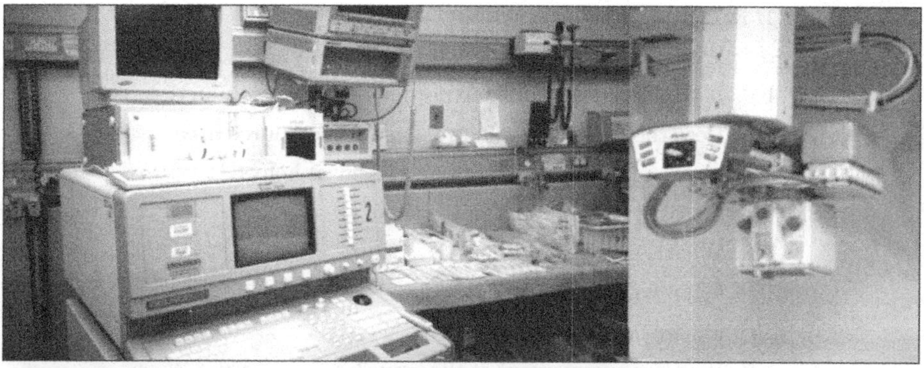

22 INDUSTRIAL AND MACHINERY ACCIDENT

For details on triage see Chapter 34, Triage in a Nutshell.

PATIENT'S STORY – INTERVIEW QUESTIONS

1. When was the accident?
2. Where are the injuries?
   a. Are any other symptoms associated with the chief complaint, e.g., pain with no obvious injury, nausea, vomiting, headache, sweating, or irregular heartbeat?
   b. For symptoms of pain with no obvious injury:
      i. Where is the pain or discomfort located?
      ii. Does it radiate?
      iii. How does the patient describe the severity of the symptoms?
3. Consider the nature of the emergency.
   a. If the patient was electrocuted, consider chapter #15 Electrocution.
   b. If there is an isolated head injury, consider chapter #32 Traumatic Injury and Head Injury.
   c. If the patient fell > 6 feet, consider chapter #17 Falls and Spinal Injury.
4. What type of machinery was involved?
   a. Was the patient trapped or caught in the machinery?
   b. How long was the patient caught or trapped?
5. Is the cause of the incident known?
   a. Was the incident preceded by an event related to mechanical failure?
   b. Was the incident preceded by an event or symptom related to the patient, e.g., fainted, slipped, tripped, fell asleep?

6. How do the injuries affect normal function?
    a. What is the appearance of the injured area?
    b. Is neurovascular function normal distal to the injury?
    c. Does the patient have normal use of the injured areas?
7. Has any treatment been initiated, and has it helped?
8. Has the patient had injury in the same area before?
    a. What was the injury?
    b. What was the treatment?
9. Is unlawful activity suspected?
    a. Was law enforcement at the scene?
    b. What agency?

Medical personnel are obligated to notify law enforcement if unlawful activity is suspected.

10. Does the patient have any pertinent past history?
11. Does the patient take any routine medications?
    a. What is the name, dosage, route, and frequency of each medication?
    b. When was the last dose?
12. Does the patient take any complementary or alternative therapies, herbal products, over-the-counter medications or supplements, or natural therapies?
    a. What is the name, dosage, route and frequency of each therapy?
    b. When was the last dose or therapy?
13. Does the patient have allergies to drugs or foods?
    a. What is the name of the allergen?
    b. What was the reaction?
14. When was the patient's last tetanus immunization?
15. If the patient is female and between the ages of 10 to 50 years, when was the first day of her last menstrual period?

NURSING DOMAIN

The nursing domain, nursing diagnosis and plan of care can only be determined after an in-depth interview and consideration of the patient's story.

Domain 12. Comfort. Class 1. Physical comfort.
Domain 11. Safety/Protection Class 2. Physical injury.

ANTICIPATED MEDICAL CARE

Review of the Anticipated Medical Care of Industrial and Machinery Accidents	
Exam	Full body
Urine	Test for hematuria; pregnancy test for women of reproductive age unless they have had a hysterectomy.
Blood	Hemogram, type and screen, electrolytes, renal function studies
ECG	ECG for females and males over 35 years, and for all ages with suspected chest injury or cardiac history
X-rays	X-rays of the area of suspected bony injury
Diet	NPO
IV	Normal saline or Ringer's solution
Medications	Analgesia and prophylactic antibiotics
Disposition	Hospital admission may be required for serious injury and when observation is necessary.
Worst-case scenario	The worst-case scenario is a ruptured aorta with sudden loss of circulatory volume and shock. Treatment may include STAT vascular surgery, large bore intravenous cannula placement, fluid resuscitation, type and cross for 20 units of PRBC, consent for surgery and anesthesia, and hospital admission after surgery.

INITIAL CARE PLAN

Alcohol-based hand sanitizers are the preferred method for cleaning your hands in most clinical situations. Wash your hands with soap and water whenever they are visibly dirty, before eating, and after using the restroom.

If the patient is ambulatory, ask the patient to obtain a clean catch urine specimen in the bathroom before undressing.

1. Ask the patient to undress, remove all jewelry that might interfere with the examination and put on an exam gown. Assist as needed.
2. Obtain vital signs including pulse oximetry or test capillary refill.
3. Attach heart monitor leads, automatic blood pressure cuff, and pulse oximetry for continuous monitoring. Document the initial heart monitor strip and document changes of rhythm.
4. Obtain a 12-lead electrocardiogram if the patient has suspected injury to the chest.
5. Place on supplemental oxygen if pulse oximetry is < 94%. For serious injuries, place on oxygen 100% non-rebreather regardless of saturation levels.

6. Assure the patient that he is safe.
7. Establish intravenous access and draw laboratory blood specimens.
   a. Draw a variety of tubes that will allow the lab to perform hematology, chemistry, and coagulation studies. Patients on anticoagulants or that have cirrhosis need coagulation studies.
   b. Consider drawing other labs, e.g., type and screen, blood cultures.
8. Splint for suspected bony fractures associated with deformity, pain, bony crepitus, edema, ecchymosis, vascular compromise, open wounds, paralysis, and paresthesia.
9. For minor injuries, perform a focused physical examination.
   a. Auscultate the lungs.
   b. Examine the site of injury.
      i. Evaluate neurovascular function distal to the injury.
      ii. Evaluate normal function of the injured area.
10. For serious injuries, perform a head-to-toe assessment.

> If two nurses are at the bedside, one can ask the following questions and document the answers of the other who performs the exam. Document positive and negative findings.

   a. What is the size and reaction of the pupils?
   b. Does the patient have any head pain or injuries to the head?
      Is the tongue or mouth injured?
      Is any drainage present from the nose or ears?
   c. Is the trachea midline?
      Is jugular venous distention present (unable to detect under fluorescent light)?
   d. Does the chest expand equally?
      Is subcutaneous emphysema present?
      Are the heart tones within normal limits?
      Are the heart tones diminished?
      Are any murmurs present?
      Does the patient complain of chest pain?
      Is the chest tender to palpation?
   e. Are the lung sounds clear on the right and left?
      Are wheezes or crackles present?
      Are the lung sounds decreased or absent in any area of the lungs?
   f. Is the abdomen soft, flat, rigid, or distended?
      Are bowel sounds normal, hypoactive, hyperactive, or absent?
      Does the patient complain of abdominal pain?
      Is the patient's abdomen tender to palpation?

g. Is the patient incontinent?
Examination of the genitalia may be deferred if trauma is not suspected.
Do the genitalia appear normal?
Does the patient have bleeding from the urethral meatus or vagina?
Is priapism present?
Does the patient complain of genital pain?
Is the perineal area or genitalia tender to palpation?

h. Does the patient complain of pain when light pressure is applied to the iliac crests?
Is the pelvis stable or unstable?

i. Does the patient have normal motion and sensation in the upper and lower extremities?
Are distal pulses present in the upper and lower extremities?

j. Does the patient have normal movement of his back?
Does the patient complain of back pain?
While keeping the back immobilized, turn the patient.
Inspect the posterior surfaces.
Does the patient have obvious back injuries?
Is the back tender to palpation?

k. Does skin inspection reveal any damage to the skin, e.g., abrasions, lacerations, bruises, needle tracks, or petechiae?

l. Evaluate the level of consciousness based on the mnemonic **AVPU** or **ACDU** level of consciousness score.
AVPU: **A**lert, **V**erbal, **P**ain, **U**nresponsive.
ACDU: **A**lert, **C**onfused, **D**rowsy, **U**nresponsive.

m. In a pregnant female, inspect the perineum, assist with a pelvic examination, auscultate the fetal heart rate (normal 120 to 160), and palpate the uterus to determine, size, tenderness, contractions, and firmness.

11. For the patient with a soft tissue injury, practice the mnemonic **PRICE**.
When the injured area is not managed properly, the patient pays the **PRICE** of increased pain and disability.
Protect the injured area and keep out of harm's way. Do not leave an injured foot in the way of a passerby. Cover damaged skin with a sterile dressing.
Rest the area. Do not allow the patient to use the injured extremity. Use a sling for an upper extremity and crutches or a wheelchair to rest an injured lower extremity.
Ice the area. Use a large ice pack to saddle the area and cool the surrounding tissue.
Compress the area with light pressure from a compression bandage or ice pack to reduce the risk of swelling.
Elevate the injured area above the level of the heart.

12. If indicated, keep the patient warm with heated blankets. Place a warmed blanket like a shawl around the head, neck, and shoulders. Place another blanket over the body and tightly tuck it around the patient.
13. Administer tetanus toxoid if indicated.
14. Clean, irrigate, and dress the wounds. Consider collecting wound cultures.
15. Consider placing drains, e.g., nasogastric tube to relieve gastric distention and prevent vomiting and aspiration, indwelling Foley catheter to monitor hourly urine output.
16. Order x-rays of areas where bony injury is suspected.
17. Instruct the patient not to eat or drink and teach the patient and family the rationale of the NPO status.
18. Elevate the siderails and place the stretcher in the lowest position.
19. Inform the patient, family, and caregivers of the usual plan of care and the expected overall time in the ER.
20. Provide the patient with a device to reach someone for assistance and explain how to use it. Ask the patient to call for help before getting off the stretcher.

ONGOING CARE PLAN

Inform the medical provider of adverse changes noted during ongoing evaluation. Document that the medical provider was notified of the adverse change. Document if orders were or were not received.

1. Monitor temperature, heart rate and rhythm, blood pressure, and effectiveness of breathing.
2. Monitor therapy closely for the patient's therapeutic response.
   a. The usual time for a medication effectiveness check is 20 to 30 minutes after giving the drug.
   b. If therapy is not effective, ask the medical provider for a repeat dose or an alternative.
3. Monitor closely for the development of adverse reactions to therapy.
   a. Perform interventions to relieve the adverse reaction.
   b. Ask the medical provider for a remedy.
4. Keep the patient, family, and caregivers well informed of the plan of care and the remaining time anticipated before disposition.
5. Monitor the patient's laboratory and x-ray results and notify the medical provider of critical abnormalities. Remedy abnormalities as ordered.
6. Notify the medical provider when all diagnostic results are available for review. Ask for establishment of a diagnosis and disposition.

DISCHARGE INSTRUCTIONS

1. Provide the patient with the name of the nurse and doctor in the emergency room.
2. Inform the patient of their diagnosis or why a definitive diagnosis couldn't be made. Explain what caused the problem if known.
3. Teach the patient how to take the medication as prescribed and how to manage the common side effects. Instruct the patient not to drive or perform any dangerous tasks while taking narcotic pain medications.
4. Instruct the patient with a sutured laceration that:
   a. The laceration must be kept clean and dry.
   b. The dressing applied in the ER should be removed after one or two days and the wound left open to the air.
   c. Some lacerations of the face and scalp are not covered with a dressing in the ER. These wounds may be covered with a dry sterile dressing if needed to protect the area.
   d. Elevate the area to reduce the risk of swelling.
   e. The laceration must be kept clean with mild soap and water and an antibiotic over-the-counter ointment applied two times a day for the first three days.
   f. Follow-up is recommended for suture removal.
   g. Redness, swelling, red streaks, and pus are signs of infection. Notify the follow-up medical provider if any of these symptoms develop.
5. Instruct the patient with an unsutured laceration that:
   a. Some lacerations contaminated with dirt or bacteria are not sutured. These are considered dirty wounds and further care is necessary at home.
   b. Soak the area in warm water and prescribed solution for twenty minutes three times a day for the first three days.
   c. Keep the wound covered with a dry sterile dressing between soaks. If the wound is dry and clean after three days of soaks, stop the soaking, and keep it clean, dry, and covered.
   d. Not all dirty wounds need antibiotics. If antibiotics are prescribed, take them until the pills are gone. Do not stop when the wound looks better.
   e. Redness, swelling, red streaks, and pus are signs of infection. Notify the follow-up medical provider if any of these symptoms develop.

6. Instruct the patient with a fracture or soft tissue injury to practice the mnemonic **PRICE**.

   Protect the injured area and keep out of harm's way; do not leave a foot in the way of a passerby.
   Rest the area. Do not use or walk on an injured extremity.
   Ice the area.
   Compress the area with light pressure from a compression bandage or ice pack to reduce the risk of swelling.
   Elevate the injured area above the level of the heart.

   When the injured area is not managed properly, the patient pays the **PRICE** of increased pain and disability.

7. Instruct the patient with a fracture that splints may become too tight if swelling develops. Watch carefully for loss of the normal color in the fingers or toes and increased pain. Call the follow-up medical provider if a problem develops.

8. If the patient has been told not to bear weight, teach crutch walking as follows.

   a. Inform the patient not to bear weight on the injured leg and not to bear the body's weight on the crutches up against the armpit. This can cause serious and permanent nerve damage. Keep the arms straight and support the body's weight on the crutch handles.

   b. The two crutches serve as a support for the injured leg and swing with that leg. Move the crutches and the injured leg forward at the same time, then pick up the crutches, and step forward on the uninjured leg.

   c. Keep the rubber tips clean and tightly affixed to the crutch.

   d. Do not use crutches on wet surfaces or on ice.

   e. Depend on a wheelchair if your arms cannot support your weight on crutches.

   f. Notify the follow-up medical provider if any problems develop regarding the use of the crutches.

9. Instruct the patient that it is possible to have an internal injury or small fracture that becomes evident with the passage of time. If any unusual symptoms develop, e.g., abdominal pain, chest pain, difficulty breathing, or blood in the urine or stool, contact the follow-up medical provider immediately or return to the emergency room.

10. Recommend a medical provider for follow-up care. Provide the name, address, and phone number with a recommendation of when to schedule the care.

11. Instruct the patient to call the follow-up medical provider or return to the emergency room if the pain worsens, new symptoms develop, or if the injury is not progressing as expected. Encourage the patient NOT to IGNORE WORSENING OR PERSISTENT SYMPTOMS.
12. Ask for verbal confirmation or demonstration of understanding and reinforce teaching as needed.

COMMONLY ORDERED MEDICATIONS

DILAUDID

Dilaudid (hydromorphone)	
Indications	Moderate to severe pain
Dose	Typical dose 1 to 5 mg IV. Titrate to response No maximum dose
Onset	IV onset rapid, peak 15 to 30 minutes, duration 3 to 4 hours
Side effects	Drowsiness, dizziness, confusion, sedation, increased intracranial pressure, nausea, vomiting, urinary retention, respiratory depression
Monitor	CNS changes, respiratory effectiveness, allergic rash
Note	Dilaudid 5 mg is equivalent to Morphine 10 mg IM. Dilute to 4 or 5 ml with NS or sterile water for injection and administer slowly over at least 2 to 3 minutes Antidote is naloxone.

PHENERGAN

Phenergan (promethazine)	
Indications	Nausea, vomiting
Dose	12.5 to 25 mg IV every 4 to 6 hours. When used intravenously, promethazine injection should be given in concentration no greater than 25 mg/ml at a rate not to exceed 25 mg/min. Preferably inject through a medication port in IV tubing that is known to be functioning satisfactorily. 25 to 50 mg IM every 4 to 6 hours
Pediatric dose	More than 2 years 0.25 to 0.5 mg/kg IM or IV every 4 to 6 hours
Onset	IM onset 20 min., duration 4 to 6 hours IV onset 3 to 5 min., duration 4 to 6 hours
Side effects	Drowsiness, sedation, hypotension, palpitations, tachycardia
Monitor	Vital signs, sedation level, respiratory effectiveness

TETANUS AND DIPHTHERIA TOXOID, ABSORBED FOR ADULTS

Tetanus and Diphtheria Toxoid, Absorbed for Adults	
Indications	Immunization against tetanus and diphtheria
Dose	Adults and children 7 years and older 0.5 ml IM
Side effects	Local reactions such as erythema, induration, and tenderness are common. Systemic reactions include fever, chills, myalgias, and headache.
Monitor	Local reactions are usually self-limiting. Sterile abscess and subcutaneous atrophy may occur at the injection site.
Note	The goal is to keep tetanus immunization current not specifically to prevent tetanus infection from the current wound. Persons in the United States have a right not to be immunized. Children can receive a religious exception and be in public school without the recommended immunizations.

VERSED

Versed (midazolam hydrochloride)	
Indications	Conscious sedation.
Adult dose	1 to 2.5 mg IV over 2 min. Wait for 2 minutes to fully evaluate effect before giving another dose. A total dose of over 5 mg IV is not usually necessary. If patients receive narcotic medications before the Versed, use approximately 30% less.
Pediatric dose	Pediatric patients aged 12 to 16 years are dosed as adults. IV versed is not commonly used in pediatric patients that are not intubated. Patients less than 12 years are dosed by weight. Initial loading dose is 0.05 to 0.2 mg/kg IV administered over 2 to 3 min.
Onset	IV onset 3 to 5 minutes
Compatibility	Versed has many incompatibilities. Use normal saline in the IV line before and after the dose.
Side effects	Side effects include serious life threatening decreased respiratory tidal volume and respiratory rate.
Monitor	Continuous monitoring of the heart, blood pressure, and oxygenation is essential.
Note	Versed is a potent sedative that requires slow administration and individualization of dosage. Versed is 3 to 4 times as potent as Valium. Reversing agent is Romazicon (flumazenil).

ROMAZICON

Romazicon (flumazenil)	
Indications	Valium, Versed, benzodiazepine overdose

Romazicon (flumazenil)	
Adult dose	First dose 0.2 mg IV over 15 sec Second dose 0.3 mg IV over 15 seconds Third dose 0.5 mg IV over 30 seconds If no response, may repeat every minute until response is adequate or the maximum of 3 mg given.
Onset	IV onset 1 minute, peak 10 min., duration unknown
Side effects	Nausea, vomiting, seizures, dizziness, agitation, pain at injection site
Note	Effects of flumazenil may wear off before the benzodiazepine, repeat dose to the maximum levels.
Monitor	Monitor respiratory effectiveness

RELATED INFORMATION

AMPUTATION

Review of Amputations	
Definition	An amputation is a traumatic separation of a digit or limb from the body.
Cause	Penetrating and blunt trauma cause amputations.
Symptoms	Symptoms may include loss of a complete body part or partial tissue loss associated with bleeding, hypovolemic shock, and pain.
Tests	X-rays are done to determine the bony damage.
Management	Management in the ER includes control of bleeding with pressure dressings, elevation, cleansing of the wound, splinting, and dressing with sterile dressings.
Disposition	Prepare for hospital admission, surgical intervention, or transfer to a facility with a reclamation team.
Note	Keep the amputated part covered with saline moistened gauze in a watertight plastic bag or container. Place the watertight bag or container in ice and water. Avoid placing the amputated part in direct contact with the ice; always utilize some sort of clean, soft, moist barrier.

CRUSH INJURIES

Review of Crush Injuries	
Definition	A crush injury is destruction caused by extreme pressure against the tissue resulting in damage to skin, muscle, nerves, and bone.
Cause	The force from trauma causes crush injuries.

Review of Crush Injuries	
Symptoms	Symptoms may include pain, loss of neurovascular function distal to the injury, hemorrhage, hypovolemic shock, swelling, and ecchymosis.
Tests	Tests may include x-rays, ultrasound, CT, or MRI.
Management	Management may include control of bleeding, fluid resuscitation with normal saline to increase urinary output and facilitate excretion of myoglobin, elevation, cleansing and irrigation of wounds, monitoring of urine for presence of myoglobin in urine and neurovascular function.
Disposition	Hospital admission may be required for possible surgical débridement, fasciotomy, or amputation.

COMPARTMENTAL SYNDROME

Review of Compartmental Syndrome	
Definition	Compartmental syndrome is a condition in which tissue is severely constricted in its space causing damage to the tissue.
Cause	Compartmental syndrome occurs when trauma causes more tissue inflammation and swelling than can be contained within the compartment resulting in tissue damage.
Symptoms	Symptoms may include progressive pain, sensory deficits, muscle weakness, and a tense swollen area. It usually occurs in the forearm and lower leg.
Tests	Tests may include measurement of muscle compartment pressure. A reading of greater than 35 to 45 mmHg is indicative of the need for a fasciotomy.
Management	Management includes elevation TO the level of the heart to assure venous outflow (elevation above the heart decreases perfusion) and ongoing monitoring of size and tenseness of the injured area.
Disposition	Hospital admission may be required for a surgical fasciotomy and repair of neurovascular damage.

FAT EMBOLUS

Review of Fat Emboli	
Definition	Fat emboli are emboli made of fat that lodge in the vessels and obstruct blood flow.
Cause	The emboli are fat globules from bone marrow released into injured veins following fractures of pelvic and long bones.

Review of Fat Emboli	
Symptoms	A petechial rash may develop 12 to 96 hours after an injury caused by fat globules obstructing the capillaries of the skin and subcutaneous tissue. When a petechial rash is associated with breathing problems, it may be a sign of pulmonary embolism due to fat emboli.
Tests	Tests may include hematology, serum lipase, ABG, chest x-ray, ventilation perfusion scan, and pulmonary arteriogram.
Management	The management goal is maintenance of adequate oxygenation to the tissues.
Disposition	Hospital admission may be required for observation and supportive treatment.

FEMUR FRACTURES

Review of Femur Fractures (Hip Fracture)	
Definition	A femur fracture is a disruption of the long bone in the thigh.
Cause	Causes include major trauma, falls, motor vehicle crashes, and slip-and-fall injuries in the elderly.
Symptoms	Symptoms may include pain, inability to bear weight, and shortening and rotation of the leg. Hypovolemic shock may be present.
Tests	Tests may include x-ray and preoperative laboratory studies if surgery is anticipated. Pre-operative laboratory studies may include CBC, electrolytes, glucose, renal studies, type and screen, coagulation studies if on anticoagulants or cirrhotic, chest x-ray, and electrocardiogram for females over 45 and males over 35 years.
Management	Management includes immobilization and support of the leg (traction splint or traction pin), ice pack, fluid-resuscitation with normal saline, and ongoing monitoring of sensation, movement, and circulation distal to the fracture.
Disposition	Hospital admission is commonly required for open surgical reduction and internal fixation or continued traction.

FRACTURES

Review of Fracture Types	
Closed	Closed fracture means the skin over the site is intact.
Comminuted	Comminuted fracture means the bone is splintered into fragments.
Complete	Complete fracture means the bony continuity is interrupted.
Displaced	Displaced fracture means the proximal and distal segments of bone are not aligned.

Review of Fracture Types	
Greenstick	Greenstick fracture means the bone is bent.
Impacted	Impacted fracture means the distal and proximal fracture sites are wedged together.
Open	Open fracture means the skin over the site is not intact.

FRACTURE MANAGEMENT

Review of ER General Management of Fractures	
Expose	Expose the site by removing all clothing and jewelry near the suspected fracture.
Perform a physical assessment	Inspect for color, position, disrupted skin, bleeding, deformity, and differences as compared to the uninjured side. Assess the extremity for pain, pallor, pulses, paresthesia, and paralysis (five Ps).
When to splint	Splint for deformity, pain, bony crepitus, edema, ecchymosis, vascular compromise, open wounds, paralysis, and paresthesia.
Immobilize	Immobilize with a splint that effectively immobilizes the joints below and above the injury. Avoid manipulation of the bone. Rigid splints (plastic and metal) are used for lower extremity fractures. Soft splints, such as pillows and slings, are used for upper extremity fractures. Traction splints are used for femur and proximal tibial fractures.
PRICE	Protect, rest, ice, compress, and elevate the site. Ice and elevation are essential ER procedures.
Medications	Administer analgesics.
Diagnostic testing	Order x-rays. The views should include the joints above and below the injury.
On-going monitors	Frequently reassess the five Ps (pain, pallor, pulses, paresthesia, and paralysis).
Anticipate	Anticipate definitive stabilization, traction, internal or external fixation, and hospitalization for closed or open reduction.

JOINT DISLOCATIONS

Review of Joint Dislocations	
Definition	A joint dislocation is a displacement of a bone from its normal position in the joint.

Review of Joint Dislocations	
Cause	The cause of joint dislocations is commonly a traumatic force that moves the bone beyond its normal range of motion.
Symptoms	Symptoms may include pain, deformity, swelling, inability to move the joint, and neurovascular compromise.
Tests	Tests may include x-ray, CT, and MRI.
Management	Management is EMERGENT if circulation is absent distal to the dislocation (threat to a limb is second only to a threat of life). Temporarily immobilize the joint, prepare for conscious sedation and immediate reduction.
Disposition	Joint dislocations are commonly admitted to the hospital for observation and supportive treatment.
Comments	A dislocation of the knee and elbow are considered EMERGENT. In the knee, the peroneal nerve and vein can be permanently damaged. An angiogram is necessary to evaluate vascular compromise post reduction.

OPEN FRACTURES

Review of Open Fractures	
Definition	An open fracture is a bony fracture with disruption of the skin either from external or internal forces.
Cause	The cause of a bony fracture is most often a traumatic force.
Symptoms	Symptoms include disrupted skin near the fracture site, possible protrusion of the bone, pain, and may include neurovascular compromise and bleeding.
Tests	Tests may include x-rays, CT, and MRI.
Management	Management includes a wound culture, cleansing and irrigation of the wound, dressing with a sterile dressing, and a splint if indicated.
Disposition	Hospital admission may be required for surgery or transfer to a facility that can provide the necessary care.

PELVIC FRACTURES

Review of Pelvic Fractures	
Definition	A pelvic fracture is a break in the pelvic bone.
Cause	The cause of pelvic fractures is usually a traumatic force.
Symptoms	Symptoms may include deformity and swelling at the site of fracture, shortening or abnormal rotation of the leg, and pain.
X-ray	Tests may include x-ray, CT, and cystogram.

Review of Pelvic Fractures	
Management	Management may include splinting with pressurized trousers if the patient is hemodynamically unstable and fluid resuscitation with normal saline. Up to 4.5 liters of blood can be lost with unstable pelvic fracture.
Disposition	Hospital admission may be required for an unstable fracture or transfer to a facility that can surgically repair the fracture.
Associated injury	Associated injuries are common in the perineum, genitalia, and rectum.

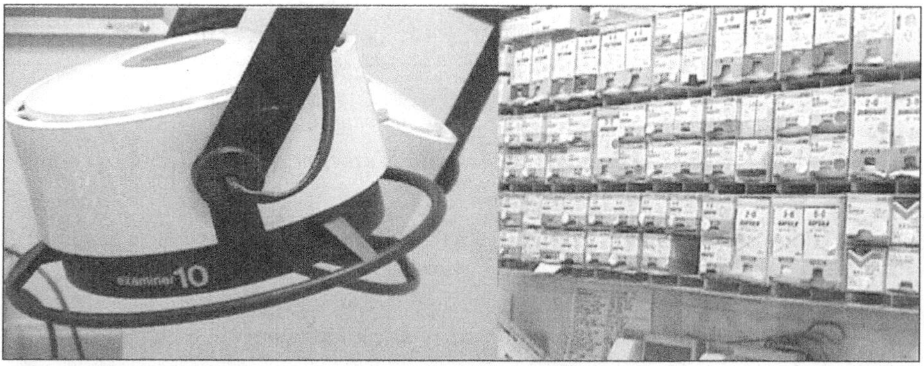

23 LACERATION AND SHARP TRAUMA

For details on triage see Chapter 34, Triage in a Nutshell.

PATIENT'S STORY – INTERVIEW QUESTIONS

1. When did the patient sustain the injury?
2. Where is the injury and are any associated symptoms present?
3. What caused the laceration, e.g., slip and fall, syncope?
   a. If the patient suffered a syncopal episode, consider #33 Weakness, Unconscious or Altered Consciousness, Syncope and Near Syncope as the nature of the emergency.
   b. If the patient was assaulted, consider #04, Assault, Rape, and Survivor of Violence as the nature of the emergency.
4. How does the injury affect the patient's normal function?
   a. What is the initial impression of the severity of the laceration, e.g., injury of skin and subcutaneous tissue, injury of muscle, tendons?
   b. Is any bleeding present?
   c. Does the patient have normal neurovascular function distal to the laceration?
   d. Does the patient have normal use of the injured area?
5. Has any treatment been initiated, and has it helped?
6. Has the patient had serious injury to the same area in the past?
   a. When was the injury?
   b. What was the diagnosis and treatment?
7. Is unlawful activity suspected?
   a. Was law enforcement at the scene?
   b. What agency?

Medical personnel have a legal obligation to report crime. Assault is a crime.

8. Does the patient have any pertinent past history?
9. Does the patient take any routine medications?
    a. What is the name, dosage, route, and frequency of each medication?
    b. When was the last dose?
10. Does the patient take any complementary or alternative therapies, herbal products, over-the-counter medications or supplements, or natural therapies?
    a. What is the name, dosage, route and frequency of each therapy?
    b. When was the last dose or therapy?
11. Does the patient have allergies to drugs or foods?
    a. What is the name of the allergen?
    b. What was the reaction?
12. When was the patient's last tetanus immunization?
13. If the patient is female and between the ages of 10 to 50 years, when was the first day of her last menstrual period?

NURSING DOMAIN

The nursing domain, nursing diagnosis and plan of care can only be determined after an in-depth interview and consideration of the patient's story.

Domain 12. Comfort. Class 1. Physical comfort.
Domain 11. Safety/Protection Class 3. Violence.

ANTICIPATED MEDICAL CARE

Review of the Anticipated Medical Care of Blunt and Sharp Injuries	
Exam	Local examination of the injuries area
Urine tests	If the injury will require surgery for repair, pregnancy test for women of reproductive age unless they have had a hysterectomy.
Blood tests	Anticipate a hemogram if bleeding was excessive and a PT if the patient is taking anticoagulants.
X-ray	None unless bony damage is suspected.
Diet	NPO until the extent of the injury is known and treatment is determined.
IV	None
Medications	Tetanus toxoid if last immunization was > 5 years ago.

Review of the Anticipated Medical Care of Blunt and Sharp Injuries	
Disposition	Hospital admission may be required for surgery.
Worst-case scenario	The worst-case scenario is an arterial bleed in a non-compressible area then a patient is on anticoagulants.

INITIAL CARE PLAN

Alcohol-based hand sanitizers are the preferred method for cleaning your hands in most clinical situations. Wash your hands with soap and water whenever they are visibly dirty, before eating, and after using the restroom.

1. Ask the patient to remove clothes and jewelry near the laceration.
2. Obtain vital signs.
3. Position the patient in a relaxed anatomically correct position that allows easy access to the lacerated area for irrigation and repair.
4. Perform a focused examination of the laceration.
    a. Assess the injury size and depth.
    b. Evaluate neurovascular function distal to the laceration.
    c. Evaluate motor function distal to the laceration.
5. Clean, irrigate, and cover the injury with sterile saline moistened gauze.
6. Give tetanus toxoid if indicated.
7. Set up suture equipment on a stand within easy access of the laceration.
    a. Suture tray with washing solutions
    b. Sterile gloves in the proper size for the person doing the suturing.
    c. Local anesthesia in a syringe placed within easy reach.
    d. Kick bucket for waste placed within easy reach.
    e. A spotlight placed behind the shoulder of the person suturing and directed down towards the laceration.
    f. Suture material if known. The usual practice is to have the person doing the suturing select the suture material and the needle size and shape.
8. Instruct the patient not to eat or drink and teach the patient and family the rationale for the NPO status.
9. Elevate the siderails and place the stretcher in the lowest position.
10. Inform the patient, family, and caregivers of the usual plan of care and the expected overall time in the ER.
11. Provide the patient with a device to reach someone for assistance and explain how to use it. Ask the patient to call for help before getting off the stretcher.

ONGOING CARE PLAN

Inform the medical provider of adverse changes noted during ongoing evaluation. Document that the medical provider was notified of the adverse change. Document if orders were or were not received.

1. Monitor vital signs.
2. Monitor therapy closely for the patient's therapeutic response.
   a. The usual time for a medication effectiveness check is 20 to 30 minutes after giving the drug.
   b. If therapy is not effective, ask the medical provider for a repeat dose or an alternative.
3. Monitor closely for the development of adverse reactions to therapy.
   a. Perform interventions to relieve the adverse reaction.
   b. Ask the medical provider for a remedy.
4. If not NPO, provide the patient with food at mealtimes and fluids during the stay.
5. Keep the patient, family, and caregivers well informed of the plan of care and the remaining time anticipated before disposition.
6. Monitor the patient's laboratory and x-ray results and notify the medical provider of critical abnormalities. Remedy abnormalities as ordered.
7. Notify the medical provider when all diagnostic results are available for review. Ask for establishment of a diagnosis and disposition.

DISCHARGE INSTRUCTIONS

1. Provide the patient with the name of the nurse and doctor in the emergency room.
2. Inform the patient of their diagnosis or why a definitive diagnosis couldn't be made. Explain what caused the problem if known.
3. Teach the patient how to take the medication as prescribed and how to manage the common side effects. Instruct the patient not to drive or perform any dangerous tasks while taking narcotic pain medications.
4. Instruct the patient that:
   a. After an injury is sutured, keep it clean and dry.
   b. After one or two days, the dressing applied in the ER may be removed and the wound left open to the air.
   c. Some injuries of the face and scalp are not covered with a dressing in the ER.
   d. The wound may be covered with a dry sterile dressing if needed to protect the area.
   e. Elevation of the area when possible will reduce the risk of swelling.

f. After the dressing is removed, the injury should be kept clean with mild soap and water and an antibiotic over-the-counter ointment be applied two times a day for the first three days.

g. Follow-up is recommended for suture removal.

5. Some injuries contaminated with dirt or bacteria are not sutured. These are considered dirty wounds and further care is necessary at home.

    a. Soak the area in warm water and prescribed solution for twenty minutes three times a day for the first three days.

    b. The wound should be covered with a dry sterile dressing between soaks. If the wound is dry and clean after three days of soaks, stop the soaking, and keep it clean, dry, and covered.

    c. Not all dirty wounds need antibiotics. If antibiotics are prescribed, take them until the pills are gone. Do not stop when the wound looks better.

    d. Redness, swelling, red streaks, and pus are signs of infection. Notify the follow-up medical provider if any of these symptoms develop.

6. For the patient with soft tissue injury teach the mnemonic **PRICE**. When the injured area is not managed properly, the patient pays the PRICE of increased pain and disability.
   Protect the injured area and keep out of harm's way. Cover skin that is not intact with a sterile dressing when in a dirty environment.
   Rest the area. Do not use or walk on an injured extremity.
   Ice the area.
   Compress the area with light pressure from a compression bandage or ice pack to reduce the risk of swelling.
   Elevate the injured area above the level of the heart.

7. Recommend a medical provider for follow-up care. Provide the name, address, and phone number with a recommendation of when to schedule the care.

8. Instruct the patient to call the follow-up medical provider immediately or return to the emergency room if the pain or problem worsens in any way or any unusual symptoms develop. Encourage the patient NOT to IGNORE WORSENING OR PERSISTENT SYMPTOMS.

9. Ask for verbal confirmation or demonstration of understanding and reinforce teaching as needed.

COMMONLY ORDERED MEDICATIONS

TETANUS AND DIPHTHERIA TOXOID, ADSORBED FOR ADULTS

Tetanus and Diphtheria Toxoid Adsorbed for Adult	
Indications	Immunization against tetanus and diphtheria
Dose	Adults and children 7 years and older 0.5 ml IM

Tetanus and Diphtheria Toxoid Adsorbed for Adult	
Side effects	Local reactions, such as erythema, induration, and tenderness, are common. Systemic reactions include fever, chills, myalgias, and headache.
Monitor	Local reactions are usually self-limiting. Sterile abscess and subcutaneous atrophy may occur at the injection site.
Note	The goal is to keep tetanus immunization current not specifically to prevent tetanus infection from the current wound. Persons in the United States have a right not to be immunized. Children can receive a religious exception and be in public school without the recommended immunizations.

RELATED CONDITIONS AND INFORMATION

LOCAL ANESTHESIA

Local Anesthesia is usually done by local infiltration or regional block. Sedation or conscious sedation can be used.

AVULSION

An avulsion is a full-thickness skin loss and approximation of the skin edges is impossible.

CONTROL OF EXTERNAL HEMORRHAGE

For hemorrhage of the extremities, elevate the extremity as high as possible above the heart level and compress the area. With the elevation of the extremity maintained, a compression bandage will control the bleeding.

CONTUSION

A contusion is an altered area of skin integrity caused by blunt trauma.

FACIAL LACERATIONS

Keep the tissue moist with saline gauze before cleaning, after cleaning, and before suturing to minimize devitalization of the tissue. Keeping the tissue vital is beneficial for skin layer matching and to minimizing scarring. Betadine and peroxide can be caustic to tissue. Facial sutures should be removed in 3 to 5 days to further minimize scarring.

HEMOPHILIA

Even minor trauma can cause major bleeding in the patient with hemophilia. Hemorrhage can occur anywhere in the body. The partial thromboplastin time (PTT) is prolonged. Bleeding into a joint is extremely painful and leads to severe disability. The patients and family are knowledgeable about the disease. Therapy is FFP for hemophilia A and von Willebrand's disease and factor VII for hemophilia B. Patients often have factor VIII at home but are unable to give it because of difficult intravenous access from repeated transfusions.

In the past, the concentrate was made from fractionated freeze-dried antihemophilic factor and contained 250 to 1500 UV of factor VIII:C in a reconstituted volume. Factor VIII is also produced by recombinant DVA techniques and is considered to be the replacement of choice. Cryoprecipitate derived from fresh frozen plasma was once the mainstay of hemophilia A and may be used when noninfectious factor VIII concentrates are not available.

Most hemophiliac patients require large doses of narcotic analgesia because they have built a tolerance from frequent use. Most patients know the amount of medication necessary to relieve their pain. Patients are often under-treated by medical providers for fear of contributing to an addiction.

A hemophilia patient should not be given an IM injection unless factor replacement was given within the past several days.

Intraosseous infusion of intravenous fluids and blood products can be administered into the sternum on adults and the anterior tibia on children.

June 11, 1975, the Governing Body of Jehovah's Witnesses adjusted its previous position and agreed it was acceptable for hemophiliacs to accept repeated treatment. Prior to this date, the hemophiliacs were only allowed treatment once as medicine.

The Jehovah's Witness (JW) doctrine does not believe in accepting homologous or autologous blood transfusions, and acute normovolemic hemodilution. The following procedures may also be refused but are at the discretion of each individual's interpretation of the JW doctrine: autologous blood salvage or cell-saver scavenging, closed-circuit acute normovolemic hemodilution, epidural blood patch, heart-lung machine, hemodialysis, labeling or tagging, platelet gel, and plasmapheresis.

LACERATION

Lacerations are wounds caused by blunt force trauma. Superficial lacerations are through the epidermis and dermis. Deep lacerations involve the deep muscle layers.

LOCAL ANESTHESIA DURATION

Review of Local Anesthesia Duration	
Lidocaine (Xylocaine)	Lasts for 30 to 60 minutes
Lidocaine with epinephrine	Lasts 60 to 90 minutes
Marcaine 0.5% (bupivacaine)	Lasts for 3 to 6 hours. Marcaine can be used as a regional block and injection directly into the wound that impairs matching of the wound edges can be avoided.

PRESSURE POINTS

Pressure Points to Stop Arterial Hemorrhage	
Axillary	To control an axillary artery hemorrhage, apply pressure to the head of the humerus. Press high in the axilla against the upper part of the humerus.
Brachial	To control a brachial artery hemorrhage, apply pressure to the shaft of the humerus. Press against the humerus by pulling aside the biceps and pressing deep against the bone.

Pressure Points to Stop Arterial Hemorrhage	
Carotid	To control a carotid artery hemorrhage, apply pressure against the cervical vertebra. Press one inch to the side of the prominence of the windpipe. Hold pressing deeply towards the back.
Facial	To control a facial artery hemorrhage, apply pressure against the lower part of the jaw. Press an inch in front of the angle of the jaw.
Femoral	To control a femoral artery, apply pressure to the rim of the pelvis or the shaft of the femur. Press against the pelvis midway between the iliac spine and symphysis pubis or press high on the inner thigh about 3 inches below the rim of the pelvis.
Posterior tibial	To control a posterior tibial hemorrhage, apply pressure against the inner side of the tibia towards the ankle. Press against the tibia above the hemorrhage. For hemorrhage of the foot, press behind the inner ankle.
Subclavian	To control a subclavian artery hemorrhage, apply pressure against the first rib behind the clavicle. Press deep down and backward over the center of the clavicle after depressing the shoulder.
Temporal	To control a temporal artery hemorrhage, apply pressure against the temporal bone. Press against the bony prominence in front of the ear or temple.

SUTURE REMOVAL

Review of Anticipated Suture Removal Times	
Face	3 to 5 days
Scalp, trunk, hands, feet	7 to 10 days
Arms and legs	10 to 14 days
Over joints	14 days

TETANUS PRONE WOUNDS

Wounds greater than six hours old, avulsed, crushed with devitalized tissue, or contaminated with dirt, feces, or salvia are considered tetanus prone.

TYPES OF WOUNDS

Review of Types of Wounds

Review of Types of Wounds	
Open	An abrasion is a superficial wound in which the topmost layers of the skin are scraped off. An avulsion is a wound with a full-thickness skin loss and approximation of the skin edges is impossible. A gunshot wound is caused by a projectile driving into or through the body. An incision is caused by a sharp-edged object. A laceration is a rough, irregular wound caused by blunt force trauma. A puncture is caused by an object puncturing the skin. A penetrating wound is caused by an object entering the body.
Closed	A contusion (bruise) is caused by blunt force trauma that damages the tissue under the skin. A crush injury is caused by an extreme amount of force applied over a long period of time. A hematoma is caused by damage to a blood vessel that causes blood to collect under the skin.

WOUND MANAGEMENT

Review of Wound Management
Control bleeding with pressure
Ask that local anesthesia be initiated. Clean the wound. Scrub if necessary. If contaminated, irrigate for five to 30 minutes with normal saline. Soak puncture wounds for 15 to 30 minutes.
Set up for debridement of devitalized tissue and approximation of wound edges with sutures, staples, or Steri-Strips by assembling and arranging instruments, light, sutures, and a kick bucket.
After the wound is débrided and approximated, apply a thin layer of antibiotic ointment and dress with a dry sterile dressing. DO NOT USE PLASTIC BAND-AIDS. Plastic coverings macerate the skin and prevent healing. Facial injuries are covered with ointment and normally no dressing is applied.
Instruct the patient in proper home wound care. Recommend the time and place for suture or staple removal.

WOUND AGE

Wound age is a critical factor in deciding whether a wound should undergo primary closure. A wound more than six hours old is considered a high risk for infection.

WOUND CLOSURES

Review of Wound Closures

Review of Wound Closures	
Tape closures (Steri-Strips®)	Tape closures are used for superficial wounds under minimal tension. An anesthetic is not necessary, and a lower rate of infection is associated with tape closures than no closure. No follow-up visit is required for tape removal
Sutures	Sutures approximate wound edges, decrease infections, promote wound healing, and minimize scarring. A local anesthetic is required. A follow-up visit is required for suture removal.
Staples	Staples approximate the wound edges, have a low rate of infection, but do not approximate the wound edges close enough to minimize scarring. A follow-up visit is required to remove the staples.
Tissue adhesive (Dermabond®)	Dermabond® is a cyanoacrylate tissue adhesive that forms a strong bond across apposed wound edges providing a flexible water-resistant protective coating and eliminates the need for suture removal. Tissue adhesive should not be used on jagged wounds, animal bites, severely contaminated wounds, ulcers, puncture wounds, mucous membranes (including mucocutaneous junctions) or areas of high moisture content, such as the groin or axillae. The adhesive may be used for sutures of 5-0 or smaller to selected wounds on the face, torso and extremities.

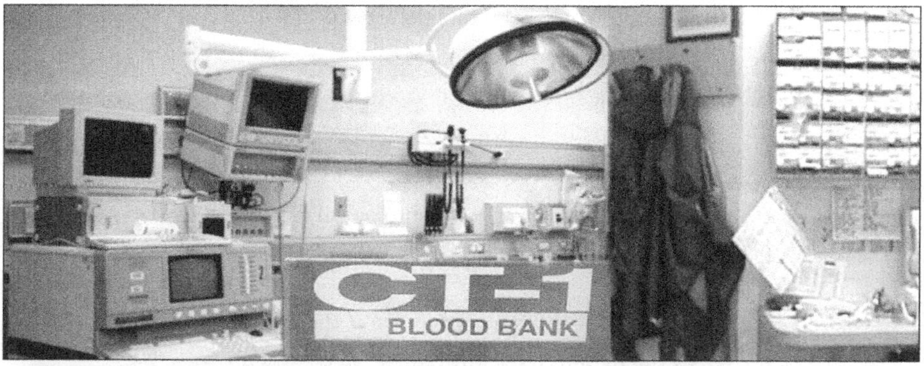

24 MOTOR VEHICLE COLLISION

For details on triage see Chapter 34, Triage in a Nutshell.

PATIENT'S STORY – INTERVIEW QUESTIONS

1. When did the crash occur?
2. Describe the crash.
   a. What type of vehicle was involved; e.g., ground vehicle (auto, bicycle, motorcycle), marine vehicle (personal watercraft, boat), or aircraft (plane, helicopter, balloon)?
   b. What was the point of impact to the vehicle; e.g., front driver, passenger side, the rear? Be specific.
   c. What was the patient's location within the vehicle; e.g., driver, front-passenger, rear-passenger behind the driver?
3. Were any deformities present inside the vehicle; e.g., dash, side-windows, steering wheel, mirror?
   a. Did the patient have any protection; e.g., seatbelt, shoulder strap, helmet or airbag and did the air bag deploy?
   b. Was the patient trapped or thrown from the vehicle? If trapped, what was the extrication time?
   c. Was a fire or explosion involved?
   d. Were chemicals or hazardous materials involved? If yes, consider HAZMAT (hazardous material protocol). Is the placard number or chemical ID known?
4. Where are the patient's injuries?
   a. Where are the injuries and what type of injuries were sustained, e.g., right arm abrasion, left foot amputation, face soft tissue, left leg bony, chest blunt trauma, left foot burn?
   b. Are any associated symptoms present?

5. How is the patient's normal function affected?
    a. Was the patient unconsciousness at the scene?
    b. For how long?
    c. Does the patient have amnesia for the events of the incident?
    d. Have any drugs been used that affect the level of consciousness?
    e. Does the patient have any neurological deficits?
    f. Does the patient have normal neurovascular function distal to the injuries?
    g. Does the patient have normal use of the injured areas?
    h. Does the patient have any pain?
        i. Where is the pain or discomfort located?
        ii. Does it radiate?
        iii. How does the patient describe the severity of the pain?
        iv. It is appropriate to use the terms mild, moderate, or severe or the words of the patient.
        v. Does the patient have any associated symptoms; e.g., nausea, vomiting, headache, sweating, irregular-heartbeat, or the urge to urinate or defecate?
6. What caused the crash?
    a. Did a mechanical problem or another vehicle cause the crash?
    b. Did a medical problem cause the incident; e.g., chest pain, shortness of breath, seizure, or syncope?
7. Is unlawful activity suspected?
    a. Was law enforcement at the scene?
    b. What agency?

> Medical personnel are obligated to notify law enforcement if unlawful activity is suspected.

8. Was any treatment started before coming to the hospital and has it helped?
9. Has the patient had a history of prior injury to the same area?
    a. What was the diagnosis?
    b. What was the treatment?
10. Does the patient have any pertinent past history?
11. Does the patient take any routine medications?
    a. What is the name, dosage, route, and frequency of each medication?
    b. When was the last dose?

12. Does the patient take any complementary or alternative therapies, herbal products, over-the-counter medications or supplements, or natural therapies?
    a. What is the name, dosage, route and frequency of each therapy?
    b. When was the last dose or therapy?
13. Does the patient have allergies to drugs or foods?
    a. What is the name of the allergen?
    b. What was the reaction?
14. When was the patient's last tetanus immunization?
15. If the patient is female and between the ages of 10 to 50 years, when was the first day of her last menstrual period?

NURSING DOMAIN

The nursing domain, nursing diagnosis and plan of care can only be determined after an in-depth interview and consideration of the patient's story.

Domain 12. Comfort. Class 1. Physical comfort.
Domain 11. Safety/Protection. Class 1. Infection. Class 2. Physical injury.

ANTICIPATED MEDICAL CARE

Review of the Anticipated Medical Care of Motor Vehicle Crash Anticipated Medical Care of Patients	
Exam	Full body
Urine tests	Dip urine for blood; pregnancy test for women of reproductive age unless they have had a hysterectomy
Blood tests	Hemogram, electrolytes, renal studies, type and screen for serious blood loss
ECG	ECG for females and males over 35 years with complaints of chest pain and for all ages if chest trauma is suspected.
Radiographic studies	Anticipate x-rays of the cervical spine to include cross table lateral, anterior to posterior, odontoid, and obliques, x-rays of chest, pelvis, and thoracic and lumbar spine, CT scan or MRI of injured spinal areas, and x-rays of areas of suspected bony damage
Diet	NPO
IV	Normal saline or Ringer's solution
Medications	Pain medications and intravenous steroids for patients with spinal cord involvement

Review of the Anticipated Medical Care of Motor Vehicle Crash Anticipated Medical Care of Patients	
Other	A nasogastric tube to reduce the risk of vomiting and aspiration in a non-alert patient, an indwelling urinary catheter to decompress the bladder and monitor urinary output
Disposition	Hospital admission is required for moderate or severe body injury. Anticipate transfer to a trauma center if serious multiple traumas are present.
General indicators for transfer to a trauma center	• Glasgow coma scale < 13 or systolic blood pressure < 90 or respiratory rate < 10 or > 29 • Penetrating injury to trunk or head • Flail chest • Two or more long bone fractures • Burns > 15% total body surface area or to the face or airway • Evidence of high impact, vehicle deformity with passenger compartment intrusion • Ejection from vehicle • Rollover • Death of same car occupant • Pedestrian stuck at speeds of 20 miles per hour or more • Age < 5 or > 55 years • Known history of cardiac or respiratory disease • When in doubt, call the trauma center and speak with the trauma surgeon. Level one trauma centers are staffed 24 hours a day and serve as an educational resource for emergency personnel. Appropriate interfacility transfer includes the following: • Acceptance by the receiving facility • Copies of the medical record • Qualified personnel with the level of skill and equipment need to care for the patient in transport
Worst-case scenario	The worst-case scenario is sudden circulatory volume loss from an undiagnosed internal bleed. Management is arrangement for STAT surgery and blood replacement.

INITIAL CARE PLAN

Alcohol-based hand sanitizers are the preferred method for cleaning your hands in most clinical situations. Wash your hands with soap and water whenever they are visibly dirty, before eating, and after using the restroom.

1. For the patient in C-spine immobilization, remove shoes, socks, and jewelry that will interfere with the examination and x-rays.
2. Obtain vital signs including pulse oximetry or test capillary refill.
   a. Attach heart monitor leads, automatic blood pressure cuff, and pulse oximetry for continuous monitoring. Document the initial heart monitor strip and document changes of rhythm.
   b. Core temperature is essential. If the patient is unable to cooperate, obtain a rectal temperature.
   c. For a pregnant female, place on fetal monitor.
3. Place on oxygen, 100% by non-rebreather mask.
4. Assure the patient that he is safe, and he will receive attention based on his needs. Instruct the patient that pain medications will be administered as soon as it is safe. Instruct the patient that early pain medications are not always considered safe because they may mask important signs and symptoms of worsening.
5. Establish intravenous access with two large bore intravenous cannulas and draw laboratory blood specimens.
   a. Draw a variety of tubes that will allow the lab to perform hematology, chemistry, and coagulation studies. Patients on anticoagulants and cirrhotic patients need coagulation studies.
   b. Consider drawing other labs; e.g., type and screen, blood cultures.
6. Perform a head-to-toe physical examination.

If two nurses are at the bedside, one can ask the following questions and document the answers of the other who performs the exam. Document positive and negative findings.

   a. What is the size and reaction of the pupils?
   b. Does the patient have any head pain or injuries to the head?
      Is the tongue or mouth injured?
      Is any drainage present from the nose or ears?
   c. Is the trachea midline?
      Is jugular venous distention present (unable to detect under fluorescent light)?

d. Does the chest expand equally?
Is subcutaneous emphysema present?
Are the heart tones within normal limits?
Are the heart tones diminished?
Are any murmurs present?
Does the patient complain of chest pain?
Is the chest tender to palpation?

e. Are the lung sounds clear on the right and left?
Are wheezes or crackles present?
Are the lung sounds decreased or absent in any area of the lungs?

f. Is the abdomen soft, flat, rigid, or distended?
Are bowel sounds normal, hypoactive, hyperactive, or absent?
Does the patient complain of abdominal pain?
Is the patient's abdomen tender to palpation?

g. Is the patient incontinent?
Examination of the genitalia may be deferred if trauma is not suspected.
Do the genitalia appear normal?
Does the patient have bleeding from the urethral meatus or vagina?
Is priapism present?
Does the patient complain of genital pain?
Is the perineal area or genitalia tender to palpation?

h. Does the patient complain of pain when light pressure is applied to the iliac crests?
Is the pelvis stable or unstable?

i. Does the patient have normal motion and sensation in the upper and lower extremities?
Are distal pulses present in the upper and lower extremities?

j. Does the patient have normal movement of his back?
Does the patient complain of back pain?
While keeping the back immobilized, turn the patient.
Inspect the posterior surfaces.
Does the patient have obvious back injuries?
Is the back tender to palpation?

k. Does skin inspection reveal any damage to the skin; e.g., abrasions, lacerations, bruises, needle tracks, or petechiae?

l. Evaluate the level of consciousness based on the mnemonic **AVPU** or **ACDU** level of consciousness score.
AVPU: **A**lert, **V**erbal, **P**ain, **U**nresponsive.
ACDU: **A**lert, **C**onfused, **D**rowsy, **U**nresponsive.

m. In a pregnant female, inspect the perineum, assist with a pelvic examination, auscultate the fetal heart rate (normal 120 to 160), and palpate the uterus to determine size, tenderness, contractions, and firmness.

7. Keep the patient warm. Place a warmed blanket around the head, neck, and shoulders like a shawl. Place another blanket over the body and tightly tuck it around the patient.
8. Position the patient, e.g., to enhance normal body function and comfort. Elevate head of stretcher after C-spine immobilization is removed. For a pregnant female, position on the left side if greater than 20 weeks gestation or tilt the backboard.
9. Give initial medications covered by hospital protocols, e.g., tetanus toxoid.
10. Consider collecting wound cultures before cleaning. Clean, irrigate, and dress wounds with sterile saline moistening dressings.
11. Consider placing drains.
    a. Gastric tube to decompress the stomach and prevent vomiting and aspiration
    b. Indwelling urinary catheter to decompress the bladder and monitor urinary output
12. Initiate orders for appropriate x-rays of suspected bony damage.
13. Instruct the patient not to eat or drink and teach the patient and family the rationale for the NPO status.
14. Elevate the siderails and place the stretcher in the lowest position.
15. Inform the patient, family, and caregivers of the usual plan of care and the expected overall time in the ER.
16. Provide the patient with a device to reach someone for assistance and explain how to use it. Ask the patient to call for help before getting off the stretcher.

ONGOING CARE PLAN

Inform the medical provider of adverse changes noted during ongoing evaluation. Document that the medical provider was notified of the adverse change. Document if orders were or were not received.

1. Monitor temperature, heart rate and rhythm, respiratory rate and rhythm, blood pressure, temperature, and effectiveness of breathing.
2. For the pregnant female:
    a. Monitor fetal heart rate and movement.
    b. Monitor for uterine contractions.
3. Monitor therapy closely for the patient's therapeutic response.
    a. The usual time for a medication effectiveness check is 20 to 30 minutes after giving the drug.
    b. If therapy is not effective, ask the medical provider for a repeat dose or an alternative.
4. Monitor physical status:

   a. Monitor neurovascular function in extremities
   b. Monitor extremity movements by asking the patient to gently wiggle toes and fingers and gently lift arms and legs. Compare with baseline.
   c. Monitor extremity sensation with a gentle touch on all extremities and compare with baseline.
5. Monitor closely for the development of adverse reactions to therapy.
   a. Perform interventions to relieve the adverse reaction.
   b. Ask the medical provider for a remedy.
6. Keep the patient, family, and caregivers well informed of the plan of care and the remaining time anticipated before disposition.
7. Monitor the patient's laboratory and radiographic results and notify the medical provider of critical abnormalities. Remedy abnormalities as ordered.
8. Notify the medical provider when all diagnostic results are available for review. Ask for establishment of a diagnosis and disposition.

DISCHARGE INSTRUCTIONS

1. Provide the patient with the name of the nurse and doctor in the emergency room.
2. Inform the patient of their diagnosis or why a definitive diagnosis couldn't be made. Explain what caused the problem if known.
3. Teach the patient how to take the medication as prescribed and how to manage the common side effects. Instruct the patient not to drive or perform any dangerous tasks while taking narcotic pain medications.
4. Instruct the patient that:
   a. People involved in motor vehicle crashes often have pain and stiffness that worsens over the next one to two days.
   b. It is possible to have an internal injury, glass foreign body, or minor fracture become evident over time.
   c. If any unusual symptoms develop (e.g., abdominal or chest pain, difficulty breathing, or blood in the urine or stool), contact the follow-up medical provider immediately or return to the emergency room.

5. For the patient with a soft tissue injury teach the mnemonic **PRICE**.
   Protect the injured area and keep out of harm's way; do not leave an injured foot in the way of a passerby. Cover skin that is not intact with a sterile dressing when in a dirty environment.
   Rest the area. Do not use the injured extremity. Use crutches or a wheelchair to rest an injured lower extremity.
   Ice the area.
   Compress the area with light pressure from a compression bandage or ice pack to reduce the risk of swelling.
   Elevate the injured area above the level of the heart.
   When the injured area is not managed properly, the patient pays the PRICE of increased pain and disability.
6. For the patient with a fracture, inform the patient that splints can become too tight if swelling develops. Watch carefully for loss of the normal color in the fingers or toes and increased pain. Call the follow-up medical provider if a problem develops.
7. Instruct the patient that must not bear weight that:
   a. Crutches can be used to support your weight. Do not bear weight on the injured leg and do not bear the body's weight on the crutches up against the armpit. This can cause serious and permanent nerve damage. Keep the arms straight and support the body's weight on the crutch handles.
   b. The two crutches should serve as a support for the injured leg and swing with that leg. Move the crutches and the injured leg forward at the same time, then pick up the crutches and step forward on the uninjured leg.
   c. The rubber tips must be kept clean and tightly affixed to the crutch. Do not use on wet surfaces or on ice.
   d. If the arms cannot support your weight on crutches, a wheelchair can be used.
8. Notify the follow-up medical provider if any problems develop regarding the use of the crutches.
9. Instruct the patient with an injury caused by blunt or sharp trauma that:
   a. An injury must be kept clean and dry.
   b. The dressing applied in the ER must be removed after one to two days and the wound left open to the air.
   c. Some injuries of the face and scalp are not covered with a dressing in the ER. These wounds may be covered with a dry sterile dressing if needed to protect the area.
   d. Elevation of the area will reduce the risk of swelling.
   e. The injury should be kept clean with mild soap and water and antibiotic over-the-counter ointment should be applied two times a day for the first three days.

f. Follow-up is recommended for suture removal.

10. Some injuries contaminated with dirt or bacteria are not sutured. These are considered dirty wounds and further care is necessary at home.
    a. Soak the area in warm water and prescribed solution for twenty minutes three times a day for the first three days.
    b. Keep the wound covered with a dry sterile dressing between soaks. If the wound is dry and clean after three days of soaks, stop the soaking, and keep it clean, dry, and covered.
    c. Not all dirty wounds need antibiotics. If antibiotics are prescribed, take them until the pills are gone. Do not stop when the wound looks better.
    d. Signs of infection are redness, swelling, red streaks, and pus. Notify the follow-up medical provider if any of these symptoms develop.
11. Recommend a medical provider for follow-up care. Provide the name, address, and phone number with a recommendation of when to schedule the care.
12. Instruct the patient to call the follow-up medical provider immediately or return to the emergency room if the pain or problem worsens in any way or any unusual symptoms develop. Encourage the patient NOT to IGNORE WORSENING OR PERSISTENT SYMPTOMS.
13. Ask for verbal confirmation or demonstration of understanding and reinforce teaching as needed.

COMMONLY ORDERED MEDICATIONS

DILAUDID

Dilaudid (hydromorphone)	
Indications	Moderate to severe pain
Dose	Typical dose 1 to 5 mg IV. Titrate to response. No maximum dose.
Onset	IV onset rapid, peak 15 to 30 minutes, duration 3 to 4 hours
Side effects	Drowsiness, dizziness, confusion, sedation, increased intracranial pressure, nausea, vomiting, urinary retention, respiratory depression
Monitor	CNS changes, respiratory effectiveness, allergic rash
Note	Dilaudid 5 mg equivalent to Morphine 10 mg IM. Dilute to 4 or 5 ml with NS or sterile water for injection and administer slowly over at least 2 to 3 minutes Antidote is naloxone.

PHENERGAN

Phenergan (promethazine)	
Indications	Nausea, vomiting
Dose	12.5 to 25 mg IV every 4 to 6 hours. When used intravenously, promethazine injection should be given in concentration no greater than 25 mg/ml at a rate not to exceed 25 mg/min. Preferably inject through a medication port in IV tubing that is known to be functioning satisfactorily. 25 mg IM every 4 to 6 hours
Pediatric dose	More than 2 years 0.25 to 0.5 mg/kg IM or IV every 4 to 6 hours
Onset	IV onset 3 to 5 min., duration 4 to 6 hours IM onset 20 min., duration 4 to 6 hours
Side effects	Drowsiness, sedation, hypotension, palpitations, tachycardia
Monitor	Vital signs, responsiveness, respiratory effectiveness

TETANUS AND DIPHTHERIA TOXOID, ADSORBED FOR ADULTS

Tetanus and Diphtheria Toxoid, Adsorbed for Adult	
Indications	Immunization against tetanus and diphtheria
Dose	0.5 mg for adults and children 7 years and older
Side effects	Local reactions such as erythema, induration, and tenderness are common. Systemic reactions include fever, chills, myalgias, and headache.
Monitor	Local reactions are usually self-limiting. Sterile abscess and subcutaneous atrophy may occur at the injection site.
Note	The goal is to keep tetanus immunization current not specifically to prevent tetanus infection in the current wound. Persons in the United States have a right not to be immunized. Children can receive a religious exception and be in public school without the recommended immunizations.

RELATED CONDITIONS AND INFORMATION

ABDOMINAL TRAUMA

Review of Abdominal Trauma	
Definition	Abdominal trauma is a blunt or penetrating force to the abdomen.
Symptoms	Symptoms may include abdominal pain, distention, and hypovolemia shock.
Blood tests	Common blood tests include serum amylase, urine for hematuria, nasogastric tube drainage for blood, and a pregnancy test for females able to conceive.

Review of Abdominal Trauma	
Radiographic studies	Ultrasound of the abdomen identifies bleeding. CT of the abdomen identifies solid organ lacerations. IVP, cystogram, or urethrogram identifies damage to the kidneys, ureter, or bladder. Plane x-rays visualizes foreign objects and free air.
Other	Diagnostic peritoneal lavage may be done to determine if peritoneal bleeding is present. Normal saline is instilled into the peritoneal cavity and aspirated. The aspirate is tested for blood. A positive test is > 100,000 red blood cells/mm3 in the aspirate and may indicate an injury to the bowel is positive for fecal matter and blood. This procedure cannot determine if a retroperitoneal bleed is present. It is contraindicated if the patient has a history of multiple abdominal surgeries (adhesions can prevent the bowel from moving and increase the risk of bowel puncture), cirrhosis, coagulopathy, and in the extremely obese patient.
Ongoing Monitoring	Monitoring includes vital signs, urinary output, gastric-tube drainage, and frequent inspection of the abdomen for signs of injury. Look for Gray Turner's sign (bruising of the flank), Cullen's sign (periumbilical bruising), and distention. Auscultate for a change in abdominal bowel sounds. Percuss the abdomen for a change from baseline and palpate for tenderness.
Diet	NPO
IV	Intravenous access with two large bore cannulas (14 or 16 gauge), fluid resuscitation with normal saline, blood replacement.
Procedures	Procedures may include stomach decompression with a gastric tube to reduce the risk of aspiration, urinary bladder decompression with a urinary catheter and monitoring of urinary output, dressing of wounds, and stabilization of impaled objects.
Medications	Prophylactic antibiotics are often ordered to reduce the risk of peritonitis.
Disposition	Prepare the patient for possible surgery and hospital admission or transfer. Obtain consents for surgery and anesthesia.

ABRASIONS

Abrasions are injuries of the skin caused by a mechanical scraping away of a portion of the skin. When the abrasion is caused by scraping against pavement, the injury is commonly called road rash. A thorough scrubbing is necessary to remove the road particles and debris. The procedure is painful. Lidocaine jelly can be spread over the area and left for approximately 5 minutes to lessen the discomfort.

The area can also be infiltrated with Lidocaine or a regional block can be performed.

AEIOU TIPS

AEIOU TIPS Mnemonic of Potential Causes of Loss of Consciousness			
A	Alcohol	T	Trauma and tumors
E	Epilepsy	I	Infections
I	Insulin	P	Psychiatric
O	Overdose	S	Stroke
U	Uremia		

AMPUTATION

Review of Amputations	
Definition	An amputation is a traumatic separation of a digit or limb from the body.
Symptoms	Symptoms include loss of the part or tissue and may include bleeding, hypovolemic shock, and pain.
Tests	X-rays are ordered to determine bony damage.
Management	Management includes control of bleeding with pressure dressings, elevation, cleansing of the wound, splinting, and a sterile dressing.
Disposition	Prepare for hospital admission and surgical intervention or transfer to a facility with a reclamation team.
Note	Keep the amputated part covered with saline moistened gauze in a watertight plastic bag or container. Place the bag or container in ice and water.

BLOOD LOSS

	Class I	Class II	Class III	Class IV
Blood loss	Up to 750 cc	750 to 1500 cc	1500 to 2000 cc	> 2000
HR	< 100	> 100	> 120	> 140
BP	Normal	Normal	Decreased	Decreased
RR	14 to 20	20 to 30	30 to 35	> 35
Cap refill	Normal	Slight delay	from 2 to 3 seconds	No filling
Skin	Pink and cool	Pale and cold	Pale, cold, moist	Mottled
Urine	> 30 cc/hr	20 to 30 cc/hr	5 to 15 cc/hr	< 5 cc/hr
Behavior	Slight anxiety	Mild anxiety	Anxious, confused	Lethargic, confused

	Class I	Class II	Class III	Class IV
Fluid	Crystalloid	Crystalloid	Crystalloid and blood	Crystalloid and blood

BLOOD TRANSFUSIONS

Massive blood transfusions require 1 to 2 units of fresh frozen plasma for every five units of blood transfused to treat dilutional coagulopathy.

Type and screen: The patient's blood sample is tested for ABO, Rh, and unexpected antibodies. The derived information is stored in the blood bank for immediate cross matching if transfusion becomes necessary.

Cross match: The patient's serum is tested with donor red cells to check the ABO compatibility when the patient's medical provider orders a transfusion of red cells.

CHEST TRAUMA

Review of Chest Trauma	
Definition	Chest trauma is defined as a blunt trauma or penetrating force to the chest.
Symptoms	Symptoms may include pain, swelling, ecchymosis, laceration or puncture of the thorax, shortness of breath, difficulty swallowing, and hoarseness.
Assessment	Assessment includes the following: • Inspection of the chest for ecchymosis and asymmetrical movements • Inspection of the neck for swelling, ecchymosis, and to establish a baseline • Listening to the movement of air through the airways to establish a baseline • Auscultation of lung sounds • Palpation of the chest wall for the presence of crepitus and subcutaneous emphysema
Note	A fracture of the scapula, 1st rib, and 2nd rib has a high probability of underlying tissue damage. Although rare, clavicular fractures near the sternum carry the potential of damage to the underlying structures.
Tests	Tests may include cardiac enzymes, ABG, Swan-Ganz catheter or CVP, chest x-ray, ultrasound study of the aorta, esophagoscopy, CT scan, bronchoscopy, laryngoscopy, electrocardiogram, and echocardiography.

Review of Chest Trauma	
Airway and breathing	Airway management may include securing the airway with endotracheal intubation or a surgical airway and providing 100% oxygen with ventilator support. At a minimum, supplemental oxygen by 100% via non-rebreather mask is required.
Pulmonary contusion	Pulmonary contusion is the most common cause of impaired gas exchange in blunt chest trauma and best indicated on chest x-ray as patchy infiltrations initially and progressing later to consolidation. Approximately 75% of motor vehicle crash patients with blunt chest trauma have some degree of pulmonary contusion because of the amount of mechanical energy transferred to the chest.
Pneumo-thorax	If pneumothorax is suspected, anticipate possible chest tube insertion or needle thoracentesis for tension pneumothorax. Have ready a 12 to 16-gauge needle for insertion into the second intercostal space in the midclavicular line (the intercostal artery and vein are located under the third rib) or the fifth intercostal space in the midaxillary line on the injured side of the pneumothorax (opposite the tracheal deviation).
Fluids	Anticipate intravenous access with two large bore (14 or 16 gauge) cannulas and fluid resuscitation without over-hydration with normal saline and blood products.
General	Drains may be necessary (e.g., indwelling urinary catheter, a nasogastric tube) to decompress the stomach and prevent aspiration. Fluid resuscitation is usually with normal saline. A thoracotomy may be necessary in the ER. Cover open wounds with nonporous dressings and stabilize impaled objects.
Disposition	Hospital admission may be required for surgical intervention and support.

COMMON HEAD INJURIES

Review of Common Head Injuries	
Anatomical location	The brain is covered with three fibrous membranes. The pia mater is the thick membrane covering nearest the brain, the arachnoid mater is a thinner membrane between the pia and dura, and the dura is the outermost covering. A mnemonic is PAD starting from the brain the Pia, Arachnoid and Dura membranes form a pad to protect and hold the brain. To define the location of a hematoma or bleed, use the prefix *epi* (above) or the prefix *sub* (below) with the name of the membrane.

Review of Common Head Injuries	
Cerebral concussion	A cerebral concussion is a mild closed head injury with a history of loss of consciousness. Amnesia and headache are common symptoms.
Cerebral contusion	A cerebral contusion is a closed head injury with bruising of the brain.
Epidural hematoma	An epidural hematoma is a hematoma located above (epi) the dura usually from an arterial source. Rapid surgical intervention is considered the best treatment.
Hemorrhage	Intracerebral hemorrhage is a hemorrhage inside the brain.
Penetrating head injury	A penetrating head injury is a wound from a missile that has penetrated the skull.
Scalp laceration	A scalp laceration causes profuse bleeding and is seldom life threatening but causes a great deal of anxiety.
Skull fracture	Skull fractures may have obvious deformity or be visible only on x-ray or CT. The skull may need to be repaired. The threat to life is the damage to the brain and surrounding tissue caused by the fracture.
Subarachnoid hematoma	A subarachnoid hematoma is located below (sub) the arachnoid membrane usually from an arterial bleed.
Subdural hematoma	A subdural hematoma is located below (sub) the dura usually from a venous source and can develop days or weeks after an injury.

COMPARTMENTAL SYNDROME

Review of Compartmental Syndrome	
Definition	Compartmental syndrome is a condition in which tissue is severely constricted in its space causing damage to the tissue. The condition commonly occurs hours or days after the injury.
Cause	The cause of compartmental syndrome is a trauma that causes inflammation and swelling of the tissue. More swelling than can be contained within the compartment without constriction damage of the tissue.
Symptoms	Symptoms may include progressive pain, sensory deficits, muscle weakness, and a tense swollen area. The syndrome usually occurs in the forearms and lower legs.
Tests	Tests may include measurement of muscle compartment pressure. A reading of greater than 35 to 45 mmHg is indicative of the need for fasciotomy.

Review of Compartmental Syndrome	
Management	Management includes elevation to the level of the heart to assure venous outflow (elevation above the heart decreases perfusion) and ongoing monitoring of size and tenseness of the injured area.
Disposition	Hospital admission may be required for potential surgical fasciotomy or repair of neurovascular damage.

CONTROL OF EXTERNAL HEMORRHAGE

For hemorrhage of the extremities, elevate the extremity as high as possible above the heart level and compress the area. With the elevation of the extremity maintained, a compression bandage will control the bleeding.

CORD FUNCTION LEVELS

Level of Injury Related to Level of Function	
C1 to C3	Usually fatal, requires immediate and continuous respiratory support
C4	Respiratory difficulty, no function in all extremities, head and neck control, shoulder shrug
C5	Shoulder control and shrug, elbow flexion, wrist rotation
C6	Shoulder control, elbow flexion, wrist rotation and extension
C7	Shoulder control, elbow flexion and extension, wrist rotation and extension
C8 to T1	Neck weakness, limited or natural hand function
T2 to T6	Normal upper extremity function, increased control of trunk muscles
T7 to T12	Normal upper extremity function, increased abdominal muscle control
L1 to L5	Movement of hips and knees
S1 to S5	Increasing return of bladder, bowel, and sexual functions

CRUSH INJURIES

Review of Crush Injuries	
Definition	A crush injury is destruction caused by extreme pressure against the tissue resulting in damage to skin, muscle, nerves, and bone.
Cause	The cause of a crush injury is a traumatic force.
Symptoms	Symptoms may include pain, loss of neurovascular function distal to the injury, hemorrhage, hypovolemic shock, swelling, and ecchymosis.
Tests	Tests may include x-rays and CT.

Review of Crush Injuries	
Management	Medical management includes control of bleeding, fluid resuscitation with normal saline to increase urinary output and facilitate excretion of myoglobin, elevation, cleaning, and irrigation of the wounds, monitoring of urinary output volume and urinary myoglobin, and monitoring of neurovascular function distal to the wound.
Disposition	Hospital admission may be required for possible surgical débridement, fasciotomy, or amputation.

CULLEN'S SIGN

Cullen's sign is bruising around the umbilicus caused from free blood in the abdomen.

EYE BLUNT TRAUMA

Injuries Caused by Blunt Trauma	
Iris Injury	An iris injury is an inflammation to the iris and ciliary bodies from a contusion. Treatment may include cycloplegic and steroidal agents. Complications can include vision loss and loss of the eye.
Lens Injury	Lens injuries may include total and partial dislocation and opacification. Treatment may include surgery. Consents must be obtained for surgery and anesthesia. Repair is not emergent unless the injury is causing acute angle-closure glaucoma.
Subconjunctival hemorrhage	Bleeding beneath the conjunctiva is a hemorrhage making the white part of the eye bright red. Trauma, simple sneezing, or coughing can cause a subconjunctival hemorrhage. This painless benign problem heals spontaneously without treatment.

CHEMICAL BURNS TO THE EYE

Review of Chemical Burns of the Eye	
Acuity	EMERGENT A chemical burn of the eye takes first priority after a threat to life.
Causes	Chemical eye burns are caused by an alkaline, acid, or chemical irritant that denature the tissue. The cornea appears white. Some chemicals are neutralized on impact. Alkaline burns from concrete, lye, and drain cleaners continue to burn the eye until the substance is removed.

Review of Chemical Burns of the Eye	
Management	Initial management is immediate copious irrigation with normal saline or at an eyewash station. Irrigation continues until the pH reaches 7.40. Irrigation is commonly 2 liters over 30 minutes. For severe cases, irrigation can last as long as 2 to 4 hours. When the pH reaches 7.40, medical management may include topical antibiotics, cycloplegic, steroids, bilateral eye patches, and systemic analgesia.
Disposition	Ophthalmology consultation is essential.

EYE THERMAL BURNS

Review of Thermal Burns of the Eye	
Acuity	EMERGENT
Causes	Eye globe burns are commonly caused by heat, hot metal, steam, or ignited gasoline.
Management	Medical management may include analgesia, sedation, eye irrigation, antibiotics, and bilateral eye patches.
Disposition	Ophthalmology consultation is recommended.

EYE EXTERNAL EXAMINATION AND EVALUATION OF EYE MOTILITY

Review of External Examination and Evaluation of Eye Motility
Begin the exam away from the eye and gradually move closer.
Inspect for lacerations, bruises, and differences between the eyes.
Inspect the eyelids, lashes, and how the eyes lay in the sockets.
Inspect the conjunctiva and sclera for colors
Evaluate the patient's ability to move the eyes through the six positions of gaze by asking the patient to follow a finger moved around the eye. Asking the child to follow a toy is more apt to be successful.

EYE MEDICATION INSTILLATION AND APPLICATION OF PATCHES

Review of Eye Medication Instillation and Application of Patches
Pull the lower eyelid downward and ask the patient to look up.
Instill eye drops or a thin line of ointment into the cul-de-sac of the lower eyelid. When eye drops are placed in the inner canthus the solution drains immediately into the lacrimal duct and then into the nose. If more than one drug is administered, wait several minutes between drugs.
Ask the patient to blink several times and roll his eyes gently to expose the entire eye surface to the medications.
Ask the patient to apply pressure for the next few minutes to the tear duct near the nose to minimize systemic absorption.

Review of Eye Medication Instillation and Application of Patches
Instruct the patient not to tightly squeeze eyelids together causing the medication to leak out.
Ask the patient to close both eyes and place a horizontally folded eye patch over the lid. The folded patch fills the indention between the brow and the cheek and when taped will apply a light pressure on the globe. Place a second patch unfolded over the first patch and tape obliquely with paper tape.

EYE PENETRATING INJURIES

Review of Penetrating Eye Injuries	
Conjunctival laceration	A fingernail is a common cause of conjunctival laceration. Lacerations < 5 mm are treated with antibiotics and patching. Lacerations > 5 mm require suturing.
Corneal abrasion	Corneal abrasions occur when a foreign body denudes the epithelium. Diagnosis is made by fluorescein stain. Treatment may include pressure patching for 24 to 48 hours to prevent the eyelid from scraping against the denuded area.
Corneal laceration	Corneal lacerations are the next step above abrasions. Small lacerations are treated the same as corneal abrasions. Large lacerations may require suturing in surgery.
Corneal ulcer	A corneal ulceration is often caused by irritation from contact lenses left in the eye too long. The ulcer appears as a white spot on the cornea. Symptoms may include pain, photophobia, vascular congestion, and profuse tearing. Fluorescein stain is used for diagnosis. Treatment may include local and systemic antibiotics, warm compresses, and an eye patch.
Eyelid wounds	Wounds to the eyelids often mean an eye injury. Careful examination of the eye is essential. The eyelids are vascular, and edema develops quickly preventing good approximation of the wound edges. A plastic surgeon is recommended for closure.
Foreign body	Foreign bodies consist of anything that will fit into the eye. Symptoms may include pain, hypersensitivity to light, and excessive tearing. Treatment may include local anesthesia to facilitate examination and removal of the foreign object. A needle should never be used to facilitate removal of an object imbedded in the cornea. Special ophthalmic tools are available. Antibiotic ointment is essential, and patching is often necessary to prevent further damage from scraping of the eyelid and for comfort. Organic materials have a high incidence of infection. Metallic objects can cause rust rings if left in the eye for over 12 hours. Ocular burr drills are used to remove rust rings. Topical anesthetics retard healing and are not for long-term use.

Review of Penetrating Eye Injuries	
Globe rupture	EMERGENT Globe rupture can result from blunt or penetrating trauma. Symptoms may include altered light perception, a deep anterior chamber, hyphema, and occasionally vitreous hemorrhage. AVOID EYE MANIPULATION DO NOT REMOVE CONTACTS DO NOT USE LOCAL EYE MEDICATIONS If the penetrating object is still present, stabilize it and loosely patch both eyes to decrease eye movement. Treatment commonly includes surgery for repair or enucleation.
Intraocular foreign bodies	EMERGENT Small projectiles striking the eye at a high rate of speed can penetrate the eye and come to rest in the anterior chamber. The most common is a metal fragment from a metal drill. Symptoms may be only minor discomfort. A good history is essential. X-rays of the eye are used to identify the size and position of the fragment if it is metal. CT is used for non-metal objects. Treatment may include surgical removal of the object, antibiotics, tetanus toxoid, and patching is often necessary to prevent further damage from scraping of the eyelid and for comfort.

FACIAL INJURIES

Review of Facial Injuries	
Definition	Facial injury is damage to the bones and soft tissues of the face.
Symptoms	Symptoms may include pain, swelling, ecchymosis, and a deformity of the face.
Ongoing monitoring	Monitoring includes observing for increasing edema, a compromised airway, bleeding, decreased level of consciousness, changes in pupil and eye movement, and for signs of impending shock. A reliable indicator of impending shock is a decreased hourly urine output.
Management	Management includes positioning in a high sitting position to maintain a clear airway, manage secretions, and decrease edema. Ice and elevation are essential ER procedures. Prophylactic antibiotics may be given. Hospital admission may be required for treatment and airway support.

FEMUR FRACTURES

Review of Femur Fractures	
Definition	Fracture of the femur is a disruption of the continuity of the femur.

Review of Femur Fractures	
Cause	Causes of a fractured femur include major trauma, falls, motor vehicle crashes, and slip-and-fall injuries in the elderly.
Symptoms	Symptoms may include pain, inability to bear weight, shortening and rotation of the leg, and hypovolemic shock.
Tests	Tests include x-ray.
Management	Management may include immobilization of the leg (traction splint or traction pin), fluid resuscitation with normal saline, ongoing monitoring of sensation, movement, and circulation distal to the fracture, and pre-operative laboratory studies to include type and screen and coagulation studies if on anticoagulants or cirrhotic. Hospital admission may be required for open surgical reduction and internal fixation or continued traction.

FLAIL CHEST

Paradoxical chest wall movement characterizes a flail chest when (1) three-or-more adjacent ribs are fractured in two or more sites or (2) one rib fracture is associated with a costochondral separation or a fractured sternum. The free-floating ribs move inward during inspiration and outward during expiration and pain, shock, and hypoventilation result. Hypercapnia, hypoxia and dyspnea are indicators that ventilatory support is needed. Management may include frequent low-dose narcotics and ventilatory support. The most efficient method of pain control is intercostal nerve block or thoracic epidural analgesia.

FLUORESCEIN STAINING

Review of Fluorescein Staining Technique
Moisten the end of a fluorescein strip with sterile normal saline solution.
Pull down the patient's lower eyelid.
Touch the strip to the fluid inside the lower eyelid and remove the strip.
Ask the patient to blink several times to distribute the stain over the eye.
Examine the cornea with a cobalt blue light (Wood's lamp). Denuded areas of the cornea will show as a bright yellow spot.

FRACTURES

Types of Fractures	
Closed	The skin over the fracture site is intact.
Comminuted	The bone is splintered into fragments.
Complete	The bony continuity is interrupted.
Compression	Seen in the spinal column, usually the lumbar region and is the collapse of the bone tissue of the vertebral body. It may be caused by osteoporosis, tumor or trauma.
Displaced	The proximal and distal segments of bone are not aligned.

Types of Fractures	
Greenstick	The bone is bent.
Impacted	The distal and proximal fracture sites are wedged together.
Open	The skin over the site or near the site is not intact.

FRACTURE MANAGEMENT IN THE ER

Review of the ER Management of Fractures	
Expose	Remove all clothing and jewelry near the suspected fracture site.
Perform a physical assessment	Inspect for color, position, and obvious differences as compared to the uninjured side. Look for a break in the skin and assess for bleeding and deformity. Assess the extremity for pain, pallor, pulses, paresthesia, and paralysis (Five Ps).
Need for splinting	Splint for deformity, pain, bony crepitus, edema, ecchymosis, vascular compromise, open wounds, and paralysis or paresthesia.
Immobilize	Splint with the appropriate splint to immobilize the joints below and above the injury. Avoid manipulations of the bone. Rigid splints, such as plastic devices and metal splints, are used for lower extremity fractures. Soft splints, such as pillows and slings, are used for upper extremity fractures. Traction splints are used for femur and proximal tibial fractures. A thumb spica splint is applied as if the hand were holding a soda can.
PRICE	Protect, rest, ice, compress, and elevate the site. Ice and elevation are essential ER procedures.
Medications	Administer analgesics.
Diagnostic Testing	Order x-rays. The views should include the joints above and below the injury.
On-going monitors	Frequently reassess the five Ps (pain, pallor, pulses, paresthesia, and paralysis).
Disposition	Hospital admission for definitive stabilization, traction, or open reduction and internal fixation. Navicular fractures require immobilization for 12 weeks. They usually occur after a fall on an outstretched hand.

GRAY TURNER'S SIGN

Gray Turner's sign is bruising in the flank area from bleeding into the retroperitoneal space usually caused by trauma.

HEAD INJURY

Review of Head Injury	
Definition	A head injury is damage to the brain or craniofacial area.
Causes	Causes of head injury are blunt acceleration and deceleration forces causing injury as the brain moves within the skull, blunt blows to the head, and penetrating missiles. Associated secondary injury includes hypoxemia, cerebral edema, hypercapnia, hypotension, and increased intracerebral pressure.
Symptoms	Early signs may include headache, nausea, vomiting, a change in the patient's normal level of consciousness, speech, mentation and amnesia of both past and current events. Late signs may include dilated and nonreactive pupil, unresponsiveness, posturing, increased systolic blood pressure, bradycardia, and changes in respiratory rate and rhythm.
Ongoing monitoring	The Glasgow Coma Scale is used as a baseline and for ongoing monitoring. Monitor the pupil's size, shape, equality, and reaction to light and eye motility. Inspect for contusions, development of ecchymosis, and for drainage from the ears or nose. Perform ongoing evaluation of sensation and motor ability and compare to the baseline obtained on initial exam. Monitor vital signs including core temperature.
Tests	Tests may include CT scan of the brain, skull x-rays, MRI, and ABG. If cerebral spinal fluid leak is suspected, test the drainage for glucose. Glucose is a normal finding in spinal fluid. Spinal fluid should not be draining from any orifice.
Airway and breathing	Intubation is considered when the Glasgow Coma Scale is less than 8 as the patient's level of consciousness is acutely decreased and the patient may be unable to clear his airway. Hyperventilation may be done to maintain a PaCO2 between 26 and 30 mmHg with 100% oxygen. A bag-valve mask with an attached reservoir may be used if the patient is not intubated.
Fluids	Support with normal saline to maintain stability. Do not over-hydrate.
Drainage	Medical management may include an oral gastric or nasogastric tube for decompression of the stomach to reduce the risk of vomiting and aspiration and an indwelling urinary catheter for monitoring the urinary output.
Position	The position of choice is to keep the head positioned midline. Rotation of the head can increase intracranial pressure.

Review of Head Injury	
Medications	Medical management may include administration of Mannitol, a diuretic, to decrease intracranial pressure. Monitoring of urine output hourly is essential. Sedatives may be used for restlessness.
Temperature	Maintain a normal core temperature with heating or cooling blankets. Give antipyretic medications as ordered.
Disposition	Hospital admission may be required for surgery (obtain consents for anesthesia and surgery), further diagnostic workup, treatment, and support. Trauma center transfer may be indicated.

HEMOPHILIA

Even minor trauma can cause major bleeding in the patient with hemophilia. Hemorrhage can occur anywhere in the body. The partial thromboplastin time (PTT) is prolonged. Bleeding into a joint is extremely painful and leads to severe disability. The patients and family are knowledgeable about the disease. Therapy is FFP for hemophilia A and von Willebrand's disease and factor VII for hemophilia B. Patients often have factor VIII at home but are unable to give it because of difficult intravenous access from repeated transfusions.

In the past, the concentrate was made from fractionated freeze-dried antihemophilic factor and contained 250 to 1500 UV of factor VIII:C in a reconstituted volume. Factor VIII is also produced by recombinant DVA techniques and is considered to be the replacement of choice. Cryoprecipitate derived from fresh frozen plasma was once the mainstay of hemophilia A and may be used when noninfectious factor VIII concentrates are not available.

Most hemophiliac patients require large doses of narcotic analgesia because they have built a tolerance from frequent use. Most patients know the amount of medication necessary to relieve their pain. Patients are often under-treated by medical providers for fear of contributing to an addiction.

A hemophilia patient should not be given an IM injection unless factor replacement was given within the past several days.

Intraosseous infusion of intravenous fluids and blood products can be administered into the sternum on adults and the anterior tibia on children.

June 11, 1975, the Governing Body of Jehovah's Witnesses adjusted its previous position and agreed it was acceptable for hemophiliacs to accept repeated treatment. Prior to this date, the hemophiliacs were only allowed treatment once as medicine.

The Jehovah's Witness (JW) doctrine does not believe in accepting homologous or autologous blood transfusions, and acute normovolemic hemodilution. The following procedures may also be refused but are at the discretion of each individual's interpretation of the JW doctrine: autologous blood salvage or cell-saver scavenging, closed-circuit acute normovolemic hemodilution, epidural blood patch, heart-lung machine, hemodialysis, labeling or tagging, platelet gel, and plasmapheresis.

HEMORRHAGIC SHOCK

Review of Hemorrhagic Shock	
Definition	When the circulating blood volume is decreased to a point that it is no longer effective for organ and tissue perfusion, the patient is in hemorrhagic shock.
Signs	Signs may include decreasing arterial pressure, tachycardia, cold and clammy skin, pallor, altered mental status, and decreased kidney function.
Ongoing Monitoring	Hypovolemic shock is best evaluated by the hourly urine output. A mean arterial pressure 80 to 100 is needed to perfuse organs. As the shock develops, the urinary output drops.
Management	Management may include fluid resuscitation with intravenous isotonic fluids, replacement of lost blood, and elevation of the legs to increase circulatory volume to the trunk. Determining the source of the bleeding is a priority. Diagnostic bedside ultrasound study of the abdomen can rule out internal hemorrhage needing immediate surgery. Consents must be obtained for anesthesia and surgery. Hospital admission may be required for further fluid resuscitation and treatment of the underlying cause.

IRRIGATION OF THE EYE

Review of the Technique for Eye Irrigation
Wash the entire area about the eye
Assemble the equipment: • Warmed irrigating solution of normal saline • IV tubing • IV cannula with the needle removed attached to the tubing. A nasal cannula attached to the tubing and placed over the bridge of the nose for bilateral irrigation is not recommended.
Place the patient on the affected side or on his back for bilateral irrigation. Pad well with towels.
Run a gentle stream of solution over the eye from the inner canthus to the outer.
Ask the patient to occasionally blink, look up, down, and side-to-side to assure that the irrigating solution reaches all surfaces of the eye.
Evert (turn inside out) the upper eyelid by placing a cotton swab over the eyelid, pulling the eyelashes down, and then up over the swab to irrigate under the upper lid.

INJURY PATTERNS

Review of Body Injury Patterns Related to Vehicle Damage

Review of Body Injury Patterns Related to Vehicle Damage	
Body injury patterns related to vehicular damage	Injury patterns are usually consistent with the vehicular damage. Body injury first occurs to the part of the body facing the vehicular damage and then to the side of the body facing away from it.
Vehicular front-end damage	First injury is to the front of the body that faces the front of the vehicle. The body is then thrown away from the damaged area often injuring the neck and back.
Vehicular side damage	First injury is to the side of the body facing the side of the vehicle; and then, as the body is thrown away from the damage, injury can occur on the opposite side.
Vehicular inside damage	The person inside the car most often causes the damage inside the car. Ask about windshields and side windows broken from the inside outward. Broken inside mirrors could be caused by a head striking the mirror.

INTERNAL HEMORRHAGE, ER MANAGEMENT

Generic ER Management of Hemorrhage
Establish venous access with two large bore (18 to 14 gauge) cannulas or a central venous catheter.
Monitor the heart, blood pressure, pulse oximetry, and hourly urine output.
Administer intravenous fluid with isotonic IV solution (normal saline or Ringer's), albumin, fresh frozen plasma in patients with coagulopathy, and PRBC to maintain a hematocrit of 25 to 30.
Administer vitamin K 10 mg SC in patients with a coagulopathy.
Administer drug therapy specific to the problem.
An exploratory emergency surgery may be required for uncontrolled or prolonged bleeding. Consents must be obtained for anesthesia and surgery.

INTRAOSSEOUS INFUSIONS

Intraosseous infusions are often necessary when venous access is impossible to obtain. Use the sternum on adults and the anterior tibia on children for intraosseous infusion of both intravenous fluids and blood products.

JOINT DISLOCATIONS

Review of Joint Dislocations	
Definition	A joint dislocation is a displacement of a bone from its normal position in the joint.
Cause	The cause of a joint dislocation is usually traumatic movement beyond the normal range of motion.
Symptoms	The symptoms may include pain, deformity, swelling, inability to move the joint, and neurovascular compromise.
Tests	Tests include x-ray of the joint.

Review of Joint Dislocations	
Management	Management may be EMERGENT. Temporarily immobilize the joint. Prepare for conscious sedation and immediate reduction. Hospital admission may be required for observation and supportive treatment.
Comments	A dislocation of the knee and elbow are considered emergent. In the knee, the peroneal nerve and vein may be permanently damaged. An angiogram is necessary to evaluate vascular compromise.

LACTATED RINGER'S SOLUTION

Lactated Ringer's solution (Hartmann's solution) contains sodium lactate similar to the serum plasma. It is isotonic and used to treat losses from burns and the lower gastrointestinal tract. It does not contain free water or calories.

LIVER INJURY

Review of Liver Injuries	
Definition	Liver injury is damage to the liver tissue caused by an external force. Force may be to the entire abdomen or to the right side and often associated with rib fractures on the lower right side.
Causes	Liver injuries are caused by blunt or penetrating trauma to the abdomen. The liver is vascular. The tissue is friable. The blood supply is extensive.
Symptoms	Symptoms may include right upper quadrant pain with rebound tenderness, abdominal rigidity, guarding, hypoactive or absent bowel sounds, and hypovolemic shock.
Tests	Tests may include peritoneal lavage, and ultrasound or CT of the abdomen.
Management	Management may include: • Intravenous access with two large bore (14 or 16 gauge) cannulas • Fluid resuscitation with normal saline or Ringer's solution • Blood replacement • Insertion of gastric tube to decompress the stomach and to reduce the risk of vomiting and aspiration • Insertion of indwelling urinary catheter for decompression of the bladder and monitoring of urinary output • STAT arrangements for definitive surgical exploration and measures to stop the hemorrhage

MECHANISM OF INJURY

Mechanism of injury (MOI) is the exchange of forces that results in an injury to the patient

PREDICTABLE INJURIES FOR UNRESTRAINED DRIVERS

Review of Predictable Injuries for Unrestrained Drivers
Cardiac contusion
Facial injuries
Head injuries
Lacerated great vessels
Lacerated liver and/or spleen
Larynx, clavicle, femur, patella, and sternum fractures
Pulmonary contusion (75% of patient with blunt chest trauma experience some degree of pulmonary contusion from the mechanical energy transferred to the chest)

PREDICTABLE INJURIES FOR RESTRAINED DRIVERS

Review of Predictable Injuries for Restrained Drivers
Clavicle and sternum contusions
Cardiac injuries
Diaphragmatic rupture (tear)
Liver, spleen, and pancreas bruising or laceration
Pelvic injuries
Abdomen, breast, shoulder bruising

MONOCULAR AND BIOCULAR VISION

The causes of monocular vision loss include ischemia from vascular occlusion and retinal detachment. Biocular changes indicate a neurological problem.

NEUROGENIC SHOCK

Neurogenic shock is associated with sympathetic blockade due to spinal cord injury and managed with interventions to increase vascular tone, such as Dopamine. Patients have bradycardia and vasodilation. The skin is warm and dry due to the vasodilation compared to the cool and clammy skin characteristic of hypovolemic shock. Bradycardia, not tachycardia, occurs in neurogenic shock due to the sympathetic blockade associated with hypotension.

O-NEGATIVE BLOOD

O-negative blood can be administered in an emergency until typed and cross-matched blood is available. O-negative is considered the universal donor.

OPEN FRACTURES

Review of Open Fractures	
Definition	An open fracture is a fracture associated with a disruption of the skin near the fracture site either from external or internal forces.
Cause	The cause of an open fracture is usually trauma.

Review of Open Fractures	
Symptoms	Symptoms include disrupted skin near the fracture site; and may include protrusion of the bone, pain, neurovascular compromise, and bleeding.
Tests	Tests may include x-rays, CT, and MRI.
Management	Management includes a wound culture, cleansing and irrigation of the wound, dressing with a sterile dressing, and splinting.
Disposition	Hospital admission may be required for surgery or transfer to a facility that can provide the necessary care.

ORGAN PROCUREMENT ORGANIZATION (OPO)

Studies have shown that the consent rate for donation increased 50% when Organ Procurement Organizations are involved with the hospital staff.

Organs that can be donated include the heart, intestines, kidneys, lungs, liver, and pancreas. Tissues that can be grafted include bones, femoral veins, great saphenous veins, heart valves, skin, tendons, cornea.

Under U.S. law, the states regulate organ donations within the limitations of the National Organ Transplant Act of 1968. Each state has a Uniform Anatomical Gift Act that governs organ donation for the purpose of transplantation and the use of one's cadaver to be studied by medicine.

ORTHOSTATIC VITAL SIGNS

Review of Orthostatic Vital Signs	
Definition	Orthostatic vital signs are sequential blood pressure readings and pulse obtained with the patient lying, sitting, and standing. There should be less than one minute between readings.
Rationale	A patient with a clinically significant circulatory volume loss will have objective findings of a decrease in blood pressure >20 mmHg and an increase in pulse > 20 beats/min. Subjective findings include light-headedness, nausea, and sweating.

PELVIC FRACTURES

Review of Pelvic Fractures	
Definition	A pelvic fracture is a bony disruption to the pelvis.
Cause	The cause of a pelvic fracture is trauma.
Symptoms	Symptoms may include deformity and swelling at the site of fracture, shortening or abnormal rotation of the leg, and pain. A pelvic fracture in males is the most common cause of injury to the posterior urethra.
Tests	Tests may include x-ray, CT, and cystogram.

Review of Pelvic Fractures	
Management	Management may include splinting with pressurized trousers if the patient is hemodynamically unstable, and fluid resuscitation with normal saline or Ringer's solution. Large blood loss can accompany an unstable pelvic fracture.
Disposition	Hospital admission may be required or transfer to a facility that can surgically repair an unstable pelvis.
Associated injury	Injuries to the perineum, genitalia, and rectum are associated with pelvic fracture.

PERITONEAL LAVAGE

Diagnostic peritoneal lavage is done to determine if bleeding is present in the peritoneal space. Normal saline is instilled into the peritoneal cavity and aspirated. The aspirate is tested for blood. The retroperitoneal space is separate from the peritoneal cavity and this procedure is unable to determine if bleeding is present in the retroperitoneal space. Peritoneal lavage is contraindicated in the patient with a history of cirrhosis, coagulopathy, or multiple abdominal surgeries (adhesions can prevent the bowel from moving and increase the risk of bowel puncture), and in the patient with extreme obesity.

PREGNANCY AND TRAUMA

Review of Anatomical and Physiological Changes in the Pregnant Female	
Gastrointestinal	The stomach and intestines are displaced upward. Gastric emptying is delayed
Hemodynamic	Hemodynamic changes include a cardiac output increase of approximately 40%, a systolic blood pressure increase of 5 to 15 mmHg, a heart rate increase of 15 to 20 beats per minute, and hematocrit results increase by 30 to 35%, and a decreased clotting time.
Renal	Renal blood flow is increased.
Respiratory	The diaphragm is displaced upward by about 1½ to 2 inches. The air passages are engorged because of the increased blood flow. The respiratory rate is increased. Basal metabolism and oxygen consumption are increased. The pCO_2 is decreased to 30 mmHg.
Uterus	The uterus that is normally the size of a pear increases to contain the fetus and about 1 liter of amniotic fluid.

CRITICAL SIGNS ASSOCIATED WITH PREGNANT FEMALES

Review of the Critical Signs Associated with Pregnant Females	
Vaginal bleeding	Vaginal bleeding in a pregnant female may indicate separation of the placenta from the wall of the uterus or penetration of the uterus.

Review of the Critical Signs Associated with Pregnant Females	
Decreased fetal heart rate and movement	Decreased fetal heart rate and movement may indicate fetal distress.
Taut fundus	A taut fundus may indicate intrauterine hemorrhage.
Hypovolemic shock	Hypovolemic shock may indicate intrauterine hemorrhage.

PRESSURE POINTS TO STOP ARTERIAL HEMORRHAGE

Pressure Points to Stop Arterial Hemorrhage	
Axillary	To control an axillary artery hemorrhage, apply pressure to the head of the humerus. Press high in the axilla against the upper part of the humerus.
Brachial	To control a brachial artery hemorrhage, apply pressure to the shaft of the humerus. Press against the humerus by pulling aside the biceps and pressing deep against the bone.
Carotid	To control a carotid artery hemorrhage, apply pressure against the cervical vertebra. Press one inch to the side of the prominence of the windpipe. Hold pressing deeply towards the back.
Facial	To control a facial artery hemorrhage, apply pressure against the lower part of the jaw. Press an inch in front of the angle of the jaw.
Femoral	To control a femoral artery, apply pressure to the rim of the pelvis or the shaft of the femur. Press against the pelvis midway between the iliac spine and symphysis pubis or press high on the inner thigh about 3 inches below the rim of the pelvis.
Posterior tibial	To control a posterior tibial hemorrhage, apply pressure against the inner side of the tibia towards the ankle. Press against the tibia above the hemorrhage. For hemorrhage of the foot, press behind the inner ankle.
Subclavian	To control a subclavian artery hemorrhage, apply pressure against the first rib behind the clavicle. Press deep down and backward over the center of the clavicle after depressing the shoulder.
Temporal	To control a temporal artery hemorrhage, apply pressure against the temporal bone. Press against the bony prominence in front of the ear or temple.

RUPTURED DIAPHRAGM

A ruptured diaphragm is characterized by auscultation of bowel sounds in the chest.

SPLENIC INJURIES

Review of Splenic Injuries	
Causes	Blunt trauma or penetrating trauma to the left upper quadrant of the abdomen and fractures of the 8th, 9th, or 10th rib on the left side are associated with splenic damage.
Acuity	Injuries range from minor to serious. The most serious is a fractured spleen or a vascular tear that produces splenic ischemia and extensive blood loss.
Symptoms	Symptoms may include signs of hemorrhage or hypovolemic shock, tenderness in the left upper quadrant, Kehr's sign (pain in the left shoulder), abdominal guarding, and rigidity.
Diagnostic testing	Tests may include peritoneal lavage to look for red blood cells in the peritoneal fluid and ultrasound or CT to look for densities consistent with hemorrhage or hematoma.
Management	Medical management may include: Intravenous access with two large bore (14 or 16 gauge) cannulas Fluid resuscitation with normal saline or Ringer's solution Blood replacement Insertion of gastric tube to decompress the stomach and reduce the risk of vomiting and aspiration Insertion of indwelling urinary catheter for decompression of the bladder and to monitor urinary output STAT arrangements for definitive surgical exploration and measures to stop the hemorrhage

SUCKING CHEST WOUND

A sucking chest wound is an open pneumothorax that allows air to go in and out of the chest cavity through the chest wall causing a sucking sound.

VERTEBRAL FRACTURES AND DISLOCATIONS

Vertebral Fractures and Dislocations	
Burst	A vertebral burst fracture is a comminuted fracture of the vertebral body. The mechanism of injury is axial loading. Compression of the cord may or may not be present.
Compression	A vertebral compression fracture is a fracture of the vertebral body. The mechanism of injury is compression, hyperflexion, and anterior or lateral flexion. The spinal column is compressed and can be wedged. Compression of the cord may or may not be present.

Vertebral Fractures and Dislocations	
Simple	A vertebral simple fracture is a linear fracture of the transverse process or pedicles. Mechanism of injury is acceleration or deceleration. The spinal column maintains its alignment. Spinal cord injury is rare.
Teardrop	A vertebral teardrop fracture is a small fracture most commonly of the anterior edge of the vertebra. The fracture may be associated with posterior locations. The mechanism of injury is hyperflexion. Fragmentation of the vertebra may impinge the cord.

GERIATRIC CONSIDERATIONS

SHOCK IN OLDER ADULTS

An older adult's loss of reserve volume and catecholamine response prevent compensation mechanism found in younger adults. Shock is poorly tolerated in older adults because of the lack of compensatory reserve.

PEDIATRIC CONSIDERATIONS

PEDIATRIC BLUNT TRAUMA

Pediatric blunt abdominal trauma most commonly causes injuries to the spleen, liver, kidneys, and intestine. Fifty percent of all pediatric trauma victims have a head injury. Ninety percent of pediatric trauma deaths are secondary to head trauma. The hemodynamic effects of head injury with increased intracranial pressure are hypertension, bradycardia, abnormal posturing, abnormal respirations, and unilateral pupillary dilatation. Shock is most always from volume loss. The circulating volume must be restored. Normal urinary output in a child is 1 to 2 ml/kg per hour.

CAR SEATS

After a motor vehicle crash, a child should not be discharged until a seat appropriate for the child is available for the ride home.

- Infants under 1 year and less than 20 pounds face the rear only
- Infants less than 1 year, over 20 pounds, ride in a seat approved for heavier infants and face the rear
- Child over 1 year and 20 pounds or more face the front

CONSIDERATIONS FOR AN INJURED CHILD

Cardinal Considerations for an Injured Child
The child's oropharynx is relatively small and is easily obstructed by the tongue.
Vocal cords are short and concave and collapse easily if the head is hyper flexed or extended.
Lower airway passages are smaller and easily obstructed by mucus and swelling.
The mediastinum is more mobile allowing more great vessel damage.

Cardinal Considerations for an Injured Child
Crying children swallow air and gastric distension can prevent free respiratory movement.
Lungs sounds can be difficult to auscultate because of crying.
The child's blood volume is less than an adult, but more on a ml/kg basis.
Hypotension is usually not present until the child has lost 20 to 25% of their blood volume.
Low blood pressure is a late sign of hypovolemia in a child and is a sign of imminent cardiac arrest.
Bradycardia is a late sign of cardiac decompensation.
The head is larger and heavier. The skull offers less protection for the brain as it yields readily to external pressure. The scalp is vascular and bleeds more readily.
Brain tissue is more easily damaged.
The child is more vulnerable to spinal injuries because of the heavy head and less developed bony structure.
The protuberant abdomen of the child makes it vulnerable to injury. The internal organs are close together and multiple injuries occur at once.
The pliable rib cage offers little protection for the lungs.
The liver is vulnerable to injury because of its large size.
The large kidneys are not protected well because of less perinephric fat.
Bones are stronger, thicker, and bend more easily. Even though bones are strong, fractures occur more frequently than sprains. A growth plate fracture can be present and not be seen on x-ray.
The child has a larger ratio of body surface area and less subcutaneous fat. Therefore, they are more prone to heat loss.

PEDIATRIC HYPOVOLEMIC SHOCK

A fluid bolus in a child with hypovolemic shock is an initial bolus of 20 ml/kg over twenty minutes. Additional fluid boluses of 20 ml/kg can be given based on the child's hemodynamic response. The 4-2-1 rule for maintenance fluids is 4 ml/kg for the first 10 kg of body weight, 2 ml/kg for the next 10 kg of weight, and 1 ml/kg for the rest of the weight.

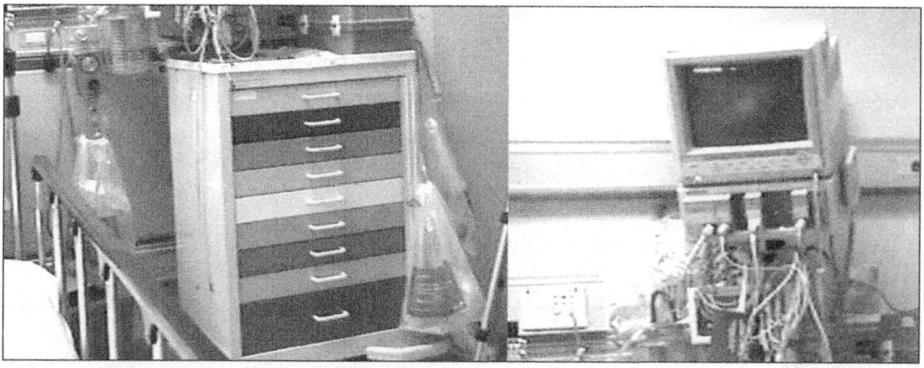

25 OVERDOSE AND POISONING

For details on triage see Chapter 34, Triage in a Nutshell.

PATIENT'S STORY – INTERVIEW QUESTIONS

1. When was the poison encountered or ingested?
2. What body system is involved?
3. What is the cause of the poisoning?
   a. What drug or poison was involved; e.g., name of the medication, insecticide, or plant?
   b. What was the quantity involved; e.g., number of pills, amount of liquid?

For a prescription medication, the maximum possible amount consumed can often be determined by finding out if any pills are left in the bottle and when it was last filled.

Information on hazardous materials is readily available in the ER in the Material Safety Data Sheets (MSDS).

   c. Over what length of time did the patient encountered or ingested the poison?
      i. Was the substance encountered or ingested all at once?
      ii. Was the substance encountered or ingested over time; e.g., over an hour, a day, or a week?
4. Is the overdose or poisoning considered accidental or a suicide attempt?
   a. Has the patient's behavior been cooperative?
   b. Are any other symptoms associated with the poisoning; e.g., nausea, vomiting, headache, sweating, or heart irregularity?

i. Has the patient vomited?

ii. Does the patient have any pain?

1. Where is the pain or discomfort located?
2. How does the patient describe the severity of the pain?

5. Is unlawful activity suspected?
   a. Was law enforcement at the scene?
   b. What agency?

Medical personnel are obligated to notify law enforcement if unlawful activity is suspected.

6. Was the Poison Control Center notified prior to coming to the hospital?
7. Has any treatment been initiated, and has it helped?
8. Does the patient have any pertinent past history and has the patient had an overdose before?
9. Does the patient take any routine medications?
   a. What is the name, dosage, route, and frequency of each medication?
   b. When was the last dose?
10. Does the patient take any complementary or alternative therapies, herbal products, over-the-counter medications or supplements, or natural therapies?
    a. What is the name, dosage, route and frequency of each therapy?
    b. When was the last dose or therapy?
11. Does the patient have allergies to drugs or foods?
    a. What is the name of the allergen?
    b. What was the reaction?
12. When was the patient's last tetanus immunization?
13. If the patient is female and between the ages of 10 to 50 years, when was the first day of her last menstrual period?

NURSING DOMAIN

The nursing domain, nursing diagnosis and plan of care can only be determined after an in-depth interview and consideration of the patient's story.

Domain 12. Comfort. Class 1. Physical comfort.
Domain 11. Safety/Protection Class 3. Violence.
Domain 5. Perception/Cognition Class 1. Self-concept.

ANTICIPATED MEDICAL CARE

Review of the Anticipated Medical Care of Overdoses and Poisonings	
Exam	Full body
Urine tests	Urine for toxicology screening; pregnancy test for women of childbearing years unless they have had a hysterectomy
Blood tests	Serum blood levels of suspected ingested toxins
ECG	12-lead electrocardiogram for females over 45 years, males over 35 years, and for all ages if the drug is cardiotoxic.
Poison Control Center	Place a call to the Poison Control Center. In all cases, it is essential to consult the experts. When a case is referred to the Poison Control Center, a toxicologist is available for consult and the case will be followed after discharge from the ER.
Diet	NPO
IV	Normal saline or Ringer's solution is the initial solution of choice. The maintenance solution is dependent on the type of poison. For alcohol intoxication, D5W or D10W is considered the appropriate solution. The rationale is that the dextrose facilitates the metabolism of the alcohol.
Medications	Medications may include specific antidote, activated charcoal, and magnesium citrate.
Management	Management may include gastric lavage, forced diuresis, hemodialysis, skin decontamination, and soft or leather restraints.
Disposition	If admission is necessary for the patient's safety, a medical provider must complete legal documentation to secure the patient's commitment to a psychiatric hospital for treatment.
Worst-case scenario	The worst-case scenario is aspiration during vomiting. If vomiting is intractable or the patient is obtunded, endotracheal intubation is necessary to protect the airway.

INITIAL CARE PLAN

> Alcohol-based hand sanitizers are the preferred method for cleaning your hands in most clinical situations. Wash your hands with soap and water whenever they are visibly dirty, before eating, and after using the restroom.

1. Ask the patient to undress, remove all jewelry that might interfere with the examination, and put on an exam gown. Assist as needed.

Consider the need for a urine specimen while the patient is dressed and able to collect a clean catch in the bathroom. Observe the person who is considered an attempted suicide patient to keep him safe and for the accidentally poisoned patient, observation will assure a non-contaminated specimen.

2. Obtain vital signs including pulse oximetry or test capillary refill.
3. Attach heart monitor leads, automatic blood pressure cuff, and pulse oximetry for continuous monitoring. Document the initial heart monitor strip and document changes of rhythm.
4. Obtain a 12-lead electrocardiogram if the poison is cardiotoxic.

The latest and most effective methods of treatment are available from a Poison Control Center. When the history is obtained and initial vital signs completed, call the Poison Control Center where the latest treatment information is available.

5. Position the patient in the high Fowler's position to protect the airway.
6. Establish intravenous access and draw laboratory blood specimens.
    a. Draw a variety of tubes that will allow the lab to perform hematology, chemistry, and coagulation studies. Patients on anticoagulants and cirrhotic patients need coagulation studies.
    b. Consider drawing other laboratory tests, e.g., serum drug or poison levels, type and screen.
7. Perform a focused physical examination.
    a. Assess the pupils.
    b. Auscultate lungs.
    c. Auscultate the abdomen for bowel sounds.
    d. Evaluate the level of consciousness based on the mnemonic **AVPU** or **ACDU** level of consciousness score.
AVPU: **A**lert, **V**erbal, **P**ain, **U**nresponsive.
ACDU: **A**lert, **C**onfused, **D**rowsy, **U**nresponsive.
8. Give initial medications covered by hospital protocol; e.g., ipecac, activated charcoal. Note: The American Academy of Clinical Toxicology and the European Association of Poisons Centre and Clinical Toxicology jointly published a paper regarding the use of ipecac in which they stated that the routine use of ipecac administration in the emergency room should be abandoned. The poison center has the most recent treatment information regarding the use of ipecac for each specific case.
9. Consider placing drains, e.g., indwelling urinary catheter for hourly urine output.
10. Instruct the patient not to eat or drink and teach the patient and family the rationale for the NPO status.
11. Elevate the siderails and place the stretcher in the lowest position.

12. Inform the patient, family, and caregivers of the usual plan of care and the expected overall time in the ER.
13. Provide the patient with a device to reach someone for assistance and explain how to use it. Ask the patient to call for help before getting off the stretcher.

ONGOING CARE PLAN

> Inform the medical provider of adverse changes noted during ongoing evaluation. Document that the medical provider was notified of the adverse change. Document if orders were or were not received.

> The Poison Control Center will outline the recommended ongoing monitoring specific to the drug or poison.

1. Monitor temperature, heart rate and rhythm, blood pressure, and effectiveness of breathing according to the Poison Control Center's instructions.
2. Monitor serum drug levels and diagnostic tests specific to the poison.
3. Establish security measures, as necessary, to assure the safety of the patient and the staff.
4. Provide emotional support for the patient and family.

> The emergency room is not the place for psychoanalysis.

5. Monitor therapy closely for the patient's therapeutic response.
   a. The usual time for a medication effectiveness check is 20 to 30 minutes after giving the drug.
   b. If therapy is not effective, ask the medical provider for a repeat dose or an alternative.
6. Monitor closely for the development of adverse reactions to therapy.
   a. Perform interventions to relieve the adverse reaction.
   b. Ask the medical provider for a remedy.
7. Keep the patient, family, and caregivers well informed of the plan of care and the remaining time anticipated before disposition.
8. Monitor the patient's laboratory and x-ray results and notify the medical provider of critical abnormalities. Remedy abnormalities as ordered.
9. Notify the medical provider when all diagnostic results are available for review. Ask for establishment of a diagnosis and disposition.

DISCHARGE INSTRUCTIONS

1. Provide the patient with the name of the nurse and doctor in the emergency room.

2. Inform the patient of their diagnosis or why a definitive diagnosis couldn't be made. Explain what caused the problem if known.
3. Teach the patient how to take the medication as prescribed and how to manage the common side effects. Instruct the patient not to drive or perform any dangerous tasks while taking narcotic pain medications.
4. Instruct the patient with accidental overdose that:
   a. The medical provider has determined that the ingestion was minor.
   b. If vomiting was induced or a tube placed, a mild sore throat, residual vomiting, and intestinal discomfort may be present over the next day.
   c. Severe vomiting, vomiting of blood, or more than mild abdominal pain should be reported to the follow-up medical provider.
   d. If activated charcoal was given, stools may be watery and black for the next few days.
   e. If severe sore throat, difficulty swallowing or breathing, seizures, fainting, or unexpected symptoms develop, call the follow-up medical provider immediately. If the medical provider is unavailable or contact is delayed, return to the emergency room.
5. Instruct the patient with a toxic inhalation that:
   a. Occasionally symptoms do not arise for 12 to 24 hours after inhalation.
   b. If new or unexpected symptoms develop (e.g., vomiting, diarrhea, difficult breathing, sore throat, or difficult swallowing) report the symptoms to the follow-up medical provider immediately.
   c. If the medical provider is unavailable or contact is delayed, return to the emergency room.
6. Recommend a medical provider for follow-up care. Provide the name, address, and phone number with a recommendation of when to schedule the care.
7. Inform the patient, if the pain or problem worsens in any way or any unusual symptoms develop, call the follow-up medical provider immediately or return to the emergency room. Encourage the patient NOT to IGNORE WORSENING OR PERSISTENT SYMPTOMS.
8. Ask for verbal confirmation or demonstration of understanding and reinforce teaching as needed.

COMMONLY ORDERED MEDICATIONS

ACTIVATED CHARCOAL

Activated Charcoal	
Indications	Poisonings that are absorbed in the gastrointestinal tract. Activated charcoal is not given for an overdose of a heavy metal (lithium, iron), a sustained-release medication, or alcohol.

Activated Charcoal	
Adult and child dose	5 to 10 times the weight of the substance ingested PO, minimum dose 30 gm. Severe poisoning may require 20 to 40 gm every 6 hours for 1 to 2 days. Obtain specific drug-related dose from a Poison Control Center.
Onset	PO onset 1 min., peak unknown, duration 4 to 12 hours
Compatibility	Ipecac, laxatives, and dairy products decrease the effectiveness of the activated charcoal
Side effects	Nausea, vomiting, diarrhea or constipation, black stools
Note	Give after vomiting. Mix with 8 ounces of water or fruit juice. Do not mix with dairy products. Repeat the dose if the medication is vomited. May give through a nasogastric or an orogastric tube if the patient is unable or unwilling to swallow.

NARCAN

Narcan (naloxone)	
Indications	Respiratory and neurological depression due to opioid overdose
Dose	0.4 to 2 mg IV every 2 to 3 min. A maximum dose has not been established. However, if the patient does not respond after 10 mg of Narcan, the diagnosis of an opioid overdose must be questioned.
Pediatric dose	< 5 years or > 20 kg 0.1 mg/kg IV > 5 years or > 20 kg 2.0 mg IV
Onset	IV onset 1 min., duration 45 min.
Side effects	Nervousness, ventricular tach, increased systolic blood pressure in high doses
Monitor	Return of pre narcotic status

MAGNESIUM CITRATE

Magnesium Citrate	
Indications	Laxative
Adult dose	10 fluid ounces
Pediatric Dose	6 to 12 years 7 fluid ounces 2 to 6 years 3 fluid ounces
Onset	½ to 6 hours
Ingredient	Active ingredient 1.745 grams of magnesium citrate per ounce
Side effects	Loose stools

Magnesium Citrate	
Note	Keep at 46° to 86° F

GoLYTELY

GoLYTELY	
Indications	Bowel cleansing and is not usually used for overdoses of sustained-release medications or those containing heavy metals (lithium, iron)
Adult dose	8 ounces PO every 10 min. until four liters have been ingested. Nasogastric tube administration rate is 20 to 30 ml per min.
Pediatric dose	Safety and effectiveness in children have not been established
Onset	PO onset one hour
Compatibility	Mix with water
Side effects	Nausea, bloating
Note	GoLYTELY is an isosmotic solution and has the same total concentration of ions in solution as the body fluid. Large volumes can be administered without significant change in fluid or electrolyte balance. Mix powder with four liters to reconstitute.

RELATED CONDITIONS AND INFORMATION

ACETAMINOPHEN

Acetaminophen is rapidly absorbed in the intestine and broken down by the liver where a toxic metabolite is formed. The liver is damaged as the metabolite increases. In therapeutic amounts, the liver enzymes detoxify this toxin. Serum levels of >140 mg/kg are considered toxic. Symptoms at 0 to 24 hours post ingestion may include lethargy, nausea, vomiting, and diaphoresis. At 24 to 48 hours, abnormal liver studies are present. At 72 to 96 hours, massive liver damage is present, and the patient may not survive. Management may include induced emesis, gastric lavage, activated charcoal, a cathartic, and Mucomyst (N-acetylcysteine) that replenishes the liver's essential enzymes and allows removal of the metabolites. Activated charcoal is not given if the Mucomyst is given orally because the charcoal binding with the Mucomyst and deactivates it. Hemodialysis removes the acetaminophen but does not reverse the damage already done to the liver.

ACTIVATED CHARCOAL

Activated charcoal dose is one gram per kilogram. When the ingested agents are adsorbed to charcoal, activated charcoal alone is the recommended gastrointestinal decontamination procedure of choice. Most ingested drugs and chemicals are absorbed to charcoal and absorption in the gastrointestinal tract is prevented. Ipecac and lavage can remove some drug from the stomach but does not prevent drug absorption from the small bowel, the primary site of absorption. One study has demonstrated that ipecac and lavage could move drugs from the stomach into the small bowel and increase absorption.

ALCOHOL

Common alcohol poisons are ethanol, methanol (antifreeze, Sterno), isopropanol (rubbing alcohol, nail polish remover), and ethylene glycol (antifreeze, paints, coolants). Alcohol can be ingested or absorbed topically. The liver converts the alcohol to toxic metabolites. A diagnostic finding of methanol ingestion is metabolic acidosis. Isopropanol ingestion may show an elevated serum acetone. Ethylene glycol ingestion often presents with a metabolic acidosis. Management is by gastric emptying. Activated charcoal is usually ineffective because of the fast absorption rate of the alcohol. Endotracheal intubation and mechanical ventilation can maximize respiratory excretion. Dialysis will remove the alcohol.

Ethanol IV may be given to the methanol overdose because it competes with methanol at the receptor sites and prevents the conversion of the methanol to formaldehyde.

ANTICHOLINERGIC SYNDROME

Review of Anticholinergic Syndrome	
Causes	Antihistamines, antiparkinson medication, atropine, scopolamine, amantadine, antipsychotic agents, antidepressant agents, antispasmodic agents, cyclic antidepressants, mydriatic agents, over-the-counter sleep preparations, skeletal relaxants, jimsonweed
Signs and symptoms	Delirium with mumbling speech, tachycardia, dry flushed skin, dilated pupils, myoclonus, slightly elevated temperature, urinary retention, decreased bowel sounds, seizures, arrhythmias in severe cases

ANTIDOTES

Drug/Toxin	Antidote
Acetaminophen	N-Acetylcysteine (Mucomyst)
Anticholinergics	Physostigmine
Anticholinesterases (organophosphates and carbamates)	Atropine, pralidoxime
Benzodiazepines	Flumazenil
Beta Blockers	Glucagon
Botulism	Botulinum antitoxin
Bromide	Sodium chloride
Calcium channel blockers	Calcium
Carbon monoxide	Oxygen
Cardiac glycosides (Digoxin)	Fab antibody therapy
Cyanide	Nitrites, sodium thiosulfate

Drug/Toxin	Antidote
Ethylene glycol	Ethanol, fomepizole, hemodialysis
Gyri metra mushrooms	Pyridoxine
Heavy metals (lead, mercury, arsenic,	Dimercaprol (BAL) Penicillamine Disodium EDTA DMSA (Chelating agents)
Heparin	Protamine
Hydrofluoric acid	Decontamination, calcium gluconate, calcium chloride
Iron	Deferoxamine
Isoniazid	Pyridoxine
Lead	BAL, EDTA, DMSA
Methanol	Ethanol, fomepizole, hemodialysis
Methemoglobinemia	Methylene Blue
Nitrites	Methylene Blue
Opiates	Naloxone
Organophosphates	Atropine Pralidoxime
Tricyclic antidepressants	Sodium bicarbonate
Warfarin	Vitamin K

ARSENIC

Symptoms of arsenic poisoning may include hair loss, abdominal pain, vomiting, bloody diarrhea, dehydration, hypovolemic shock, and coma. Symptoms can be delayed for several hours post ingestion. Shock is secondary to hemorrhagic gastroenteritis. Diagnostic findings may include abnormal liver function studies. Emergency management may include emesis, gastric lavage, supportive measures, and chelating therapy. Antidote is BAL (dimercaprol).

ASPIRIN (SALICYLATE) OVERDOSE

Salicylate serum levels over 150 mg/kg are considered toxic. Toxic salicylates levels cause tachypnea, tinnitus, altered mental status, metabolic acidosis, direct gastric irritation, electrolyte abnormalities, and bleeding disorders. Peak serum levels occur 2 to 4 hours after ingestion. Symptoms may include nausea and vomiting, hyperventilation, upper gastrointestinal bleeding with abdominal pain, shock, and hyperthermia. Diagnostic studies may include ABG, serial salicylates levels until a drop to nontoxic levels are reached (<40 mg/dl), serum potassium, PT, and aPTT. Management may include gastric decontamination with lavage or induced vomiting and activated charcoal, forced diuresis, and alkalinization. Hemodialysis is used to remove the salicylates, correct acidosis, and potassium levels.

CHARACTERISTIC ODORS CAUSED BY SUBSTANCES

Characteristic Odors caused by Substances	
Acetone	Ethyl alcohol, isopropyl alcohol, lacquer
Bitter Almond	Cyanide, apricot pits, amygdalin, laetrile
Burnt rope	Marijuana
Garlic	Arsenic, arsine gas, organophosphates, dimethyl sulfoxide, phosphorus, selenium, thallium
Mothballs	Para dichlorobenzene, naphthalene
Peanuts	Rodenticides
Pear	Chloral hydrate, paraldehyde
Pungent aromatics	Ethchlorvynol
Rotten egg	Hydrogen sulfide, mercaptans, sewer gas
Shoe polish	Nitrobenzene
Violets	Turpentine
Wintergreen	Methyl salicylates

CHOLINERGIC SYNDROMES

Review of Cholinergic Syndromes	
Causes	Organophosphates and carbamate insecticides, physostigmine, edrophonium, some mushrooms, severe black widow spider bite
Signs and symptoms	Confusion, CNS depression, weakness, salivation, lacrimation, urinary and fecal incontinence, gastrointestinal cramping, emesis, diaphoresis, muscle fasciculation, pulmonary edema, miosis, bradycardia or tachycardia, seizures
Mnemonic	SLUDGE Salivation, lacrimation, urination, defecation, GI upset (cramps), emesis

COMMON POISONS

Common Poisons	
Adults	Children

Common Poisons	
Adults	Children
Pain medicine sedatives	Cosmetics and personal care products
Hypnotics	Cleaning substances
Antipsychotics	Pain medicine and fever-reducers
Cleaning substances	Coins, thermometers
Antidepressants	Plants
Bites and envenomations	Diaper care products
Alcohols	Acne preparations
Food products and food poisoning	Antiseptics
Cosmetics and personal care products	Cough and cold preparations
Chemicals	Pesticides
Pesticides	Vitamins
Cardiovascular drugs	Gastrointestinal preparations
Fumes, gases, vapors	Antimicrobials
Hydrocarbons	Arts, crafts, and office supplies
Antihistamines	Antihistamines
Anticonvulsants	Hormones and hormone antagonists
Antimicrobials	Diabetes medications
Stimulants and street drugs	Contraceptives
Plants	Hydrocarbons (lamp oil, kerosene, gasoline, lighter fluid)
Cough and cold preparations	

DON'T Mnemonic

Mnemonic for Treatment for Altered Mental Status
Dextrose
Oxygen
Narcan
Thiamine

Drug Information Guide

Review of Drugs with Associated Symptoms and Duration

Review of Drugs with Associated Symptoms and Duration	
Alcohol	Puffiness of face, red eyes, disorientation, shallow respirations, depression, aggression, blurred vision and lack of coordination. Duration 1 to 12 hours. Alcohol abuse is defined as a pattern of drinking that results in one or more alcohol related problems in a 12-month period, such as failure to fulfill major responsibilities, drinking in dangerous situations (driving, operating machinery) being arrested, and disputes that are worsened or caused by drinking.
Amphetamines (uppers, speed, black beauties, dexies)	Unusual increase in activity, increased heart rate, breathing and blood pressure, high doses can cause tremors. Duration ½ to 2 hours
Barbiturates, Methaqualone, Quaaludes, (ludes, yellow jackets, red devils)	Slurred speech, drunken behavior without odor of alcohol, unsteady gait, poor and/or slow judgment, and slow reflexes. Duration 1 to 16 hours
Cocaine (coke, snow, blow, gold dust and lady)	Apathy, anxiety, sleeplessness, paranoia, cocaine hunger, constant sniffing, dilated pupils, increased body temperature, blood pressure, and heart rate. Duration ½ to 2 hours
Crack cocaine (crack, rock)	Same as cocaine but gets to the brain quicker. Duration 5 to 10 minutes
Gasoline and glue (rush, locker room), aerosol cans of amyl nitrate, gasoline, lighter fluid inhaled through a saturated cloth covering the nose and mouth	Keen senses, hallucinations, scrambled words and disconnected sentences, an odor of the substance used, risk is cardiac arrhythmias. Duration variable
Hallucinogens (LSD, mescaline, peyote, mushrooms)	Dilated pupils, nausea, increased blood pressure, stomach cramps, flashbacks, beady eyes, nervous erratic behavior, laughing, crying, personality changes, a sense of seeing smells and hearing colors, and marked depersonalization. Duration 3 to 12 hours

Review of Drugs with Associated Symptoms and Duration	
Heroin (Mexican brown, China white, Persian porcelain, H)	The triad of symptoms in heroin induced pulmonary edema is hypoxia, stupor, and miosis. Watery eyes, runny nose, yawning, irritability, panic, chills, miosis (contraction of the pupil), repeated use can lead to infections of the heart and valves, skin abscesses, and lung congestion. Duration 12 to 24 hours
Inhalants	Common substances sniffed or huffed to give the user an immediate mind-altering effect or high and include solvents, gases, and nitrates. National Inhalant Prevention Coalition http://www.inhalants.org
Marijuana (pot, reefer, grass, RHC, hash and hash oil)	Euphoria, relaxed inhabitation, disoriented behavior, staring into space, laughing without cause, time disorientation, bloodshot eyes, impaired memory, perception and judgment. Duration 2 to 4 hours
MDMA (Adam, ecstasy, X-TC days, a designer drug)	Increased heart rate and blood pressure, blurred vision, chills, sweating, confusion, sleep problems, anxiety, paranoia, muscle tension, involuntary teeth clenching. Duration variable, up to days.
Mescaline/peyote	Psychedelic effects, nausea, vomiting, mydriasis, hyperreflexia, ataxia, nystagmus, tremors. Duration 8 to 12 hours
Methamphetamine (Meth, amp, crank, devil's dandruff, ice, redneck cocaine)	Tachycardia, hypertension, vasoconstriction, bronchodilation, hyperglycemia, decreased appetite, jaw clenching, hyperkalemia, agitation, hyperthermia Duration varies Schedule II drug, pharmaceutical drug Desoxyn
PCP or phencyclidine (angel dust, killer weed, crystal cyclone, elephant tranquilizer, rocket fuel)	Increased heart rate and blood pressure, sweating, dizziness, hallucinations, confusion, violence and aggression, or silence and withdrawal. The patient has decreased pain sensation and decreased judgment. Duration variable

Review of Drugs with Associated Symptoms and Duration	
Prescription Drugs	Prescription drug abuse is widespread and on the rise. The most common are: Narcotics: Fentanyl, Ketamine, OxyContin, Vicodin, Percocet Depressants: Xanax, Valium, Librium Stimulants: Ritalin, Dexedrine, Meridia
Steroids (anabolic androgenic)	Used illicitly by body builders and other athletics to give them a competitive advantage and improve their appearance. Severe health consequences. High doses promote aggression and harmful psychological effects.
Tobacco	Number one on the top-ten list. Over 400,000 deaths per year, or one in every five deaths. It is the biggest killer. Estimated 46.5 million adults in the U.S. smoke cigarettes. Electronic source: Retrieved Street Drugs. November 2010. http://www.streetdrugs.org/html%20files/Tobacco.html

HEAVY METALS

Heavy metals including lead are deposited in body systems and excreted slowly. The kidneys are especially susceptible to these deposits. Diagnostic tests may include 24-hour urine studies and x-rays of the long bones and abdomen to identify deposits.

OPIATE, SEDATIVE, OR ETHANOL INTOXICATION

Review of Opiate, Sedative, or Ethanol Intoxication	
Causes	Narcotics, barbiturates, benzodiazepines, ethanol, meprobamate, clonidine
Signs and symptoms	Coma, respiratory depression, miosis, hypotension, bradycardia, hypothermia, pulmonary edema, decreased bowel sounds, hyporeflexia, seizures

PARAQUAT

Paraquat (herbicide) causes skin rash and ulcerations if not washed off. There is a low incidence of permeability through skin causing systemic effects.

RESPIRATORY DEPRESSION

Respiratory depression is particularly pronounced with opiate overdose and the respiratory rate commonly becomes diminished before the blood pressure or pulse.

RHUBARB

Rhubarb leaves contain oxalic acid causing localized pain and swelling of the lips, mouth, and tongue.

SYMPATHOMIMETIC SYNDROMES

Review of Sympathomimetic Syndromes

Review of Sympathomimetic Syndromes	
Causes	Cocaine, amphetamine, methamphetamine, over-the-counter decongestants, caffeine, theophylline
Signs and symptoms	Delusions, paranoia, tachycardia (or bradycardia if the drug is a pure adrenergic agonist), hypertension, hyperpyrexia, diaphoresis, piloerection, mydriasis and hyperreflexia, seizures, hypotension in severe overdose

TOXIN REMOVAL

ER Interventions used for Overdoses	
Alkalinization	Alkalinization therapy is endotracheal intubation and mechanical ventilation with administration of sodium bicarbonate to elevate pH to 7.5.
Antidotes	Antidotal therapy is the administration of antidotes. Antidotes may be ineffective and cause dangerous adverse reactions.
Chelation	The use of chelating agents to bind metals that are present in toxic concentrations so they can be excreted (usually in urine) from the body
Decontamination	Decontamination therapy is removal of the toxic substance by vomiting, gastric lavage, absorption with activated charcoal, and irrigation for dermal and eye decontamination.
Elimination	Elimination therapy includes cathartics (Magnesium citrate or GoLYTELY) and repeated doses of activated charcoal to decrease serum concentration after absorption. Activated charcoal may also decrease serum drug levels of therapeutic drugs, e.g., Dilantin and Aminophyllin.
Forced diuresis	Forced diuresis therapy is useful in removing alcohols. Over-hydrating with normal saline can increase elimination of toxin excreted by the kidneys. Dextrose solutions theoretically provide calories that burn the alcohol.
Hemodialysis	Hemodialysis therapy is useful to remove toxins and correct acid-base imbalance.

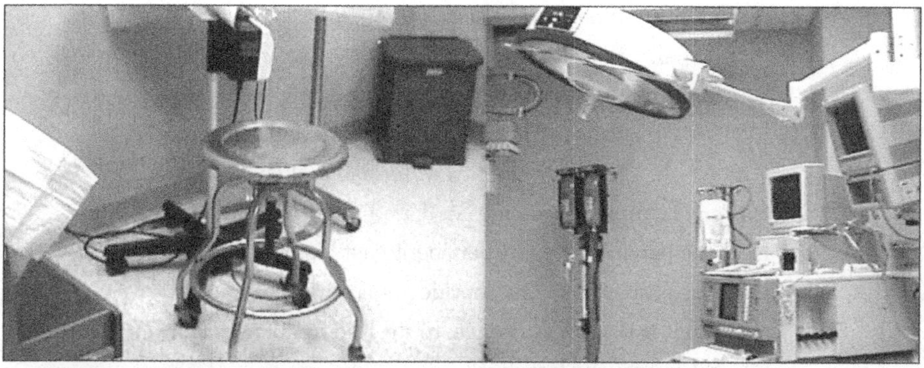

26 PREGNANCY AND DELIVERY EMERGENCY

For details on triage see Chapter 34, Triage in a Nutshell.

PATIENT'S STORY – INTERVIEW QUESTIONS

1. When did the symptoms begin?
   a. If the symptoms are no longer active, how long did they last?
   b. If the symptoms were intermittent, how long did each episode last and how frequent were they?
2. Identify the facts about the pregnancy and any associated symptoms.
   a. What was the first day of the patient's last period?
   b. How many months or weeks pregnant is the patient?
   c. What is the expected date of birth?
   d. Has the patient received any prenatal care?
   e. Is this the first pregnancy?
   f. How many deliveries, term deliveries, pre-term deliveries, abortions or miscarriages?
   g. How many living children?
   h. Are any other symptoms associated with the chief complaint, e.g., breaking of the water bag, vaginal bleeding, or passage of tissue vaginally?
3. Is the cause of the problem known?
   a. What was the patient doing when the symptoms began?
   b. Did a specific event cause the symptoms, e.g., a fall, motor vehicle crash, running, or sexual intercourse?
4. How does the problem affect normal function?
   a. Is the patient having any pain?

        i. Where is the pain located?
        ii. Does it radiate?
    b. Is the patient in labor?
        i. How many minutes apart are the labor pains?
        ii. Has the patient's water bag broken?
5. Has any treatment been initiated, and has it helped?
6. Does the patient have any pertinent past history?
7. Does the patient take any routine medications?
    a. What is the name, dosage, route, and frequency of each medication?
    b. When was the last dose?
8. Does the patient take any complementary or alternative therapies, herbal products, over-the-counter medications or supplements, or natural therapies?
    a. What is the name, dosage, route and frequency of each therapy?
    b. When was the last dose or therapy?
9. Does the patient have allergies to drugs or foods?
    a. What is the name of the allergen?
    b. What was the reaction?

NURSING DOMAIN

The nursing domain, nursing diagnosis and plan of care can only be determined after an in-depth interview and consideration of the patient's story.

Domain 12. Comfort. Class 1. Physical comfort.
Domain 8. Sexuality. Class 3. Reproduction.

ANTICIPATED MEDICAL CARE

Review of the Anticipated Medical Care of Pregnancy and Delivery Emergencies	
Exam	Full body
Urine tests	Clean catch or catheterized urine specimen for urinalysis
Tests	Hemogram, type and screen, Rh factor, cervical cultures, wet prep
ECG	ECG for females over 35 years with chest discomfort
X-rays	None
Other	Obstetrical ultrasound (indwelling urinary catheter often required)
Diet	NPO

Review of the Anticipated Medical Care of Pregnancy and Delivery Emergencies	
IV	Normal saline or Ringer's solution
Disposition	If an obstetrical emergency is found, hospitalization may be required for observation and treatment.
Worst-case scenario	The worst-case scenario is when an infant does not survive delivery in the ER.

INITIAL CARE PLAN

If a urine specimen is needed and the patient is not bleeding, collect it before the patient gets undressed. The patient can collect a clean catch specimen in the bathroom. A woman in her third trimester may have difficulty obtaining a clean catch due to the size of her belly. A clean catch may not be absolutely necessary even though it provides a better specimen.

Alcohol-based hand sanitizers are the preferred method for cleaning your hands in most clinical situations. Wash your hands with soap and water whenever they are visibly dirty, before eating, and after using the restroom.

1. Ask the patient to undress, remove all jewelry that might interfere with the examination, and put on an exam gown. Assist as needed
2. Consider notifying labor and delivery. Often the labor and delivery unit keep a chart of all the upcoming deliveries. Also, if a labor and delivery staff member is available to assist in consultation this is a benefit especially for those specialized skills such as fetal monitoring and vaginal exams.
3. After undressing it would be appropriate to have the patient get onto a stretcher in a semi-Fowler's position or left side/tilt position, especially if she is weak or dizzy. It is important to avoid uterine pressure on the major blood vessels running near the spine, which can cause problems for the baby. So, lying flat on one's back is not an appropriate position for those in the 3rd trimester.
4. Obtain mother's vital signs and initiate heart, noninvasive blood pressure, and pulse oximetry monitoring.
5. Initiate fetal monitoring or listen to fetal heart tones and assess fetal movement.
6. Place on oxygen if gas exchange is compromised.
7. Establish intravenous access and draw laboratory blood specimens.
    a. Draw a variety of tubes that will allow the lab to perform hematology, chemistry, and coagulation studies.
    b. Consider drawing other labs, e.g., type and screen and blood cultures if rupture of membranes has been established.

8. Perform a focused physical examination
    a. Auscultate the lungs.
    b. Examine the abdomen and mark the level of the uterus as it relates to the mother's umbilicus. An example of this is as follows. The top of the fundus is 2-finger widths above the umbilicus which would roughly indicate 22-week gestation. At 20-week gestation the fundus is at the umbilicus.
    c. Attach a fetal monitor if available and palpate the uterus for contractions. Palpating a contraction involves placing one's hand on the fundus or top of the uterus. When a contraction begins, the fundus gets noticeably rigid, not unlike wood. Upon completion, it remains firm but less so than during the contraction. The patient will definitely be able to confirm contractions if awake.
    d. Inspect the vaginal area. Look for vaginal bleeding which could be a warning sign of placenta previa. Look for malpresentation (e.g., foot or cord presentation). Note bulging membranes and ask again if the patient has experienced any leaking from her vaginal area that she thinks is not urine. If she states, she has found her panties wet or has fluid running down her leg(s) then 1) test for ruptured membranes with Nitrazine paper or a fern test and 2) note the color of the fluid. Green fluid, even pale, could mean ruptured membranes with meconium staining. Meconium indicates that the infant has defecated in utero, a sign of stress. When meconium is observed it must be carefully evaluated.
    e. In the absence of ruptured membranes, placenta previa, or if the presenting symptoms indicate the onset of labor, a vaginal exam to determine dilatation, effacement, and station should be performed by personnel trained in this skill using sterile technique. Transfer to labor and delivery may be appropriate.
9. Start a pad count if the patient is bleeding vaginally. One saturated pad holds about 30 ml of bleed. Inspect frequently to see if blood is collecting under the patient.
10. Instruct the patient not to eat or drink and teach the patient and family the rationale for the NPO status.
11. Elevate the side rails and place the stretcher in the lowest position. Remember to leave the patient in semi-Fowler's position or a left side tilt position to diminish uterine pressure on the major blood vessels supplying not only the mother but the baby with oxygen.
12. Inform the patient, family, and caregivers of the usual plan of care and the expected overall time in the ER.
13. Provide the patient with a device to reach someone for assistance and explain how to use it. Ask the patient to call for help before getting off the stretcher.

ONGOING CARE PLAN

Inform the medical provider and labor and delivery of patients in their third trimester and of adverse changes noted during the ongoing evaluation. Document that the medical provider was notified of the adverse change. Document if orders were or were not received.

1. Monitor the mother's vital signs, heart rate and rhythm, blood pressure, and effectiveness of breathing. Time contractions if the patient seems to be in labor. Note that the beginning of one contraction to the beginning of the next contraction is the time in between contractions. It can also be timed from the peak of a contraction to the peak of another contraction as the time in between contractions. An example of proper notation is as follows. Contractions are q 10 minutes lasting 45 seconds. If at all possible, place the patient on a fetal monitor.
2. Monitor the fetal heart tones and assess fetal movement.
3. Monitor blood loss volume.
4. Monitor therapy closely for the patient's therapeutic response.
    a. The usual time for a medication effectiveness check is 20 to 30 minutes after giving the drug.
    b. If therapy is not effective, ask the medical provider for a repeat dose or an alternative.
5. Monitor closely for the development of adverse reactions to therapy.
    a. Perform interventions to relieve the adverse reaction.
    b. Ask the medical provider for a remedy.
6. Keep the patient, family, and caregivers well informed of the plan of care and the remaining time anticipated before disposition.
7. Monitor the patient's laboratory and x-ray results and notify the medical provider of critical abnormalities. Remedy abnormalities as ordered.
8. Notify the medical provider when all diagnostic results are available for review. Ask for establishment of a diagnosis and disposition.

DISCHARGE INSTRUCTIONS

1. Provide the patient with the name of the nurse and doctor in the emergency room. If the patient has had a termination of pregnancy, provide the contact name and number for the pregnancy loss counselor if available in the facility.
2. Inform the patient of her diagnosis or why a definitive diagnosis couldn't be made. Explain what caused the problem if known.
3. Teach the patient how to take the medication as prescribed and how to manage the common side effects. Instruct the patient not to drive or perform any dangerous tasks while taking narcotic pain medications.
4. Instruct the patient with a spontaneous abortion that they should:

   a. Not douche or have sexual intercourse unless advised by the primary care professional.
   b. Rest in a bed for the first 24 to 48 hours or until the cramping and bleeding have stopped.
   c. Notify the follow-up medical provider for increased abdominal pain or bleeding, fever, chills, or tissue passage.
5. Instruct the patient with no specific diagnosis that:
   a. No serious problem was detectable.
   b. Follow-up is essential with an OB-GYN medical provider.
   c. Over-the-counter medications should be avoided unless recommended by a medical provider.
   d. Contact the follow-up medical provider if bleeding, elevated temperature, difficulty with urination, abdominal pain, or other unexpected symptoms arise. If follow-up arrangements cannot be made or are delayed, return to the emergency room.
6. Recommend a medical provider for follow-up care. Provide the name, address, and phone number with a recommendation of when to schedule the care.
7. Instruct the patient to call the follow-up medical provider immediately or return to the emergency room if the pain or problem worsens in any way or any unusual symptoms develop. Encourage the patient NOT to IGNORE WORSENING OR PERSISTENT SYMPTOMS.
8. Ask for verbal confirmation or demonstration of understanding and reinforce teaching as needed.

COMMONLY ORDERED MEDICATIONS

MICRHOGAM

MICRhoGAM Rho (D) immune globulin (human) ultra-filtered	
Indications	Prevention of isoimmunization in Rh females after abortion, miscarriages, and amniocentesis up to and including 12-week gestation. Over 12-week gestation use RhoGAM. NOT TO BE USED WITH ANY INDICATION OF CONTINUATION OF PREGNANCY.
Adult dose	1 vial IM given as soon as possible after termination of a pregnancy
Onset	IM onset 100% effective in 3 hours
Side effects	Irritation at injection site, fever, lethargy
Note	Made from human plasma. Products made from human plasma may contain infectious agents.

RHOGAM

RhoGAM Rho (d) immune globulin, human

RhoGAM Rho (d) immune globulin, human	
Indications	Prevention of isoimmunization in Rh females after abortion, miscarriages, and amniocentesis over 12 week's gestation. MICRhoGAM may be used for 12 weeks and less gestation.
Adult dose	1 vial IM given within 72 hours of termination of pregnancy
Onset	IM onset rapid, peak and duration unknown
Side effects	Irritation at injection site, fever, lethargy
Note	Made from human plasma. Products made from human plasma may contain infectious agents.

RELATED CONDITIONS AND INFORMATION

> 20 WEEKS GESTATION

Females >20 weeks pregnant are often seen in the labor and delivery department because the infant is considered viable. Ask the patient not to eat or drink until evaluated by the labor and delivery staff.

< 20 WEEKS GESTATION

Females < 20 weeks pregnant are commonly kept in the ER because the infant is not considered viable. Ask the patient not to eat or drink until evaluated. Assure the patient that bleeding can be normal during pregnancy.

ABORTION

Review of Abortions	
Definition	An abortion is a termination of pregnancy before the fetus is viable. The abortion can be spontaneous, induced, complete, incomplete threatened, or infected. A careful maternal history is essential to help determine the above.
Symptoms	Symptoms may include vaginal bleeding with clots, abdominal pain, and low back pain.
Tests	Tests may include serum pregnancy test, obstetrical ultrasound, pelvic examination, hemogram for evaluation of blood loss and possible infection, type and screen, and Rh factor.
Management	Medical management includes monitoring for hemodynamic changes, blood loss, and fluid resuscitation with normal saline. Make notations regarding blood clots, color and odor of discharge.
Disposition	Incomplete abortions or those with uncontrolled bleeding may require hospitalization for surgical suction curettage.
Discharge instruction	Discharge Instructions include no douches, no intercourse, resting in bed, and notifying the follow-up medical provider for increased abdominal pain, bleeding, fever, chills, and passage of tissue.

APGAR

Review of Apgar Score			
	0	1	2
Appearance	Blue	Blue limbs, pink body	Pink
Pulse	Absent	< 100 beats/min.	> 100 beat/min.
Grimace	Limp	Some flexion	Good flexion
Activity	Absent	Some motion	Good motion
Respiration	Absent	Weak cry	Strong cry
Determine the Apgar score at delivery and 5 minutes post-delivery. Assign a score to appearance, pulse, grimace, activity, and respiration. Add them together. A score 7 to 10 is good; 4 to 6 is depressed; 0 to 3 is severely depressed. Named after Virginia Apgar (1909-1974), American medical provider.			

CARDINAL SIGNS

Review of Cardinal Signs of Problems in the Pregnant Female
Vaginal bleeding may indicate placenta previa, a separation of the placenta from the wall of the uterus or penetration of the uterus. In about 20% of pregnant females, bleeding in the first trimester of pregnancy may occur. Of those with bleeding 50% go on to miscarry. Vaginal bleeding is not always an emergency but must be evaluated in pregnancy.
Decreased fetal heart rate and fetal movement may be a sign of fetal distress. The normal fetal heart rate ranges from 120 to 160 with rises during fetal movement.
Tetanic contractions may indicate intrauterine hemorrhage from a placental abruption.
Hypovolemic shock may indicate intrauterine hemorrhage.
During delivery support the perineum and the head of the baby by applying light pressure on the crown of the baby's head during contractions. This will allow for a more controlled delivery and minimize or possibly prevent vaginal lacerations from occurring on delivery.
Fluid, other than urine, leaking or gushing from the vagina is a good indicator of ruptured membranes. A fern test or Nitrazine test confirms the diagnosis. Note the color of the liquid when present. If the patient is in her third trimester delivery must be considered. Monitoring for fever and signs of infection are important.

DELIVERY

Review of ER Delivery

Review of ER Delivery
Placing a mother on a fetal heart monitor is the most accurate method of determining the fetal heart pattern. If none is available and if time permits, listen to fetal heart tones (normal 120 to 160). A heart rate outside the normal range may indicate fetal distress. Arrange for an OB consult and possible C-section.
If the fetal heart tones are normal, examine the mother's abdomen. Palpate contractions. Count them and the time in between them. To time contractions count the beginning of a contraction to the beginning of the next contraction as the time in between contractions. One can also time from the peak of a contraction to the peak of the next contraction as the time in between contractions. Also note the length of a contraction. An example of a proper notation would be contractions are q5 minutes lasting 45 seconds.
Coach the mother to relax in between contractions.
If crowning is not present and if there is no sign of ruptured membranes or previa, a sterile manual vaginal exam can be done to determine dilatation, effacement, and station of the fetus.
If delivery is not imminent (no crowning), time will allow for transport to labor and delivery. A mother often will cry out if she feels the baby coming.
If crowning is present, prepare for an ER delivery.
Use a delivery kit (available in most EDs), don a sterile gown and gloves and have a sterile towel available to support the perineum during the delivery of the head and the delivery of the baby. The vernix caseosa or cheesy material covering the baby can make the baby very slippery. Having a towel improves one's hold or grip. Support the perineum and the head of the baby by applying light pressure on the crown of the baby's head during contractions. This will allow for a more controlled delivery and minimize or possibly prevent vaginal lacerations from occurring on delivery. Encourage the mother to PUSH only with the contractions and rest in between. This makes pushing more effective.
When the head is delivered, suction the mouth, then the nose of the infant. If the cord is around the infant's neck, loosen it and slip the cord over the head or clamp it in two places and cut between the clamps. Cutting the cord should only be done when it is wrapped around the neck.
The best technique for delivery for an emergency nurse is to let the spontaneous delivery be spontaneous. Since the baby is very slippery, performing the delivery in the bed or on a stretcher reduces the risk of the baby slipping or falling to the floor.
Keep the infant parallel to the mother or in a head-dependent position to reduce the risk of aspiration. Suction the mouth and then the nose. Gently rub the back if crying or breathing is not spontaneous.

Review of ER Delivery
If the umbilical cord has not been clamped already, and when it has stopped pulsing, place two cords clamps on the cord a few inches apart. The first clamp should be, if possible, 6 inches from the baby. The length of the cord varies from baby to baby. The average length is 22 inches. Then cut between the clamps.
Dry the infant, cover and place in a warm environment. Placing her on the mother's abdomen is appropriate. Drying and wrapping the baby quickly prevents hypothermia and respiratory compromise. Determine the Apgar score.

Apgar Score			
	0	1	2
Appearance	Blue	Blue limbs, pink body	Pink
Pulse	Absent	< 100 beats/min.	> 100 beat/min.
Grimace	Limp	Some flexion	Good flexion
Activity	Absent	Some motion	Good motion
Respiration	Absent	Weak cry	Strong cry

Reassess the airway. If the airway is not clear, suction the mouth and then the nose, position the newborn, and perform a slight chin lift. Do not hyperextend the neck. If breathing is absent or the heart rate is < 80 beats/min., begin CPR.
Provide oxygen, establish effective ventilation with a bag-valve mask or endotracheal intubation, and perform chest compressions. Medications are infrequently needed. A blood glucose level of 40 mg/dl is critical in a newborn. Administer a 25% solution at 0.5 g/kg.
If the baby is well, place on the mother's abdomen and encourage the mother to breastfeed the infant. Breastfeeding stimulates the uterus to contract.
To obtain a cord blood sample for hemogram, blood type, Rh factor, and bilirubin; unclamp the cord on the side of the placenta while waiting for its delivery. Hold the appropriate tubes opened under the blood flow (then recap tube) or obtain a blood sample with a syringe from umbilical vein (largest vessel of three) in the portion of cord attached to the placenta post placental delivery. DO NOT UNCLAMP THE CORD OF THE NOW INDEPENDENT BABY FOR A CORD BLOOD SAMPLE. Parents may have contracted with a stem cell storage facility to have their baby's stem cells collected and stored for future use. Often the parents bring the collection kit and directions with them to the hospital.
Prepare for delivery of the placenta that usually occurs 5 to 10 minutes after the infant is born.

Review of ER Delivery
A sudden gush of blood occurs when the placenta separates from the uterine wall, the uterus moves upward in the abdomen, and the cord shortens. Do not yank on the cord to hasten the delivery. When the above process is complete, apply gentle traction on the cord, pushing downward on the dome of the uterus towards the supra pubis. The placenta will enter the vaginal area, continue gentle traction, and remove. Fundal checks with fundal massage should be performed regularly (q15 minutes if bleeding is normal) to determine if the uterus is contracted. Monitor the vaginal bleeding. The average blood loss in a normal spontaneous delivery is 500cc. Make notation of the amount and quality of vaginal bleeding. A small gush followed by a light flow is common when the fundus is massaged. If the fundus becomes boggy and is not responsive to massage have Methergine 0.2 mg IM on standby.

ECTOPIC PREGNANCY

Review of Ectopic Pregnancy	
Definition	An ectopic pregnancy is one in which a fertilized ovum implants anywhere outside the uterus. The fetus starts to develop there. Common locations include the fallopian tube (95% occur in the tube), ovary, and abdominal cavity. As the ovum grows, the fallopian tube may rupture typically after the twelfth week.
Symptoms	Symptoms may include amenorrhea with left or right lower quadrant intermittent mild to severe pain and vaginal bleeding. If the ectopic pregnancy is leaking or ruptured, Kehr's sign may be present as the blood irritates the diaphragm causing referred pain to the shoulder.
Tests	Tests may include serum pregnancy, CBC, type and screen, Rh factor, and ultrasonography both abdominal and transvaginal. Some hospital policies require an indwelling urinary catheter, and some do not.
Management	Medical management includes intravenous access, pelvic examination, and may include Methotrexate if rupture is not present to terminate the pregnancy. Hospital admission and immediate surgery is indicated if the ectopic pregnancy has ruptured, the patient is in shock, or non-surgical methods are not available. There are other drugs used in the treatment of an ectopic pregnancy such as mifepristone, misoprostol or a combination.
Risk factors	History of PID, previous ectopic pregnancy, IUD, induced abortion, peritubal adhesions, fertility drugs, surgical products of the fallopian tubes, exposure to diethyl stilbestrol, and in vitro fertilization

Review of Ectopic Pregnancy	
Note	Ectopic pregnancy is the leading cause of maternal death in the first trimester and the second leading cause of maternal mortality overall.

GRAVIDA, PARA, ABORTION, LIVING

Gravida is the total number of pregnancies.

Para refers to the number of delivery of infants, dead or alive, who have developed in utero to viability (birth weight of >500 g or past 20-week gestation).

Abortion refers to elective or spontaneous termination of pregnancy before the point of viability.

Living refers to the number of living children the patient has at the present time.

HELLP SYNDROME

Review of HELLP Syndrome	
Definition	HELLP Syndrome is a group of symptoms that occur in pregnant women (H) hemolytic anemia, (EL) elevated liver enzymes, and (LP) low platelet count
Cause	The syndrome occurs in about 10% of the pregnant women with pre-eclampsia or eclampsia.
Symptoms	Progressive nausea and vomiting Upper abdominal pain Headache Tenderness in the right upper quadrant of the abdomen The liver may be enlarged
Tests	Liver function tests CBC and platelets
Management	Delivery of the baby as soon as possible Severe cases are life-threatening to both mother and baby. Without treatment 1.1 to 3.5% of women die with HELLP syndrome.

HYDATIDIFORM MOLE

Review of Hydatidiform Mole	
Definition	A hydatidiform mole is a rare mass that forms inside the uterus early in pregnancy. This occurs when the trophoblast villi from a forming fetus grow very rapidly and then die. If an embryo is formed, it dies early. The cells degenerate and form a jellylike fluid. The cells become fluid filled sacs. The trophoblast secretes hCG and grows rapidly in the uterus. The uterus enlarges imitating fetal enlargement. Fetal heart tones are not detectable, and no viable fetus is seen on ultrasound.

Review of Hydatidiform Mole	
Cause	A hydatidiform mole occurs in 1 of 100 pregnancies. Most often in groups who lack protein in their diet and in mothers < 18 and > 35.
Symptoms	Symptoms may include vaginal bleeding that occurs at about 16 weeks gestation. Other symptoms may include restlessness, heat intolerance, weight loss, loose stools, edema, and trembling of extremities.
Tests	Tests include a quantitative serum pregnancy test.
Management	Hospital admission may be required for surgical intervention with dilatation and curettage to remove the mole.

HYPEREMESIS GRAVIDARUM

Hyperemesis gravidarum is pregnancy related vomiting that prevents adequate food and fluids and is a rare complication of pregnancy. Because of the potential for severe dehydration, it is generally considered an emergency. Treatment includes antiemetics, such as Zofran and IV hydration with an isotonic crystalloid IV fluid, such as NS or Ringer's solution.

NAEGELE'S RULE

Naegele's rule is a system used to estimate the date of delivery. Count back exactly 90 days from the first day of the last menstrual period, add 7 days to that date, and add one year.

Example:

Last Menstrual Period: April 7, 2010
Minus 3 months + 7 days + 1 year
January 14, 2011

NEWBORN MANAGEMENT

Review of Newborn ABCCCC Management	
A Airway	When the head is delivered, suction the mouth first and then the nose to reduce the risk of aspiration. Inspect to see if the umbilical cord is wrapped around the neck. If the cord is around the infant's neck, loosen, and slip over the infant's head. If it is impossible to slip the cord over the head, clamp the cord in two places and cut between the clamps. Suction the mouth and nose again after the baby is delivered.
B Breathing	If breathing is not spontaneous, gently rub the baby's back with a towel to stimulate breathing.

<table>
<tr><th colspan="2">Review of Newborn ABCCCC Management</th></tr>
<tr><td>C
Circulation</td><td>Move the baby to a warm environment. Placing the infant on the mother's abdomen is a warm and appropriate place. Determine the Apgar score at delivery and 5 minutes after delivery.
<table>
<tr><th colspan="4">Apgar Score</th></tr>
<tr><td></td><td>0</td><td>1</td><td>2</td></tr>
<tr><td>Appearance</td><td>Blue</td><td>Blue limbs, pink body</td><td>Pink</td></tr>
<tr><td>Pulse</td><td>Absent</td><td>< 100 beats/min.</td><td>> 100 beat/</td></tr>
<tr><td>Grimace</td><td>Limp</td><td>Some flexion</td><td>Good flexio</td></tr>
<tr><td>Activity</td><td>Absent</td><td>Some motion</td><td>Good motio</td></tr>
<tr><td>Respiration</td><td>Absent</td><td>Weak cry</td><td>Strong cry</td></tr>
</table></td></tr>
<tr><td>C
Clamp the Cord</td><td>When the cord has stopped pulsating, clamp the cord in two places, and cut between the clamps.</td></tr>
<tr><td>C
Cover</td><td>Dry the baby, cover, and place in a warm environment.</td></tr>
<tr><td>C
Continue the assessment</td><td>Continue the assessment. Reassess the airway. If the airway is not clear, suction the nose and then the mouth, position the newborn, and perform a slight chin lift. Do not hyperextend the neck. If breathing is absent or heart rate is < 80 beats/min. begin resuscitation.</td></tr>
<tr><td>R
Resuscitation</td><td>Provide oxygen, establish effective ventilation with a bag-valve mask or endotracheal intubation, and perform chest compressions. Medications are infrequently needed. A blood glucose level of 40 mg/dl is critical in a newborn. Administer a 25% solution at 0.5 g/kg.</td></tr>
</table>

NORMAL CHANGES DURING PREGNANCY

Review of the Normal Changes During Pregnancy
The stomach and intestines are displaced upward. Gastric emptying is delayed.
Hemodynamic changes include cardiac output increase of approximately 40%, systolic blood pressure increase of 5 to 15 mmHg, heart rate increase of 15 to 20 beats per minute, hematocrit increase of 30% to 35%, and a decreased clotting time.
Renal blood flow is increased.

Review of the Normal Changes During Pregnancy
The diaphragm is displaced upward by about 1½ to 2 inches. The air passages are engorged because of the increased blood flow. The respiratory rate is increased. Basal metabolism and oxygen consumption are increased. The pCO2 is decreased to 30 mmHg.
The uterus is normally the size of a plum and the shape of a pear. At delivery it weighs on average 2.2 lbs. and contains a liter of amniotic fluid.
Common discomforts of pregnancy are often present as concerns. Examples are nausea and vomiting, fatigue, hemorrhoids, varicose veins, heartburn, indigestion, bleeding gums, pica, swollen ankles and fingers, skin changes like chloasma or the mask of pregnancy, stretch marks, constipation, nasal congestion, and vaginal yeast infections. These symptoms are usually associated with normal pregnancy changes.

POSTPARTUM EMERGENCIES

Review of Postpartum Emergencies	
Postpartum DIC (disseminated intravascular coagulation)	EMERGENT DIC is characterized by the increase of clotting mechanisms. Clotting factors are consumed before the liver can replace them. Hemorrhage ensues. Causes may include amniotic fluid embolus, fetal death, abruptio placenta, and retained placenta. The diagnostic monitor is the fibrinogen level. Management may include replacement of clotting factors, platelets, fresh frozen plasma, and cryoprecipitate. Heparin may be used.
Postpartum hemorrhage	EMERGENT Postpartum hemorrhage is excessive bleeding of more than 1000 ml within 24 hours of delivery. The cause is often failure of the uterus to return to normal size, retained products of conception, and vaginal or cervical lacerations. Management may include CBC, sedimentation rate, type and cross, fluid resuscitation with normal saline and blood, vaginal examination, diagnosis, and correction of the underlying cause. Hospital admission is required for surgical repair, complete pelvic examination under anesthesia, support, and observation.

PREGNANCY AND DELIVERY EMERGENCIES

Review of Pregnancy and Delivery Emergencies

Review of Pregnancy and Delivery Emergencies	
Abruptio placenta	EMERGENT Abruptio placenta is the premature separation of the placenta during the last trimester of pregnancy. The cause is unknown. Symptoms may include vaginal bleeding, abdominal pain and tetanic contractions. Diagnostic tests include hemogram and crossmatch of 4 units of PRBC. Management includes fluid resuscitation with normal saline, fetal monitoring, and STAT C-section.
Amniotic fluid embolism	EMERGENT An amniotic fluid embolism occurs when the amniotic fluid leaks into the mother's vascular system. It is associated with abruptio placenta, placenta previa, and cases of fetal death. Symptoms may include profound hypotension, cardiopulmonary compromise, and arrest. Management may include rapid endotracheal intubation, mechanical ventilation with PEEP, fluid resuscitation with normal saline and blood products, and evaluation of coagulopathy and correction.
Breech	EMERGENT Breech presentations or malpresentations are categorized into three types. A complete breech is presentation with the infant's knees and hips flexed. An incomplete breech is presentation with one or both of the infant's feet or knees first. A front breech is presentation with the infant's hips flexed and the legs extended. Management may include a call for OB support.
Cord presentations	EMERGENT There are three variations of cord presentations: The cord is compressed by the fetus and not visible externally. The cord may not be visual but is felt in the vaginal canal. The cord is protruding from the vagina. The goal is restoration of cord patency and prevention of fetal anoxia. Management includes positioning the mother on the left side and administering 100% oxygen. If the cord is exposed, cover it with saline moistened sterile gauze. If the cervix is completely dilated, delivery might be accomplished with forceps; otherwise, STAT ER cesarean section is performed.

Review of Pregnancy and Delivery Emergencies	
Placenta previa	Placenta previa is a disorder where the placenta presents before the fetus. The amount of coverage of the cervical os is used to determine the type of placenta previa: total completely covers the os, partial partially covers the os, and marginal is beside the os. Symptoms may include hemorrhage not accompanied by labor. Diagnostic tests may include hemogram, type and crossmatch for four units of PRBC, clotting studies, and ultrasound. Management may include fluid resuscitation with normal saline, blood replacement, and transfer to labor and delivery. Pelvic examination is contraindicated.

PRE-ECLAMPSIA

PIH (pregnancy induced hypertension) aka preeclampsia and toxemia is a form of hypertension associated with pregnancy. The elevated blood pressure causes increased vascular resistance thereby restricting the blood flow to major organ systems resulting in problems in both the mother and baby such as placental abruption, intrauterine growth retardation and stillbirth. If left untreated the mother may have grand mal seizures. The cardinal signs are elevated blood pressure over 140/90, protein in the urine, edema, headaches, blurring vision, right sided upper quadrant pain, a decrease in urination, change in liver function tests. Common treatment is bedrest, possible hospitalization, magnesium sulfate therapy or other antihypertensives for PIH, fetal monitoring which may include a non-stress test, a biophysical profile, lab studies, administration of betamethasone to help with the maturation of the infant's lungs, and delivery. The problem commonly occurs in primigravida women and is associated with diabetes, hypertension, and renal disease.

RH FACTOR

The Rh factor is blood group present on the surface of erythrocytes of the rhesus monkey. It is found in variable degrees in the human population. When the factor is present a person is designated Rh+ (positive). A person without the factor is Rh- (negative). The blood of a Rh+ fetus can sensitize a pregnant female and form anti-Rh agglutinin. In subsequent pregnancies, if the fetus is Rh+ the maternal blood may cross the placenta and destroy fetal cells. RhoGAM immune globulin is prepared from the plasma of a person with high Rh antibodies.

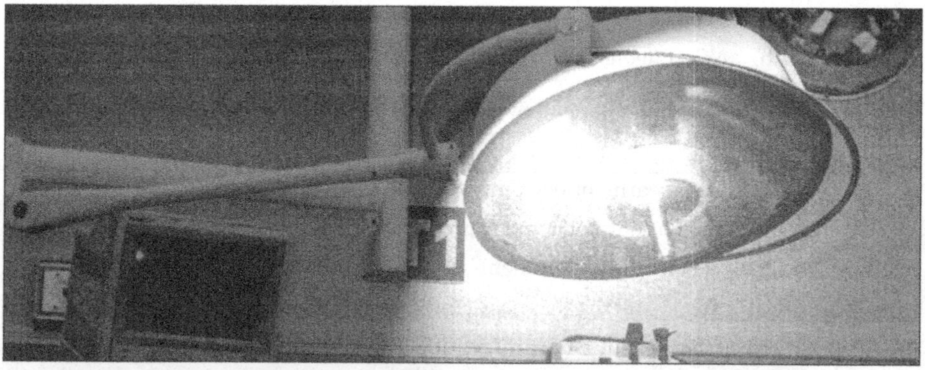

27 PSYCHIATRIC EMERGENCY AND SUICIDE ATTEMPT

For details on triage see Chapter 34, Triage in a Nutshell.

PATIENT'S STORY – INTERVIEW QUESTIONS

1. If a weapon was involved, where is the weapon?
2. Was there a suicide attempt or threat?
3. Was there violence?
4. When did the symptoms begin?
   a. If the symptoms are no longer active, how long did they last?
   b. If the symptoms were intermittent, how long did each episode last and how frequent were they?
5. Where are the physical injuries?
   a. What body system is involved?
   b. Are any other symptoms associated with the chief complaint, e.g., drug or alcohol intoxication, nausea, vomiting, headache, sweating, irregular or fast heartbeat?
6. Reconsider the nature of the emergency.
   a. Consider chapter #25 Overdose and Poisoning for an overdose.
   b. Consider chapter #8 Carbon Monoxide Inhalation and HAZMAT for a carbon monoxide poisoning.
   c. Consider chapter #29 Stabbing, Gunshot, and Penetrating Injury for injuries from a weapon.
   d. Consider chapter #23 Laceration for blunt trauma.
   e. Consider chapter #21 Hemorrhage for a laceration with hemorrhage.
7. Did an emotional crisis precede the symptoms; e.g., relationship crisis, divorce, disagreement, confrontation, or situational conflict?
8. Is unlawful activity suspected?

a. Was law enforcement at the scene?

b. What agency?

Medical personnel are obligated to notify law enforcement if unlawful activity is suspected.

9. Has any treatment been initiated, and has it helped?
10. Has the patient had similar problems before?
    a. When was the problem?
    b. What was the diagnosis and treatment?
11. Does the patient have any pertinent past history?
12. Does the patient take any routine medications?
    a. What is the name, dosage, route, and frequency of the medication?
    b. When was the last dose?
13. Does the patient take any complementary or alternative therapies, herbal products, over-the-counter medications or supplements, or natural therapies?
    a. What is the name, dosage, route and frequency of the therapy?
    b. When was the last dose or therapy?
14. Does the patient have allergies to drugs or foods?
    a. What is the name of the allergen?
    b. What was the reaction?
15. When was the patient's last tetanus immunization?
16. If the patient is female and between the ages of 12 to 50 years, when was the first day of her last menstrual period?

NURSING DOMAIN

The nursing domain, nursing diagnosis and plan of care can only be determined after an in-depth interview and consideration of the patient's story.

Domain 12. Comfort. Class 1. Physical comfort.
Domain 11. Safety/Protection. Class 3. Violence.

ANTICIPATED MEDICAL CARE

Review of the Anticipated Medical Care of Psychiatric Emergencies and Suicide Attempts	
Exam	Full body
Urine tests	Urine for toxicology

Review of the Anticipated Medical Care of Psychiatric Emergencies and Suicide Attempts	
Blood	Serum toxicology, CBC, electrolytes, renal function studies
ECG	ECG for females and males over 35 years with complaints of chest pain
Radiographic Studies	X-ray of areas where bony injury is suspected, chest x-ray if pulmonary problems are suspected.
Diet	NPO
IV	Normal saline or Ringer's solution
Medications	Anti-anxiety agents, sedatives, psychotropic medication
Other	The medical provider is responsible for the legal documentation required to commit the patient to a psychiatric facility for treatment, observation, and safety. A medical provider order is required to restrain a patient.
Disposition	Admission to a psychiatric hospital may be required.
Worst-case scenario	The worst-case scenario is suicide in the ER that was preventable with appropriate security measures, such as constant monitoring and restraints.

INITIAL CARE PLAN

Alcohol-based hand sanitizers are the preferred method for cleaning your hands in most clinical situations. Wash your hands with soap and water whenever they are visibly dirty, before eating, and after using the restroom.

1. Consider where the patient is placed within the ER.
    a. The goal is to provide a safe, harmless, and non-hostile environment. Consider if the patient needs a suicide watch? Keep the patient in an area where they can be readily observed.
    b. Does the patient show signs of agitation, aggression, or signs of immediate risk for violence?

Signs of immediate risk for violence include verbal threats of harm to self or others; the ability to carry out those threats, the influence of drugs or alcohol, agitation, yelling, use of profanity, pacing, and moving close to the staff member's face. The most important concern is for the safety of the staff and bystanders. Empathy (understanding) is the most effective tool. Keep at a safe distance and talk quietly, calmly, and keep sentences short. Evaluate the patient's response and repeat the technique that works best to quiet the patient. Give the patient as much control as possible including allowing the patient to feel in control. Offer choices whenever possible. Call for backup in a nonthreatening manner.

   c. The patient may need to move about the room.

2. Mental status exam is necessary in order to determine how best to communicate with the patient. Communicate in short concise statements while establishing rapport and trust. Psychoanalysis is not done in the ER. Resolution does not take place in the ER. The interventions started in the ER lead to resolution.
   a. Encourage the patient to vent feelings and verbalize fears. (This is not done with patient's exhibiting paranoid and psychotic symptoms.)
3. Consider the following quick mental status assessment questions.
   a. Does the patient's expression and behavior agree?
   b. Is the patient's dress appropriate for the situation?
   c. Is the patient's mood appropriate for the situation?
   d. Are the patient's interactions with the nurse appropriate?
   e. Is the patient's speech content and style appropriate for situation?
   f. Are the patient's thoughts (based on the patient's speech content) logical and appropriate for the situation?
   g. Is the patient making suicidal or homicidal statements that may require immediate interventions from you and/or law enforcement or security?

> Asking a patient about suicide plans does not introduce the idea to commit suicide. Asking if the patient is thinking about suicide is an important question. It is a necessary part of a lethality assessment to talk about the plan, including the means, location, and the time. If you don't ask , you won't know the answer.

4. Assure the patient that the symptoms will subside.
5. Obtain vital signs.
6. Perform a focused physical assessment of any areas of injury. Evaluate neurovascular function distal to the injury.
7. Evaluate the level of consciousness to use as a baseline.
8. Establish intravenous access and collect blood laboratory specimens. Draw a variety of tubes and hold for medical provider order.
9. Instruct the patient not to eat or drink and teach the patient and family the rationale for the NPO status.
10. Inform the patient, family, and caregivers of the usual plan of care and the expected overall time in the ER.
11. Provide the patient with a device to reach someone for assistance and explain how to use it.
12. Establish a set of rules for movement about the department and ask the patient to agree with the rules.

13. Try chemical restraints before physical restraints. For chemical restraints most common medications are intramuscular antipsychotic and /or benzodiazepines Physical restraints are a last resort.

ONGOING CARE PLAN

Inform the medical provider of adverse changes noted during ongoing evaluation. Document that the medical provider was notified of the adverse change. Document if orders were or were not received.

1. Consider suicide watch (constant observation with 5 to 15-minute checks)
2. Monitor temperature, heart rate, blood pressure, and effectiveness of breathing.
3. Monitor therapy closely for the patient's therapeutic response.
   a. The usual time for a medication effectiveness check is 20 to 30 minutes after giving the drug.
   b. If therapy is not effective, ask the medical provider for a repeat dose or an alternative.
4. Monitor closely for the development of adverse reactions to therapy.
   a. Perform interventions to relieve the adverse reaction.
   b. Ask the medical provider for a remedy.
5. Keep the patient, family, and caregivers well informed of the plan of care and the remaining time anticipated before disposition.
6. Monitor the patient's laboratory and x-ray results and notify the medical provider of critical abnormalities. Remedy abnormalities as ordered.
7. Notify the medical provider when all diagnostic results are available for review. Ask for establishment of a diagnosis and disposition.

DISCHARGE INSTRUCTIONS

In some states, patients admitted with a possible psychiatric diagnosis need a follow-up mental health appointment in 3 days. Make sure the patient has just enough refills to last until that visit. If you put the patient on medication in the ER, make a follow-up appointment with the patient's current provider or new provider, such as the local mental health clinic.

1. Provide the patient with the name of the nurse and doctor in the emergency room.
2. Inform the patient of their diagnosis or why a definitive diagnosis couldn't be made. Explain what caused the problem if known. If the diagnosis is psychiatric in nature, consider if it is in the best interest of the patient to discuss.
3. Teach the patient how to take the medication as prescribed and how to manage the common side effects. Instruct the patient not to drive or perform any dangerous tasks while taking narcotic pain medications.

4. Recommend a medical provider for follow-up care. Provide the name, address, and phone number with a recommendation of when to schedule the care.
5. Instruct the patient to call the follow-up medical provider immediately or return to the emergency room if the pain or problem worsens in any way or any unusual symptoms develop. Encourage the patient NOT to IGNORE WORSENING OR PERSISTENT SYMPTOMS.
6. Ask for verbal confirmation or demonstration of understanding and reinforce teaching as needed.
7. Give phone numbers for the local help and suicide hotline.

COMMONLY ORDERED MEDICATIONS

ATIVAN

Ativan (lorazepam)	
Indications	Anxiety, irritability in patients with psychiatric and organic brain disorders
Dose	1 to 2 mg IV or 2 to 6 mg PO, maximum 10 mg/d
Onset	PO onset ½ hour, IV onset 5 to 15 min., PO and IV duration 3 to 6 hours
Side effects	Dry mouth, drowsiness, tachycardia, orthostatic hypotension
Note	Give PO with food or milk

GEODON

Geodon IM	
Indications	Agitation in psychotic disorder
Dose	10 mg IM, maximum dose 40 mg per day
Onset	30 minutes
Side effects	Injection site pain, nausea, somnolence and dizziness; counter indicated with known QT interval prolongation and some cardiac problems, safety in pregnancy or in children has not been demonstrated.
Note	IM powder must be diluted and mixed

HALDOL

Haldol (haloperidol)	
Indications	Psychotic disorders
Dose	2 to 5 mg IM every 1 hour
Pediatric dose	0.05 to 0.15 mg/kg/day IM, ages 3 to 5 years
Onset	IM onset ½ hour, peak 30 to 45 minutes, duration 4 to 8 hours

Haldol (haloperidol)	
Side effects	Extrapyramidal symptoms, dystonia, seizures, neuroleptic malignant syndrome, laryngospasm, respiratory depression, cardiac arrest
Note	Haldol's therapeutic effect can be expected 30 minutes post administration of the drug. If there is no change in the patient's agitation, ask the medical provider for a second dose.

LIBRIUM

Librium (chlordiazepoxide)	
Indications	Short-term management of anxiety, acute alcohol withdrawal
Dose	50 to 100 mg IM, PO, or IV over 1 min. not to exceed 300 mg/d
Onset	PO onset 30 min., IM onset 15 to 30 min., IV onset 1 to 5 min., PO duration 4 to 6 hours, IV duration up to 1 hour
Side effects	Tachycardia, orthostatic hypotension
Note	Powder for injection with special diluents for IM injections. Do not use special diluents for IV administration, reconstitute with sterile water or normal saline.

VALIUM

Valium (diazepam)	
Indications	Anxiety, acute alcohol withdrawal
Dose	Single dose 1 to 10 mg PO, 5 to 20 mg IM, 5 to 10 mg IV
Pediatric dose	Older than 6 mo., 1 to 2.5 mg PO, 0.1 to 0.3 mg/kg IV every 15 min. times 2 doses
Onset	IV onset 5 min., peak 15 minutes, and duration 15 min. IM onset 15 min., peak ½ to 1 ½ hours, duration 1 to 1 ½ hours PO onset ½ hour, peak 1 to 2 hours, duration 2 to 3 hours
Side effects	Dizziness, drowsiness, orthostatic hypotension, blurred vision, tachycardia
Monitor	Respiratory effectiveness

ZYPREXA

Zyprexa (olanzapine) IM	
Indications	Agitation in Psychotic Disorder
Dose	Start with 10 mg may follow with 5 to 10 mg IM in 2 to 4 hr. Limit of 20 mg in 24 hr. Not to be used more than 3 days, switch to PO.
Onset	30 minutes

Zyprexa (olanzapine) IM	
Side effects	Sedation, dizziness, hypotension

RELATED CONDITIONS AND INFORMATION

AFFECTIVE DISORDERS

Affective disorders are a group of mental disorders characterized by mood disturbances, such as depression, bipolar, and dysthymic disorders. Restraints are rarely used. Most of these patients are not psychotic or violent. They need support and evaluation for suicide ideation.

ALCOHOLIC INTOXICATION

Patients with emergencies related to alcohol are common in the ER. An intoxicated patient often gives an inaccurate medical history, abnormal response to physical problems, and has the potential for violent and disruptive behavior. If restraints are needed, position the patient on his abdomen or side to reduce the risk of aspiration since vomiting and seizures are common side effects of alcohol intoxication. Haldol can be used to quiet and calm the patient. Management may include thiamine, a liter of intravenous solution, multivitamins, sleep, observation to prevent adverse physical effects, and discharge to an acute alcohol treatment center or referral to outpatient substance abuse treatment center. Evaluate for depression and suicide after the patient is sober.

DEPERSONALIZATION

Review of Depersonalization	
Definition	Depersonalization is an altered perception of the body or a sense of being outside of the body characterized by feelings that one's actions and speech cannot be controlled.
Cause	Depersonalization is usually a mechanism to protect the self.
Management	Management includes identification of the problem, relieving anxiety, and initiating a plan for psychiatric care.

DRUG INTOXICATION

In most instances, patients with acute drug intoxication present with physical symptoms or are brought in unresponsive by friends. Management includes medications to relieve symptoms (nausea, vomiting, diarrhea, agitation, dehydration) and referral to a drug program. Acute overdose treatment is aimed at the physical response to the toxin. Admission to the hospital may be required if the patient is medically unstable or if stable, to a facility to treat the drug problem.

DRUG INFORMATION GUIDE

Review of Drug Information	
Alcohol	Puffiness of face, red eyes, disorientation, shallow respirations, depression, aggression, blurred vision, lack of coordination Duration: 1 to 12 hours.

Review of Drug Information	
Amphetamines (uppers, speed, black beauties, dexies)	Unusual increase in activity, increased heart rate, breathing and blood pressure, high doses can cause tremors Duration: ½ to 2 hours
Barbiturates, Methaqualone (Quaaludes, ludes, yellow jackets, red devils)	Slurred speech, drunken behavior without odor of alcohol, unsteady gait, poor slow judgment, slow reflexes Duration: 1 to 16 hours
Cocaine (coke, snow, blow, gold dust, lady)	Apathy, anxiety, sleeplessness, paranoia, cocaine hunger, constant sniffing, dilated pupils, increased body temperature, blood pressure, and heart rate Duration: ½ to 2 hours
Crack cocaine (crack, rock)	Same as cocaine but gets to the brain quicker Duration: 5 to 10 minutes
Gasoline and glue (rush, locker room), aerosol cans of amyl nitrate, gasoline, lighter fluid inhaled through a saturated cloth covering the nose and mouth	Keen senses, hallucinations, scrambled words and disconnected sentences, an odor of the substance used, cardiac arrhythmias Duration: variable
Hallucinogens (LSD, mescaline, peyote, mushrooms)	Dilated pupils, nausea, increased blood pressure, stomach cramps, flashbacks, beady eyes, nervous erratic behavior, laughing, crying, personality changes, a sense of seeing smells and hearing colors, marked depersonalization Duration: 3 to 12 hours
Heroin (Mexican brown, China white, Persian porcelain, H)	Watery eyes, runny nose, yawning, irritability, panic, chills, repeated use can lead to infections of the heart and valves, skin abscesses, and lung congestion Duration: 12 to 24 hours
Marijuana (pot, reefer, grass, hash and hash oil)	Euphoria, relaxed inhabitation, disoriented behavior, staring into space, laughing without cause, time disorientation, bloodshot eyes, impaired memory perception and judgment Duration: 2 to 4 hours
3,4-Methylenedioxy Methamphetamine (Ecstasy, Adam, ecstasy, X-TC days, a designer drug)	Increased heart rate and blood pressure, blurred vision, chills, sweating, confusion, sleep problems, anxiety, paranoia, muscle tension, involuntary teeth clenching Duration: variable, up to days

Review of Drug Information	
PCP or Phencyclidine (angel dust, killer weed, crystal cyclone, elephant tranquilizer, rocket fuel	Increased heart rate and blood pressure, sweating, dizziness, hallucinations, confusion, violence and aggression, or silence and withdrawal Duration: variable

DYSTONIA

Haldol, Thorazine, and Compazine may cause dystonia, a reaction to medications that causes muscle spasm or contractions that usually involve the tongue, neck, and jaw. Treatment is Cogentin (benztropine mesylate).

HALLUCINATION

A hallucination is a perception of objects with no reality and may arise from a disorder of the nervous system or in response to drugs. The patient usually has a compelling sense that they are real. Orientation to reality is the supportive therapy of choice.

HYPERVENTILATION

Hyperventilation occurs when breathing is at a rate faster or deeper than the body requires and may result in a decreased carbon dioxide level. Carpopedal spasms occur as a result of decreased carbon dioxide. This causes tetany-like activity in the muscles of the hands and feet. As the carbon dioxide returns to normal the symptoms resolve. Hyperventilation can be caused by anxiety.

INFECTION

Infection of the central nervous system may produce behavioral changes that mimic psychiatric behavior.

MASLOW'S HIERARCHY OF NEEDS

Review of Maslow's Hierarchy of Needs	
Hierarchy of needs	Abraham Maslow (1908-1970) was an American psychologist and the founder of humanistic psychology. He developed a hierarchical model of human motivation, in which a higher need, ultimately that for self-actualization, is expressed only after lower needs are fulfilled.
1st Physiologic	Physiologic needs are oxygen, food, water, shelter, and sex.
2nd Safety	Safety needs are freedom from fear and physical harm.
3rd Social	Social needs are an acceptable relationship, friendship, affection, acceptance, interaction with others, and love.
4th Esteem	Esteem needs are personal feelings of achievement and self-respect, and respect and recognition from others.
5th Self-actualization	Self-actualization needs are self-fulfillment and reaching of one's potential.

Review of Maslow's Hierarchy of Needs	
Management	In the ER, recognition of unmet needs is developed from the history of the present illness and developed into a nursing diagnosis.

PANIC ATTACKS

Review of Panic Attacks	
Definition	Panic attacks are acute recurrent attacks of panic.
Cause	Panic attacks have no tangible cause.
Symptoms	Symptoms include shortness of breath, chest pain, tachycardia, sweating, nausea, vomiting, diarrhea, and a feeling of approaching death. Patients with panic level anxiety attacks may exhibit psychotic behavior. The patient may have trouble relating to others and may experience hallucinations or delusions. Hyperventilation can occur during a panic attack. It occurs when breathing is at a rate faster or deeper than the body requires and may result in a decreased carbon dioxide level. Carpopedal spasms occur as a result of decreased carbon dioxide. This causes tetany-like activity in the muscles of the hands and feet. As the carbon dioxide returns to normal, the symptoms resolve. Hyperventilation can be caused by anxiety. A return toward normal vital signs is indicative of a decrease in sympathetic stimulation and a decrease in anxiety.
Management	Management includes providing a quiet safe environment, administration of anti-anxiety mediations, encouragement to vent feelings, reinforcement of positive behavior, and referral to appropriate follow-up care.

PERSONS AT HIGH RISK FOR SUICIDE

- Older males without a spouse, unemployed, and in poor health
- People who are depressed
- Alcoholics
- Drug addicts
- Persons with spinal cord injuries, cancer, and serious debilitating illness
- Persons with mental health disorders such as schizophrenia

PHOBIAS

Review of Phobias

Review of Phobias	
Definition	A phobia is a persistent and irrational fear of a specific activity or object that results in a compelling desire to avoid the situation. Phobias are classified into three types: agoraphobias (a variety of everyday situations), social phobias (embarrassment in public), and simple phobias (specific situations, e.g., tunnels, flying, elevators).
Physical findings	Symptoms may include fear, shortness of breath, chest pain, tachycardia, sweating, nausea, vomiting, diarrhea, and a feeling that something terrible is about to happen.
Management	Management may include providing a quiet safe environment, anti-anxiety mediations, encouraging the patient to vent feelings, reinforcing positive behavior, and referral to appropriate follow-up care.

POSTTRAUMATIC STRESS DISORDER

Review of Posttraumatic Stress Disorder	
Definition	Posttraumatic stress disorder is a condition where a patient experiences recurrent dreams or thoughts about a traumatic event with feelings of detachment and estrangement from the environment. The disorder is associated with sleep disorders, hyper alertness, difficulty concentrating, and memory impairment.
Cause	The cause of posttraumatic stress disorder is commonly military combat, rape, or a disaster.
Physical findings	Symptoms may include fear, shortness of breath, chest pain, tachycardia, sweating, nausea, vomiting, diarrhea, and a feeling that something terrible is about to happen.
Management	Management includes providing a quiet safe environment, treating presenting symptom not diagnosis, anti-anxiety mediations, encouraging the patient to vent feelings, reinforcement of positive behavior, and referral to appropriate follow-up care.

ORGANIC BRAIN DISORDER

Organic disorders encompass a large group of acute and chronic mental disorders associated with brain damage (traumatic brain injury) or cerebral dysfunction. The patient may present with impaired consciousness, orientation, intellect, judgment, thought processing, or with hallucination and mood changes. Diagnosis is made by history and ruling out acute physical causes. Management may include restraints, sedatives as needed to protect the patient and staff, and admission to a psychiatric hospital.

PSYCHOTIC DISORDERS

Management is supportive. If the patient is violent, restraints and sedation may be needed to protect the patient and staff. Admission to a psychiatric hospital is often needed.

PARANOID DISORDERS

Paranoia disorder is a condition where the patient shows persistent delusions of persecution. Behavior can be consistent with the delusion or be bizarre and incoherent. The disorder usually occurs in mid or late adult life and may include anger that leads to violent behavior.

PHYSICAL CHANGES DURING STRESS

Review of Physical Changes During Stress	
Alarm stage	The alarm state is a condition where an increase in epinephrine and norepinephrine release occurs. The fight-or-flight reaction is activated. The blood pressure, pulse, respiratory rate, blood sugar, and alertness are increased.
Resistance stage	The resistance stage is a stage where hormonal levels adjust, and the patient uses coping and defensive behavior.
Exhaustion	When exhaustion occurs, the immune response decreases, the defense mechanisms are exaggerated, thinking is disorganized, sensory input is misperceived (auditory and visual illusions), reality concepts are distorted, and violent behavior can occur. Physical system failure and death can occur.

PORT OF ENTRY

The ER is the port of entry to the health care system for homeless mentally ill patients. These patients often have maladaptive behaviors that are a part of their daily existence from anxiety disorders, phobias, and posttraumatic stress syndromes. Referral to appropriate health care that will accept them is essential.

SCHIZOPHRENIA

Schizophrenia is a group of mental disorders with disordered thinking and bizarre behaviors. Clinically, patients show disturbances of thought with delusions. Speech may be coherent but unassociated with the situation, mute, completely incoherent, or catatonic. Affect may be flat or inappropriate. Perception is disordered with visual and auditory hallucinations. Management is supportive. Restraints and sedation may be needed to protect the patient and staff. Admission to a psychiatric hospital care is essential.

SOMATIZATION

Review of Somatization	
Definition	Somatization is a condition where a person has multiple somatic complaints with fifteen or more symptoms lasting over several years.
Cause	The cause of somatization is unknown usually related to psychological needs.

Review of Somatization	
Physical findings	Symptoms include multiple physical complaints, numerous surgeries, and medical consults. The condition is frequently associated with alcohol abuse.
Management	Management includes identification of the problem, objectiveness, increase in the time spent on feelings, decrease in the time spent on the physical complaint, and development of a plan for follow-up psychiatric care.

STAGES OF DEVELOPMENT

Review of Erikson's Eight Stages of Development	
E. H. Erikson is a German-born American psychoanalyst (born 1902) who proposed that people acquire mature psychosexual traits by overcoming a series of personal crises.	
Birth to 18 months	Trust vs. mistrust The ability to trust others and have a sense of hope.
18 months to 3 years	Autonomy vs. shame and doubt Self-control without loss of self-esteem. The ability to cooperate and express one's self.
3 to 5 years	Initiative vs. guilt Realistic sense of purpose and ability to evaluate one's own behavior versus self-denial and self-restriction.
6 to 12 years	Industry vs. inferiority Realization of competence, preservation versus feeling that one will never be any good and withdrawal from school and peers.
12 to 20 years	Identity vs. role diffusion Coherent sense of self; plans to actualize one's abilities versus feelings of confusion, indecisiveness, and the possibility of antisocial behavior.
18 to 25 years	Intimacy vs. isolation Capacity for love as mutual devotion, commitment to work and relationships versus impersonal relationships and prejudice.
25 to 65 years	Generatively vs. stagnation Creativity, production, concern for others versus self-indulgence and impoverishment of self.
65 years to death	Integrity vs. despair Acceptance of the worth and uniqueness of one's life versus a sense of loss and contempt for others.

SUICIDE

Asking a patient about suicide plans does not introduce the idea to commit suicide. Asking if the patient is thinking about suicide is an important question. It is a necessary part of a lethality assessment to talk about the plan, including the means, location, and the time. If you don't ask the question, you won't know the answer.

SUICIDOLOGY

The following information is taken from suicidology.org.

Facts from suicidology.org
According to the website www.suicidology.org, in 2018 (the latest year for which we have national statistics), there were 48,344 suicides in the U.S. National suicide rate (age adjusted) or 14.2 per 100,000. Firearms accounted for 24,432 suicides in 2018 (50.5%).
Suicide is the tenth leading cause of death in the US. It ranks 2nd leading cause of death for 15 to 34-year-olds.
A rate increase was seen in 2007, representing a change in the recent pattern of stability or slight decline. Since 1990, rates have ranged between 12.4 and 10.7 per 100,000.
Rates of suicide are highest in the intermountain states. Six of the top 10 states suicide rates are from those states.
Males complete suicide at a rate 3.6 times that of females. However, females attempt suicide three times more often than males.
Relative to those younger, rates of completed suicide are highest among the elderly (age 80 and over).
Suicide ranks third as a cause of death among young (15-24) Americans behind accidents and homicides.
Firearms remain the most commonly utilized method of completing suicide by essentially all groups. More than half (50.2%) of the individuals who took their own lives in 2007 used this method. Males used it more often than their female counterparts.
The most common method of suicide for all females was poisoning. In fact, poisoning has surpassed firearms for female suicides since 2001.
Caucasians (12.9 per 100,000) have higher rates of completed suicides than African Americans (4.9 per 100,000).

SUICIDE WARNING SIGNS

Warning signs of suicidal ideation (frequent suicidal thoughts):
Specific lethal plan that does not include the possibility for rescue
Depression (65% of suicides have a history of depression)
History of suicide attempts (65% of suicides have a history of attempts)
Limited psychological and social resources
Taking actions to put their lives in order

Warning signs of suicidal ideation (frequent suicidal thoughts):
Giving away possessions
Failure at work or school
Recent loss and dealing with grief
Poor work or school performance
History of alcohol abuse
History of drug abuse
More than 31,000 people kill themselves each year
More than 425,000 people with self-inflicted injuries are treated in emergency rooms each year.

TARDIVE DYSKINESIA

A neurological syndrome caused by the long-term use of neuroleptic drugs. It is characterized by repetitive involuntary, purposeless movements include grimacing, tongue protrusion, lip smacking and/or pursing, and rapid eye blinking. The extremities can be involved. There is no standard treatment. Drugs such as benzodiazepines, adrenergic antagonists, and dopamine agnostics may be helpful.

VIOLENCE

Violence in the ER is an increasing problem from both mentally disturbed and angry abusive patients and their families. A quick decision is necessary to recognize the need for security, police action, and physical or chemical restraints. Once a patient is restrained, the care time is increased. Frequent monitoring and documentation are essential. Management includes the decision to restrain, prompt action, frequent monitoring, and discharge to an appropriate medical or correctional facility.

Signs of immediate risk for violence include verbal threats of harm to self or others; the ability to carry out those threats, the influence of drugs or alcohol, agitation, yelling, use of profanity, pacing, and moving close to your face. The most important concern is for the safety of the staff and bystanders. Empathy (understanding) is the most effective tool. Keep at a safe distance and talk quietly, calmly, and keep sentences short. Evaluate the patient's response and repeat the technique that works best to quiet the patient. Give the patient as much control as possible including allowing the patient to feel in control. Offer choices whenever possible. Call for backup in a nonthreatening manner.

GERIATRIC CONSIDERATIONS

SUICIDE

The highest rate of suicide is in older adults, primarily Caucasian men who live alone.

PEDIATRIC CONSIDERATIONS

SUICIDE ATTEMPTS IN CHILDREN AND ADOLESCENTS

- Three times as many girls than boys attempted suicide.

- Of the boys who attempted suicide, they were significantly younger than girls.
- Their families demonstrated history of more psychiatric illness, alcohol and drug abuse, suicide, paternal unemployment, and paternal and/or maternal absence.
- The suicide attempts usually occurred in winter, after school or in the evening
- The attempts usually occurred at home with someone nearby.
- The usual method of attempt was overdose.

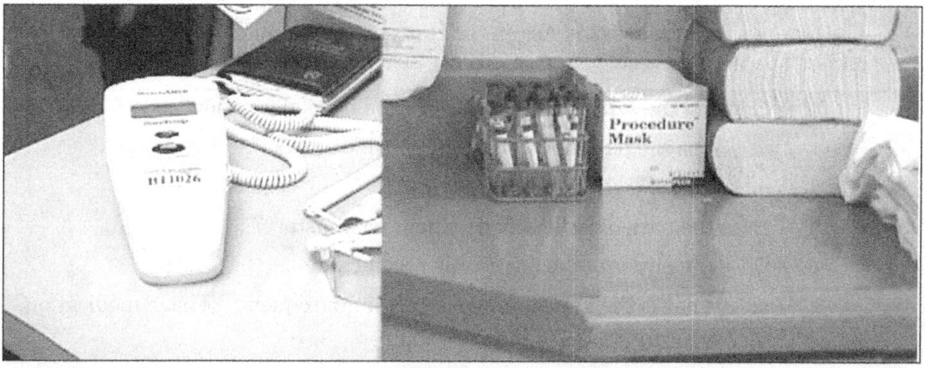

28 SEIZURE

For details on triage see Chapter 34, Triage in a Nutshell.

PATIENT'S STORY – INTERVIEW QUESTIONS

1. Have you had a recent injury?
2. When did the symptoms begin?
   a. How many seizures did the patient have today?
   b. Is there a history of seizures?
   c. When was the last seizure prior to today?
3. Describe the seizure activity if known.
   a. Did the patient lose consciousness?
   b. What part of the body was involved?
   c. What type of movement was involved?
   d. How long did the seizure last?
   e. Was the patient's head or neck injured during the seizure and are any other injuries suspected?
   f. Are any other symptoms associated with the seizure; e.g., nausea, vomiting, headache, an aura, or visual disturbance?
4. Consider chapter #26 Pregnancy and Delivery Emergency if the patient is pregnant or postpartum.
5. Is the cause of the seizure known?
   a. Does the patient take anti-seizure medications?
   b. What is the name and dosing regimen?
   c. When was the last dose?

The most common cause of recurrent seizures is noncompliance. Frequently patients do not take anti-seizure medications as prescribed.

6. How did the seizure affect the patient's normal function?
    a. Was the patient incontinent of urine or stool?
    b. Was or is the patient postictal?
7. Does the patient have any pertinent past history?
8. Does the patient take any routine medications?
    a. What is the name, dosage, route, and frequency of each medication?
    b. When was the last dose?
9. Does the patient take any complementary or alternative therapies, herbal products, over-the-counter medications or supplements, or natural therapies?
    a. What is the name, dosage, route and frequency of each therapy?
    b. When was the last dose or therapy?
10. Does the patient have allergies to drugs or foods?
    a. What is the name of the allergen?
    b. What was the reaction?
11. When was the patient's last tetanus immunization?
12. If the patient is female and between the ages of 10 to 50 years, when was the first day of her last menstrual period?

NURSING DOMAIN

The nursing domain, nursing diagnosis and plan of care can only be determined after an in-depth interview and consideration of the patient's story.

Domain 12. Comfort. Class 1. Physical comfort.
Domain 11. Safety/Protection. Class 2. Physical injury.

ANTICIPATED MEDICAL CARE

Review of the Anticipated Medical Care of Seizures	
Exam	Full body
Urine test	Toxicology screen; pregnancy test for women of reproductive age unless they have had a hysterectomy.
Blood test	CBC, electrolytes, renal function studies, serum drug levels of anticonvulsant medications
ECG	None

Review of the Anticipated Medical Care of Seizures	
Radiographic Studies	C-spine x-rays if spinal injury during seizure is suspected, x-rays of suspected bony damage, consider shoulder x-rays for posterior dislocation, CT of the brain for new onset
Diet	NPO
IV	Normal saline or Ringer's solution
Medications	Valium or Ativan for active seizures, Cerebyx, Dilantin, or other anticonvulsants in loading doses for maintenance
Other	Treatment of the underlying cause if known
Disposition	Hospital admission may be required for new seizures and for treatment of cause, such as cerebral trauma, CNS infection, cerebral tumors, and metabolic brain disorders.
Worst-case scenario	The worst-case scenario is status epilepticus with respiratory or cardiovascular insufficiency. The management may include paralyzing the patient with rapid sequence medications for endotracheal intubation and induction of pentobarbital coma or general anesthesia. The mortality rate in severe tonic-clonic status is 10%. The incidence of permanent neurological sequelae is 10 to 30%.

INITIAL CARE PLAN

NEVER FORCE AN AIRWAY OR ANY OBJECT IN A SEIZING PATIENT'S MOUTH. If the patient is seizing, stay with the patient, summon help, and protect the patient's head. Obtain an order for an anticonvulsant medication and administer. If the patient is postictal, turn the patient on his right side to protect the airway and reduce the risk of aspiration.

Alcohol-based hand sanitizers are the preferred method for cleaning your hands in most clinical situations. Wash your hands with soap and water whenever they are visibly dirty, before eating, and after using the restroom.

1. Ask the patient to undress, remove jewelry that might interfere with the examination, and put on an exam gown. Assist as needed.
2. Obtain initial vital signs including pulse oximetry or test capillary refill. Consider obtaining a rectal temperature.
3. Administer supplemental oxygen if saturation is < 94%. Severe COPD patients may be unable to maintain saturation >88% to 92%.
4. Assure the patient that he is safe.
5. Position the patient to enhance normal body function and comfort.
6. Establish intravenous access and draw laboratory blood specimens.

   a. Draw a variety of tubes that will allow the lab to perform hematology, chemistry, and coagulation studies. Patients on anticoagulants need coagulation studies.
   b. Consider drawing other labs, e.g., type and screen, blood cultures.

7. Perform a point of care finger stick blood sugar at the bedside. Treat hypoglycemia < 60.
8. Evaluate the level of consciousness based on the mnemonic **AVPU** or **ACDU** level of consciousness score.
   AVPU: **A**lert, **V**erbal, **P**ain, **U**nresponsive.
   ACDU: **A**lert, **C**onfused, **D**rowsy, **U**nresponsive.
9. Perform a focused examination.
   a. Perform a cursory assessment for stroke symptoms.
      i. Evaluate for facial droop by asking the patient to smile. Normally both sides move equally well. The smile is abnormal when one side of the face does not move as well as the other side.
      ii. Evaluate arm weakness by asking the patient to hold his arms outstretched with his eyes closed. Normally both arms move equally well. The arms are considered abnormal when one arm does not move as well as the other or one arm drifts down compared with the other.
      iii. Evaluate the speech by asking the patient to say, "You can't teach an old dog new tricks." Normally the patient uses correct words with no slurring. The speech is abnormal if the patient slurs words, uses inappropriate words, or is unable to speak.
   b. Auscultate the lungs.
   c. Auscultate the abdomen for bowel sounds.
   d. Inspect for injuries. If found, examine the site of injury and evaluate neurovascular function distal to the injury.
   e. Protect, support, elevate, and ice any injured areas.
10. Instruct the patient not to eat or drink and teach the patient and family the rationale for the NPO status.
11. Elevate the siderails and place the stretcher in the lowest position.
12. Inform the patient, family, and caregivers of the usual plan of care, and the expected overall time in the ER.
13. Provide the patient with a device to reach someone for assistance and explain how to use it. Ask the patient to call for help before getting off the stretcher.

ONGOING CARE PLAN

1. Inform the medical provider of adverse changes noted during ongoing evaluation. Document that the medical provider was notified of the adverse changes. Document if orders were or were not received.
2. Monitor temperature, heart rate and rhythm, blood pressure, and effectiveness of breathing.
3. Monitor therapy closely for the patient's therapeutic response.
    a. The usual time for a medication effectiveness check is 20 to 30 minutes after giving the drug.
    b. If therapy is not effective, ask the medical provider for a repeat dose or an alternative.
4. Monitor for seizure activity.
5. Monitor closely for the development of adverse reactions to therapy.
    a. Perform interventions to relieve the adverse reaction.
    b. Ask the medical provider for a remedy.
6. Keep the patient, family, and caregivers well informed of the plan of care and the remaining time anticipated before disposition.
7. Monitor the patient's laboratory and x-ray results and notify the medical provider of critical abnormalities. Remedy abnormalities as ordered.
8. Notify the medical provider when all diagnostic results are available for review. Ask for establishment of a diagnosis and disposition.

DISCHARGE INSTRUCTIONS

1. Provide the patient with the name of the nurse and doctor in the emergency room.
2. Inform the patient of their diagnosis or why a definitive diagnosis couldn't be made. Explain what caused the problem if known.
3. Instruct the patient not to drive or perform any dangerous tasks until the doctor specifically clears him to do so.
4. Teach the patient with a seizure that:
    a. The anticonvulsant medication must be taken as prescribed.
    b. If the serum blood level of the medication was low, the dose may be increased.
5. Recommend a medical provider for follow-up care. Provide the name, address, and phone number with a recommendation of when to schedule the care.
6. Inform the patient that if he has recurrent seizures or unusual symptoms to call the follow-up medical provider immediately or return to the emergency room. Encourage the patient NOT to IGNORE WORSENING OR PERSISTENT SYMPTOMS.

7. Ask for verbal confirmation or demonstration of understanding and reinforce teaching as needed.

COMMONLY ORDERED MEDICATIONS

CEREBYX

Cerebyx (fosphenytoin sodium)	
Indications	Short-term parenteral administration when other means of phenytoin are less advantageous
Adult dose	15 to 20 PE (phenytoin equivalents)/kg IV at a rate of <150 PE/min. May be given IM if IV is not available.
Pediatric dose	The safety of Cerebyx in pediatric patients has not been established.
Onset	Maximum phenytoin levels occur approximately 10 to 15 minutes after the end of the infusion.
Side effects	Most important and less common are cardiovascular collapse and central nervous system collapse. Hypotension can occur if the drug is infused too rapidly. Commonly observed adverse reactions are nystagmus, dizziness, pruritus, headache, paresthesia, headaches, somnolence, and ataxia.
Note	Continuous monitoring of the heart, blood pressure, and effectiveness of respiratory function is essential during the infusion and for 10 to 20 minutes post infusion until maximum serum phenytoin level occurs.

DILANTIN

Dilantin (phenytoin)	
Indications	Seizures
Adult dose	900 mg to 1.5-gram IV loading dose infused at 50 mg/min
Pediatric dose	15 mg/kg IV loading dose infused at 50 mg/min
Onset	IV onset 1 to 2 hours, duration 12 to 24 hours
Side effects	Nystagmus, hypotension, 3rd degree heart block, cardiac arrest
Note	Continuous monitoring of the heart, blood pressure, and effectiveness of respiratory function is essential during the infusion and post infusion until maximum serum phenytoin level occur. Mix with saline solution to avoid formation of crystals.

VALIUM FOR SEIZURES

Valium (diazepam)	
Indications	Active seizure activity

Valium (diazepam)	
Adult dose	5 to 10 mg IV every 10 to 15 min., maximum dose 30 mg IV
Pediatric dose	0.05 mg/kg IV or intraosseous every 10 to 15 min., maximum dose 4.0 mg IV 0.5 mg/kg rectal maximum dose 20 mg rectally. Use a 3-cc syringe without a needle and inject into the rectum.
Onset	IV onset 5 min., peak 15 min
Compatibility	Valium is not compatible with any medications or solutions. Administer into an IV line placed into a large vein to reduce the risk of venous damage.
Side effects	Central nervous system depression
Note	Continuous monitoring of the heart, blood pressure, and effectiveness of respiratory function is essential until the patient has fully returned to their pre-medication responsiveness.

RELATED CONDITIONS AND INFORMATION

ABSENCE SEIZURES

An absence seizure (formally called petit mal seizures) is a sudden brief cessation of activity with no postictal state and occurs mostly in children. Absence seizures may occur as frequently as 100 times a day.

JACKSONIAN SEIZURES

Jacksonian seizures (also called simple, partial, or focal seizures) are tonic-clonic movements on one side of the body. Todd's paralysis is a transient postictal paralysis that occurs on the same side as the seizure.

POSTICTAL STATE

A postictal state occurring post seizure is characterized by drowsiness and at times, confusion.

SEIZURES

Frequently the cause of seizures is the result of the patient not taking prescribed anticonvulsant medications. Other causes are cerebral trauma, CNS infection, cerebral tumors, and metabolic brain disorders. The definition of a seizure is an uncontrollable abnormal electrical discharge or firing of brain cells causing the signs and symptoms of a particular type of seizure. The metabolism of the involved cells is greatly increased and as a result, the serum glucose is often low after the seizure.

SEIZURES VERSUS SYNCOPE

Seizures	Syncope
Occurs day or night, regardless of the patient's posture.	Rarely occurs when recumbent.
Cyanosis or plethora may occur in seizure.	Pallor is invariable.

Seizures	Syncope
They are often heralded by an aura of localizing significance.	No advance knowledge of impending seizure.
Injury from falling is common.	Injury is rare
Return to alertness is usually slow. Postictal state may include drowsiness and confusion.	Return to alertness is prompt.
Urinary and bowel incontinence is common.	Urinary and bowel incontinence is rare.
Repeated spells of unconsciousness of several per day or per month are indicative of seizures. Not all seizures are convulsive with intense, paroxysmal, and involuntary muscular contraction.	

STATUS EPILEPTICUS

Status epilepticus is a prolonged seizure or repetitive seizures without recovery between attacks and is a life-threatening situation. The condition can occur with all kinds of seizures. The mortality rate in severe tonic-clonic status is 10%. The incidence of permanent neurological sequelae is 10 to 30%.

TONIC-CLONIC OR CONVULSIVE SEIZURES

Tonic-chronic or convulsive seizures formally called grand mal seizures, begin with sudden loss of consciousness and major contractions of major muscle groups as the arms and legs extend stiffly. As air is forced from the lungs, a loud sound or cry is often made. The patient is apneic, unresponsive with dilated pupils, and incontinent of bowel and bladder. Rhythmic contractions cause a jerky movement and a postictal state occurs as the muscles relax.

A tonic-clonic seizure can cause a sudden internal rotation of the posterior shoulder during the tonic phase and cause a posterior shoulder dislocation. Other injuries can occur from falls and/or contact with hard objects during the seizure.

TODD'S PARALYSIS

Todd's paralysis is one-sided paralysis post seizure following a Jacksonian seizure (one-sided seizure). The paralysis is usually on the same side as the seizure. A history of Jacksonian seizures, postictal state, or altered mental status with clearance in a matter of hours often supports the diagnosis.

PEDIATRIC CONSIDERATIONS

SEIZURE INCIDENCE IN THE PEDIATRIC POPULATION

The pediatric population has an incidence of seizures in 3 out of 1000 children. Febrile seizures are the most common seizure disorder in childhood. Pediatric febrile seizures are most prevalent in children 6 months to 5 years and males have a slightly (but definite) higher incidence of febrile seizures. Reassure patients that febrile seizures do not cause brain damage.

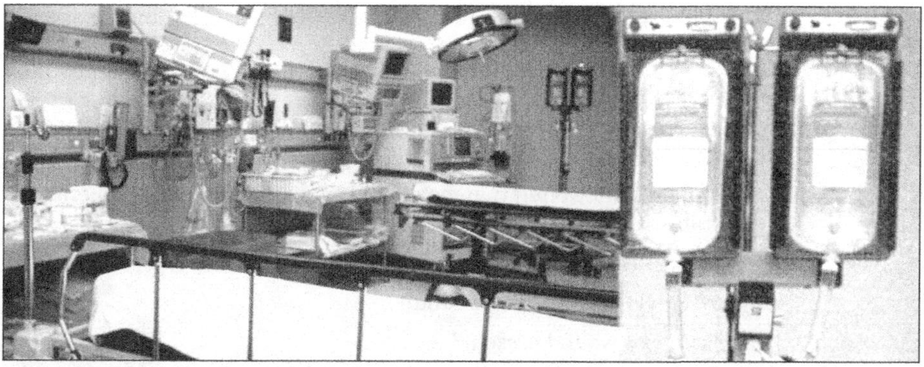

29 STABBING, GUNSHOT, AND PENETRATING INJURY

For details on triage see Chapter 34, Triage in a Nutshell.

PATIENT'S STORY – INTERVIEW QUESTIONS

1. When was the injury?
2. Where did the incident take place?
3. Where is the assailant?
4. For gunshot wounds:
    a. Where is the entrance wound?
    b. Is an exit wound present?
    c. Is more than one gunshot wound present?
    d. Is the type and caliber of the firearm known?
    e. Is the range or distance known?
    f. Is the patient's position known when the shots were fired, e.g., standing, sitting, lying, etc.?
    g. Is the angle of the projectile known; e.g., downward, upward, at a 90o angle, at a 45o angle, etc.?
5. For knife wounds:
    a. Where is the entrance wound?
    b. Is an exit wound present?
    c. Is more than one stab wound present?
    d. What was the type of weapon and what was the length of the penetrating part; e.g., a butcher knife with a 10-inch blade, an ice pick with a 4-inch awl, etc.?
    e. Was the blade curved or straight?

f. What was the patient's position when stabbed, e.g., standing, sitting, lying, etc.?

g. Was the assailant male or female?

h. Where was the assailant in proximity to the victim (in front, in back, etc.) and how close to the victim when the stabbing occurred?

i. Females more often than not stab downward, and males generally stab straight forward.

6. For penetrating objects:

   a. Where is the entrance wound?

   b. Is an exit wound present?

   c. Is more than one wound present?

   d. Is the type of projectile known; e.g., flying glass, exploding metal fragments, etc.?

   e. NEVER remove a penetrating object. Stabilize it in place until the medical provider is prepared to remove it.

7. Does the patient have any serious bleeding?

   a. Elevate the wound above the level of the heart and apply pressure.

   b. DO NOT APPLY PRESSURE IF THE IMPALING OBJECT IS IN THE WOUND.

8. Is pain present?

   a. Where is the pain?

   b. Does it radiate?

   c. What is the severity of the pain?

> It is appropriate to use the terms mild, moderate, or severe and equally appropriate to use a scale of 0 to 10. Zero typically means no pain. The meaning of a 10 is not the same for all nurses or all patients. The definition of 10 must be determined, documented, and consistently used for that patient to be an effective pain evaluation tool.

9. Are any other symptoms associated with the chief complaint; e.g., nausea, vomiting, headache, sweating, heart irregularity, etc.?

10. Is unlawful activity suspected?

    a. Was law enforcement at the scene?

    b. What agency?

> Medical personnel are obligated to notify law enforcement if unlawful activity is suspected.

11. Has any treatment been initiated, and has it helped?

12. Does the patient have any pertinent past history?

13. Does the patient take any routine medications?
    a. What is the name, dosage, route, and frequency of each medication?
    b. When was the last dose?
14. Does the patient take any complementary or alternative therapies, herbal products, over-the-counter medications or supplements, or natural therapies?
    a. What is the name, dosage, route and frequency of each therapy?
    b. When was the last dose or therapy?
15. Does the patient have allergies to drugs or foods?
    a. What is the name of the allergen?
    b. What was the reaction?
16. When was the patient's last tetanus immunization?
17. If the patient is female and between the ages of 10 to 50 years, when was the first day of her last menstrual period?

NURSING DOMAIN

The nursing domain, nursing diagnosis and plan of care can only be determined after an in-depth interview and consideration of the patient's story.

Domain 12. Comfort. Class 1. Physical comfort.
Domain 11. Safety/Protection. Class 1. Infection. Class 2. Physical injury.

ANTICIPATED MEDICAL CARE

Review of the Anticipated Medical Care of Stabbings, Gunshots, and Penetrating Injuries	
Exam	Full body
Urine tests	Test for blood; pregnancy test for women of reproductive age unless they have had a hysterectomy
Stool tests	Test for blood
Body fluid tests	Test for blood
Blood tests	Hemogram, type and screen, amylase for abdominal injuries
ECG	ECG for females and males over 35 years, and for all age patients with chest injuries

Review of the Anticipated Medical Care of Stabbings, Gunshots, and Penetrating Injuries	
Radiographic studies	Anticipate the type to be specific to the area of suspected damage, e.g., x-rays for suspected bony damage, ultrasound or CT with oral contrast for the abdominal organs, CT with intravenous contrast for the chest, arteriogram for arterial damage, and IVP, cystogram, or urethrogram for suspected renal damage. FAST's (focused assessment with sonography in trauma) primary role is in detecting free intraperitoneal blood after blunt trauma.
Diet	NPO
IV	Normal saline or Ringer's solution through two large bore (14 to 16 gauge) cannulas for fluid resuscitation, blood replacement, fresh frozen plasma or platelets for coagulopathy
Medications	Tetanus toxoid, intravenous prophylactic antibiotics
Other management	Anticipate surgical exploration to determine the distance of penetration. Cold steel and hot lights (surgery) are required for definitive treatment of a gunshot or stab wound penetrating the chest or abdominal cavity. Consents are required for both surgery and anesthesia. A penetrating trauma below the nipple line is at risk for a diaphragmatic tear allowing abdominal contents to enter the chest cavity and severe respiratory compromise. Surgery in indicated. Consents are required for both surgery and anesthesia.
Disposition	Hospital admission may be required if the wound is extensive or enters a body cavity.
Worst-case scenario	The worst-case scenario is when the assailant or his gang comes to the ER to finish the job. Call 911.

INITIAL CARE PLAN

An object lodged in the body should be left in place. Stabilize the object with a bulky dressing and tape. After medical evaluation, a determination will be made if ER removal of the object is a safe option. ALL WOUNDS OF THE TRUNK THAT ARE NOT OBVIOUSLY SUPERFICIAL ARE CONSIDERED TO ENTER THE BODY CAVITY UNTIL PROVED OTHERWISE. A medical provider must determine the depth of the wound before the patient can be considered non-urgent.

Alcohol-based hand sanitizers are the preferred method for cleaning your hands in most clinical situations. Wash your hands with soap and water whenever they are visibly dirty, before eating, and after using the restroom.

1. Ask the patient to undress, remove all jewelry that might interfere with the examination, and put on an exam gown. Assist as needed.
2. Obtain vital signs including pulse oximetry or test capillary refill to evaluate breathing effectiveness.
3. Place on continuous heart, blood pressure, and oxygenation monitoring.
4. Place on oxygen 100% non-rebreather if the wound is to the trunk or if indicated by a pulse oximetry saturation of < 94%. Severe COPD patients may be unable to maintain saturation >88% to 92%.
5. Assure the patient that he is safe.
6. Perform a head-to-toe physical examination.

> A full head-to-toe exam is essential and can be performed with the patient in C-spine immobilization.

7. Examination of the head and neck
   a. What is the size and reaction of the pupils?
   b. Does the patient have any head pain or injuries to the head?
      Is the tongue or mouth injured?
      Is any drainage present from the nose or ears?
   c. Is the trachea midline?
      Is jugular venous distention present (unable to detect under fluorescent light)?
8. Examination of the chest
   a. Does the chest expand equally?
      Is subcutaneous emphysema present?
      Are the heart tones within normal limits?
      Are the heart tones diminished?
      Are any murmurs present?
      Does the patient complain of chest pain?
      Is the chest tender to palpation?
   b. Are the lung sounds clear on the right and left?
      Are wheezes or crackles present?
      Are the lung sounds decreased or absent in any area of the lungs?
9. Examination of the abdomen
   a. Is the abdomen soft, flat, rigid, or distended?
      Are bowel sounds normal, hypoactive, hyperactive, or absent?
      Does the patient complain of abdominal pain?
      Is the patient's abdomen tender to palpation?

   b. Is the patient incontinent?
      Examination of the genitalia may be deferred if trauma is not suspected.
      Do the genitalia appear normal?
      Does the patient have bleeding from the urethral meatus or vagina?
      Is priapism present?
      Does the patient complain of genital pain?
      Is the perineal area or genitalia tender to palpation?
   c. Does the patient complain of pain when light pressure is applied to the iliac crests?
      Is the pelvis stable or unstable?

10. Examination of the extremities
    a. Does the patient have normal motion and sensation in the upper and lower extremities?
       Are distal pulses present in the upper and lower extremities?
11. Examination of the back
    a. Does the patient have normal movement of his back?
       Does the patient complain of back pain?
       While keeping the back immobilized, turn the patient.
       Inspect the posterior surfaces.
       Does the patient have obvious back injuries?
       Is the back tender to palpation?
12. Examination of the skin
    a. Does skin inspection reveal any damage to the skin, e.g., abrasions, lacerations, bruises, needle tracks, petechiae, etc.?
    b. Examine all sites of injury and evaluate the neurovascular function distal to the injury.
13. Establish intravenous access with two large bore (14 to 16 gauge) cannulas. Use normal saline for fluid resuscitation. Select tubing anticipating the use of blood products.
14. Draw laboratory blood specimens.
    a. Draw a variety of tubes that will allow the lab to perform hematology, chemistry, and coagulation studies. Patients with cirrhosis or on anticoagulants need coagulation studies.
    b. Consider drawing other labs, e.g., type and screen, blood cultures, etc.
15. Position the patient to enhance normal body function and comfort.
16. Keep the patient warm. Place a warmed blanket like a shawl around the head, neck, and shoulders. Place another blanket over the body and tightly tuck it around the patient.
17. Give initial medications covered by hospital protocol, e.g., tetanus toxoid.
18. Clean wounds by irrigating and cover them with sterile dressings.

   a. If internal body contents are visualized in the wound cover with saline moistened gauze and ask for orders before irrigating.
   b. Obtain wound cultures before cleansing.

19. Consider placing drains.
   a. Nasogastric tube to decompress the stomach and to reduce the risk of vomiting and aspiration
   b. Indwelling Foley catheter to decompress the bladder and monitor hourly urine output
20. Initiate diagnostic tests covered by hospital protocol, e.g., x-rays of areas with suspected bony damage.
21. Instruct the patient not to eat or drink and teach the patient and family the rationale for the NPO status.
22. Elevate the siderails and place the stretcher in the lowest position.
23. Inform the patient, family, and caregivers of the usual plan of care, and the anticipated overall time in the ER.
24. Provide the patient with a device to reach someone for assistance and explain how to use it. Ask the patient to call for help before getting off the stretcher.

ONGOING CARE PLAN

Inform the medical provider of adverse changes noted during ongoing evaluation. Document that the medical provider was notified of the adverse change. Document if orders were or were not received.

1. Monitor temperature, heart rate and rhythm, blood pressure, respiratory rate, and effectiveness of breathing.
2. Monitor therapy closely for the patient's therapeutic response.
   a. The usual time for a medication effectiveness check is 20 to 30 minutes after giving the drug.
   b. If therapy is not effective, ask the medical provider for a repeat dose or an alternative.
3. Monitor closely for the development of adverse reactions to therapy.
4. Perform interventions to relieve the adverse reaction.
5. Ask the medical provider for a remedy.
6. Keep the patient, family, and caregivers well informed of the plan of care and the remaining time anticipated before disposition.
7. Monitor the patient's laboratory and x-ray results and notify the medical provider of critical abnormalities. Remedy abnormalities as ordered.
8. Notify the medical provider when all diagnostic results are available for review. Ask for establishment of a diagnosis and disposition.

DISCHARGE INSTRUCTIONS

1. Provide the patient with the name of the nurse and doctor in the emergency room.
2. Inform the patient of their diagnosis or why a definitive diagnosis couldn't be made. Explain what caused the problem if known.
3. Teach the patient how to take the medication as prescribed and how to manage the common side effects. Instruct the patient not to drive or perform any dangerous tasks while taking narcotic pain medications.
4. Instruct the patient with a fracture that:
    a. Splints can become too tight if swelling develops. Watch carefully for loss of the normal color in the fingers or toes and for increased pain.
    b. The follow-up medical provider should be called if a problem develops.
5. Instruct the patient unable to bear weight on a lower extremity that:
    a. Crutches are one method for getting around. A wheelchair can be used if the patient's arms cannot support the patient's weight on crutches.
    b. The two crutches serve as a support for the injured leg and swing with that leg. Move the crutches and the injured leg forward at the same time. Then, step forward with the uninjured leg. This gives a walk that alternates the crutches with the uninjured leg.
    c. The weight of the body is not to be placed on crutches up against the armpit. This can cause serious and permanent nerve damage. Keep the arms straight and support the body's weight on the crutch handles.
    d. Care must be taken to keep the rubber tips clean and tightly affixed to the crutch. Do not use crutches on wet surfaces or on ice.
    e. If any problems develop regarding the use of the crutches, notify the follow-up medical provider.
6. Instruct the patients with a sutured laceration that:
    a. The laceration should be kept clean and dry.
    b. The dressing applied in the ER should be removed after one to two days and the wound left open to the air.
    c. Some lacerations of the face and scalp were not covered with a dressing in the ER. The wound may be covered with a dry sterile dressing if needed to protect the area.
    d. Elevation of the area, when possible, reduces the risk of swelling.
    e. The laceration should be kept clean with mild soap and water and an antibiotic over-the-counter ointment applied two times a day for the first three days.
    f. Follow-up is recommended for suture removal.

g. Redness, swelling, red streaks, and pus are signs of infection. Notify the follow-up medical provider if any of these symptoms develop.

7. Some lacerations contaminated with dirt or bacteria are not sutured. These are considered dirty wounds and further care is necessary at home.
   a. Soak the area in warm water and prescribed solution for twenty minutes three times a day for the first three days.
   b. Keep the wound covered with a dry sterile dressing between soaks. If the wound is dry and clean after three days of soaks, stop the soaking, and keep it clean, dry, and covered.
   c. Not all dirty wounds need antibiotics. If antibiotics are prescribed, take them until the pills are gone. Do not stop when the wound looks better.
   d. Redness, swelling, red streaks and pus are signs of infection. Notify the follow-up medical provider if any of these symptoms develop.
8. Recommend a medical provider for follow-up care. Provide the name, address, and phone number with a recommendation of when to schedule the care.
9. Instruct the patient to call the follow-up medical provider immediately or return to the emergency room if the pain or problem worsens in any way or any unusual symptoms develop. Encourage the patient NOT to IGNORE WORSENING OR PERSISTENT SYMPTOMS.
10. Ask for verbal confirmation or demonstration of understanding and reinforce teaching as needed.

COMMONLY ORDERED MEDICATIONS

DILAUDID

Dilaudid (hydromorphone)	
Indications	Moderate to severe pain
Dose	Typical dose 1 to 5 mg IV. Titrate to response. No maximum dose.
Onset	IV onset rapid, peak 15 to 30 minutes, duration 3 to 4 hours
Side effects	Drowsiness, dizziness, confusion, sedation, increased intracranial pressure, nausea, vomiting, urinary retention, respiratory depression
Monitor	CNS changes, respiratory effectiveness, allergic rash
Note	Dilute to 4 or 5 ml with NS or sterile water for IV injection and administer slowly over at least 2 to 3 min. Antidote is naloxone.

PHENERGAN

Phenergan (promethazine)

Phenergan (promethazine)	
Indications	Nausea, vomiting
Adult dose	12.5 to 25 mg IV every 4 to 6 hours. When used intravenously, promethazine injection should be given in concentration no greater than 25 mg/ml at a rate not to exceed 25 mg/min. Preferably inject through a medication port in IV tubing that is known to be functioning satisfactorily. 25 mg IM every 4 to 6 hours
Pediatric dose	For a child > 2 years old, 0.25 to 0.5 mg/kg IM or IV every 4 to 6 hours
Onset	IV onset 3 to 5 min., duration 4 to 6 hours IM onset 20 min., duration 4 to 6 hours
Side effects	Drowsiness, sedation, hypotension, palpitations, tachycardia
Monitor	Vital signs, level of consciousness, respiratory effectiveness

ROMAZICON

Romazicon (flumazenil)	
Indications	Valium or Versed overdose
Adult dose	First dose 0.2 mg IV over 15 seconds Second dose 0.3 mg IV over 15 seconds Third dose 0.5 mg IV over 30 seconds If no response, may repeat every minute until response is adequate or the maximum of 3 mg given.
Onset	IV onset 1 minute, peak 10 min., duration unknown
Side effects	Nausea, vomiting, seizures, dizziness, agitation, pain at injection site
Note	Effects of flumazenil may wear off before the benzodiazepine, repeat dose to the maximum levels.
Monitor	Monitor respiratory effectiveness

TETANUS AND DIPHTHERIA TOXOID, ADSORBED FOR ADULTS

Tetanus and Diphtheria Toxoid Adsorbed for Adults	
Indications	Immunization against tetanus and diphtheria
Dose	0.5 cc IM for adults and children 7 years and older
Side effects	Local reactions such as erythema, induration, and tenderness are common. Systemic reactions of fever, chills, myalgias, and headache may occur.
Monitor	Local reactions are usually mild and self-limiting. Serious local reactions include sterile abscess and subcutaneous atrophy at the injection site.

Tetanus and Diphtheria Toxoid Adsorbed for Adults	
Note	The goal is to keep tetanus immunization current not specifically to prevent tetanus infection from the current wound. Persons in the United States have a right not to be immunized. Children can receive a religious exception and be in public school without the recommended immunizations.

VALIUM

Valium (diazepam)	
Indications	Active seizure activity or agitation
Adult dose	5 to 10 mg IV every 10 to 15 min., maximum 30 mg
Pediatric dose	0.05 mg/kg IV or intraosseous every 10 to 15 min., maximum 4.0 mg 0.5 mg/kg rectally, maximum 20 mg A 3 ml syringe with an intravenous cannula (without the needle) inserted in the rectum may be used for administration.
Onset	IV onset 5 min., peak 15 min.
Compatibility	Valium is not compatible with any other medications. Administer into an intravenous line placed into a large vein to reduce the risk of venous damage.
Side effects	Central nervous system depression, serious life threatening decreased respiratory tidal volume and rate
Note	Continuous monitoring of the heart, blood pressure, and effectiveness of respiratory function is essential until the patient has fully returned to their pre-medication responsiveness.

VERSED

Versed (midazolam hydrochloride)	
Indications	Conscious sedation
Adult dose	1 to 2.5 mg IV given over at least 2 min. Wait for 2 minutes to fully evaluate effect before giving another dose. A total dose of over 5 mg IV is not usually necessary. If patients have narcotic medications before the Versed, use approximately 30% less Versed.
Pediatric dose	Pediatric patients 12 to 16 years old should be dosed as adults. Pediatric dose is weight based. Usually not given to pediatric patients unless they are intubated. IV initial loading dose is 0.05 to 0.2 mg/kg IV administered over 2 to 3 min.
Onset	IV onset 3 to 5 minutes

Versed (midazolam hydrochloride)	
Compatibility	Use normal saline in the IV line before and after the dose.
Side effects	Serious life threatening decreased respiratory tidal volume and respiratory rate
Monitor	Continuous monitoring of heart, blood pressure, and oxygenation is essential.
Note	Versed is a potent sedative that requires slow administration and individualization of dosage. Versed is 3 to 4 times as potent as Valium. Reversing agent is Romazicon (flumazenil).

RELATED CONDITIONS AND INFORMATION

ABDOMEN

Review of Penetrating Injuries of the Abdomen	
General	Penetrating wounds to the abdomen can enter through the anterior abdomen, back, flank, or lower chest. The liver, small bowel, and stomach are the most commonly injured.
Assessment	STOP — Stop and direct full attention to the abdomen. LOOK — Inspect the abdomen for injury and scars of past surgeries. LOOK — Look for Gray Turner's sign (bruising of the flank), Cullen's sign (periumbilical bruising), and distention. LISTEN — Auscultate the abdomen for bowel sounds. FEEL — Percuss the abdomen for hyper-resonance or dullness. FEEL — Palpate the abdominal for tenderness.
Tests	Blood tests may include hemogram, type and screen, and serum amylase. Other tests may include testing of urine, stool, and gastric contents for blood.
Radiographic studies	CT is indicated for suspicion of solid organ lacerations or air in the abdominal cavity. IVP is used for suspected disruption of the kidney, ureters, bladder, or urethra. Flat, upright, and lateral films are used to visualize foreign bodies or free air in the abdomen indicating laceration of the gastrointestinal tract. A cystogram or urethrogram is used to visualize the continuity of the bladder and urethra. Ultrasound visualizes the configuration of organs and hematomas.

Review of Penetrating Injuries of the Abdomen	
Other studies	Diagnostic peritoneal lavage is done to determine if peritoneal bleeding is present. Normal saline is instilled into the peritoneal cavity and aspirated. The aspirate is tested for blood. This procedure cannot test for a retroperitoneal bleed. It is contraindicated in patients with a history of multiple abdominal surgeries, cirrhosis, and coagulopathy. It is contraindicated if the patient is extremely obese.
Management	Management may include obtaining intravenous access with two large bore (14 or 16 gauge) cannulas, intravenous fluids of normal saline and blood products, oxygen via non-rebreather mask, an indwelling urinary catheter (do not insert if injury is suspected to the urethra), a nasogastric tube to decompress the stomach and reduce the risk of aspiration, prophylactic antibiotics, admission and surgery arrangements. Experienced ER nurses refer to HOT lights and COLD steel (of the operating room) as the only definitive treatment for a stab wound into the abdominal cavity.

AMPUTATION

Review of Amputations	
Definition	An amputation is a traumatic separation of a digit or limb from the body.
Symptoms	Symptoms include objective loss or partial loss of a digit or limb and may include bleeding, hypovolemic shock, and pain.
Tests	Tests include x-rays to determine bony damage.
Management	Management includes control of bleeding with pressure dressings, elevation, wound cleaning, splinting, and dressing with sterile dressings.
Disposition	Hospital admission may be required for surgical intervention or transfer to a facility with a reclamation team.
Amputated part handling	Keep the amputated part covered with saline moistened gauze in a watertight plastic bag or container. Place the bag or container in ice and water. Avoid placing the amputated part in direct contact with ice; always utilize some sort of clean, soft, moist barrier.

BLOOD LOSS

	Class I	Class II	Class III	Class IV
Blood loss	Up to 750 cc	750 to 1500 cc	1500 to 2000 cc	> 2000
HR	< 100	> 100	> 120	> 140
BP	Normal	Normal	Decreased	Decreased

	Class I	Class II	Class III	Class IV
RR	14 to 20	20 to 30	30 to 35	> 35
Cap refill	Normal	Slight delay	from 2 to 3 seconds	No filling
Skin	Pink and cool	Pale and cold	Pale, cold, moist	Mottled
Urine	> 30 cc/hr	20 to 30 cc/hr	5 to 15 cc/hr	< 5 cc/hr
Behavior	Slight anxiety	Mild anxiety	Anxious, confused	Lethargic, confused
Fluid	Crystalloid	Crystalloid	Crystalloid and blood	Crystalloid and blood

BLOOD TRANSFUSIONS

Massive blood transfusions require 1 to 2 units of fresh frozen plasma for every five units of blood transfused to treat dilutional coagulopathy.

BRAIN

Review of Penetrating Injuries to the Brain	
General	Penetrating injuries to the brain have a high mortality rate. Missile wounds from high velocity weapons can penetrate the skull. ALL PATIENTS WITH BRAIN OR FACIAL TRAUMA ARE ASSUMED TO HAVE A CERVICAL SPINE INJURY UNTIL PROVEN OTHERWISE BY A NEGATIVE X-RAY OR CT.
Assessment	Determine the level of consciousness with the Glasgow Coma Scale. Assess pupil size, shape, equality, and reaction to light. Assess eye movement. Observe for abnormal posturing. Inspect the skull for injury. Inspect the nose and ears for drainage. Palpate the craniofacial area for tenderness, swelling, and depressions. Assess motor and sensory function in all extremities.
Blood tests	Hemogram, type and screen, ABG
Radiographic studies	Computerized axial tomography (CT) scan or skull series if CT not available, facial films, MRI
IV	Fluid resuscitation with normal saline and blood products. Care must be taken not to over-hydrate. Establish intravenous access with two large bore (14 or 16 gauge) cannulas.
Positioning	Keep the head positioned midline and avoid flexing the neck or hips to facilitate venous drainage and reduce intracranial pressure.

Review of Penetrating Injuries to the Brain	
Drains	Insert an indwelling urinary catheter (do not insert if injury is suspected to the urethra) for hourly urine output monitoring. Consider placing a nasogastric tube to decompress the stomach and reduce the risk of vomiting and aspiration. DO NOT USE A NASOGASTRIC TUBE FOR PATIENTS WITH FACIAL INJURIES. THE TUBE COULD ENTER THE BRAIN THROUGH A BONY FRACTURE.
Medications	Medications may include prophylactic antibiotics, Mannitol for diuresis and decrease in intracranial pressure (ICP), anti-convulsant and antipyretic medication, Nipride to lower blood pressure, analgesics, and sedatives.
Ventilation	Start with oxygen at 100% via non-rebreather mask. Anticipate hyperventilation to maintain the pCO2 between 26 and 30 mmHg. Keeping the patient alkalotic may decrease cerebral vasoconstriction.
Other	Intracranial pressure monitoring device
Disposition	Prepare the patient for hospital admission, surgery, or transfer to another facility.

CHEST PENETRATING TRAUMA

Review of Penetrating Trauma to the Chest	
Definition	A penetrating trauma to the chest is an injury to the thorax and intrathoracic contents from a penetrating injury
Symptoms	Symptoms may include laceration or puncture of the thorax associated with pain, swelling, ecchymosis, shortness of breath, difficulty swallowing, and hoarseness.
Assessment	Assessment of the chest includes: Inspection of the chest for ecchymosis and the chest wall for asymmetrical movements Inspection of the neck for swelling and ecchymosis Listening to the movement of air through the airways Auscultation of lung sounds Palpation of the chest wall for the presence of crepitus and subcutaneous emphysema
Intervention	Interventions may include a thoracotomy in the ER. Cover open wounds with nonporous dressings and stabilize any impaled objects.

Review of Penetrating Trauma to the Chest	
Tests	Tests may include cardiac enzymes, ABG, Swan-Ganz catheter or CVP pressure monitoring, chest x-ray, ultrasound of the aorta, esophagoscopy, CT scan of the thorax, bronchoscopy or laryngoscopy, electrocardiogram, and echocardiography.
Ventilation	If indicated, secure the airway by endotracheal intubation or surgical incision, use 100% oxygen and ventilator support.
Pneumo-thorax	A needle thoracentesis may be performed for a tension pneumothorax with a 12 to 16-gauge needle inserted into the second intercostal space in the midclavicular line or the fifth intercostal space in the midaxillary line on the injured side of the pneumothorax. Prepare for chest tube insertion.
Diet	NPO
IV	Intravenous access should be established with two large bore (14 or 16 gauge) cannulas. Fluid resuscitation without over-hydration with normal saline and blood products.
Drains	Consider placing an indwelling urinary catheter for monitoring of urinary output and a nasogastric tube to decompress the stomach and reduce the risk of vomiting and aspiration.
Disposition	Hospital admission may be required for surgical intervention and support.

DIAGNOSTIC PERITONEAL LAVAGE

Diagnostic peritoneal lavage is done to determine if bleeding is present in the peritoneal space. Normal saline is instilled into the peritoneal cavity and aspirated. The aspirate is tested for blood. The retroperitoneal space is separate from the peritoneal cavity and this procedure is unable to determine if bleeding is present in the retroperitoneal space. Peritoneal lavage is contraindicated in the patient with a history of cirrhosis, coagulopathy, or multiple abdominal surgeries (adhesions can prevent the bowel from moving and increase the risk of bowel puncture). It is contraindicated in the patient with extreme obesity.

EXTERNAL EXAMINATION AND EVALUATION OF EYE MOTILITY

Review of External Examination and Evaluation of Eye Motility
Begin the exam away from the eye and gradually move closer.
Inspect for lacerations, bruises, and differences between the eyes.
Inspect the eyelids, lashes, and how the eyes lay in the sockets.
Inspect the conjunctiva and sclera for color and injury.
Evaluate the patient's ability to move the eyes through the six positions of gaze by asking the patient to follow a finger moved around the eye. In children, following a toy is more apt to be successful.

FACIAL INJURIES

Review of Facial Injuries	
Definition	Facial injuries include facial bony and soft tissue injuries.
Symptoms	Symptoms may include pain, swelling, ecchymosis, and deformity of the face.
Ongoing monitoring	Ongoing monitoring includes observation for increasing edema that might compromise the airway and bleeding (ask the patient if he is swallowing blood), for decreasing level of consciousness with a consciousness scale and the Glasgow coma scale, for changes in pupil size and equality, eye movement, vital signs, and evaluating for signs of impending shock with hourly urine output measurements. The goal in treating all forms of shock is restoration of oxygenation and tissue perfusion.
Management	Management includes positioning the patient in a high sitting position to allow for management of secretions, to decrease edema, and to maintain a clear airway. Ice and elevation are essential ER procedures. Prophylactic antibiotics may be given.
Disposition	Hospital admission is required for airway support.

FACIAL LACERATIONS

Keep the edges of a facial laceration moist with saline moistened gauze before and after cleaning and while waiting for suturing to minimize devitalization of the tissue. This will be beneficial for skin layer matching and to minimize scarring. All lacerations cause scarring; the goal is to minimize the scar. Do not use Betadine or peroxide because it can be caustic to tissue. Facial sutures should be removed in 3 to 5 days to further minimize scarring.

FEMUR FRACTURES

Review of Femur Fractures	
Definition	A fracture of the femur is a disruption of the bony continuity of the femur.
Causes	The cause of a femur fracture is usually a traumatic injury.
Symptoms	Symptoms may include pain, inability to bear weight, shortening with rotation of the leg, and hypovolemic shock. The goal in treating all forms of shock is restoration of oxygenation and tissue perfusion.
Tests	Tests include x-ray, CT, or MRI of the femur.

Review of Femur Fractures	
Management	Management includes immobilization of the leg (traction splint or traction pin), ice pack, fluid resuscitation with normal saline, and ongoing monitoring of sensation, movement, and circulation distal to the fracture. Preoperative laboratory studies may include CBC, electrolytes, BUN and creatinine, type and screen, and coagulation studies if on anticoagulants or cirrhotic.
Disposition	Hospital admission may be required for open surgical reduction and internal fixation or continued traction.

FIREARMS

Review of Firearms	
Rifle	The rifle is a high velocity weapon designed to use while holding at the shoulder. It has a rifled bore (spiral grooves) and releases a single shot but can be semi-automatic or fully automatic (capable of firing continuously until ammunition is exhausted or the trigger is released). The bullet makes a narrow and long path of injury. A bullet can deviate up to 90 degrees from a straight path after it hits the body tissue. The tissue is displaced along the path temporarily as it passes through the body. The tissue and bone are disrupted and stretched causing damage. Bullets can mushroom, deform, or fragment as they hit tissue or bone resulting in a pathway of damage larger than the bullet itself. Some bullets are designed to fragment or explode after impact.
Shotgun	The shotgun is commonly a low velocity weapon with a smoothbore barrel designed to be used at short range and classified by the diameter of the barrel, e.g., 12-gauge, 16-gauge, etc. The discharge is normally a release of multiple pellets but can discharge a single large slug. Shotguns can be semi-automatic or fully automatic (capable of firing continuously until ammunition is exhausted or the trigger is released). The path is usually wide with a short path of damage. The slugs or pellets can mushroom, deform, or fragment as they hit the body tissue or bone resulting in a larger pathway of damage than the size of the bullet. Some slugs and pellets are designed to fragment or explode after impact.

Review of Firearms	
Handguns Revolvers and auto-loading pistols	Handguns are typically low velocity weapons and designed to be held and shot with one hand. A revolver has a revolving cartridge with several chambers made to release one shot after the other. Pistols have a chamber of bullets that are auto-loading. Pistols can be semi-automatic or fully automatic (capable of firing continuously until ammunition is exhausted or the trigger is released). The path of damage is normally wide with a short path of damage. Bullets can mushroom, deform, or fragment as they hit tissue or bone resulting in a larger pathway of damage. Some bullets are designed to fragment or explode after impact.

FLAIL CHEST

Paradoxical chest wall movement characterizes a flail chest when three-or-more adjacent ribs are fractured in two or more places or detached from the sternum. The free-floating ribs move inward during inspiration and outward during expiration causing pain, shock, and hypoventilation. The goal in treating all forms of shock is restoration of oxygenation and tissue perfusion.

FRACTURES

Review of Fracture Types	
Closed	Skin over the site is intact.
Comminuted	The bone is splintered into fragments.
Complete	The bony continuity is interrupted.
Displaced	Proximal and distal segments of bone are not aligned.
Greenstick	The bone is bent.
Impacted	Distal and proximal fracture sites are wedged together.
Open	Skin over the fracture site is not intact.

FRACTURE MANAGEMENT IN THE ER

ER Management of Fractures	
Expose the area	Remove all clothing and jewelry near the suspected fracture.
Perform a physical assessment	Inspect for color, position, and obvious differences as compared to the uninjured side. Look for a break in the skin, assess for bleeding, and deformity. Palpate the extremity for pain, pallor, pulses, paresthesia, and paralysis (five Ps).
Determine the need for a splint	Splint for deformity, pain, bony crepitus, edema, ecchymosis, vascular compromise, open wounds, paralysis, or paresthesia.

ER Management of Fractures	
Immobilize	Splint with the appropriate splint to immobilize the joints below and above the injury. Avoid manipulations of the bone. Rigid splints such as plastic devices and metal splints are used for lower extremity fractures. Soft splints such as pillows and slings are used for upper extremity fractures. Traction splints are used for femur and proximal tibial fractures. A thumb spica splint is applied as if the hand was holding a soda can.
Management	Management includes protection, rest, ice, compression, and elevation of the site. Ice and elevation are essential ER procedures.
Medications	Administer analgesics.
Diagnostic Testing	The x-ray views ordered should include the joints above and below the injury.
On-going monitors	Frequently reassess the five Ps (pain, pallor, pulses, paresthesia, and paralysis).
Disposition	Hospitalization may be required for definitive stabilization, traction, and surgical open reduction with internal or external fixation.

HEMOPHILIA

Even minor trauma can cause major bleeding in the patient with hemophilia. Hemorrhage can occur anywhere in the body. The partial thromboplastin time (PTT) is prolonged. Bleeding into a joint is extremely painful and leads to severe disability. The patients and family are knowledgeable about the disease. Therapy is FFP for hemophilia A and von Willebrand's disease and factor VII for hemophilia B. Patients often have factor VIII at home but are unable to give it because of difficult intravenous access from repeated transfusions.

In the past, the concentrate was made from fractionated freeze-dried antihemophilic factor and contained 250 to 1500 UV of factor VIII:C in a reconstituted volume. Factor VIII is also produced by recombinant DVA techniques and is considered to be the replacement of choice. Cryoprecipitate derived from fresh frozen plasma was once the mainstay of hemophilia A and may be used when noninfectious factor VIII concentrates are not available.

Most hemophiliac patients require large doses of narcotic analgesia because they have built a tolerance from frequent use. Most patients know the amount of medication necessary to relieve their pain. Patients are often under-treated by medical providers for fear of contributing to an addiction.

A hemophilia patient should not be given an IM injection unless factor replacement was given within the past several days.

Intraosseous infusion of intravenous fluids and blood products can be administered into the sternum on adults and the anterior tibia on children.

June 11, 1975, the Governing Body of Jehovah's Witnesses adjusted its previous position and agreed it was acceptable for hemophiliacs to accept repeated treatment. Prior to this date, the hemophiliacs were only allowed treatment once as medicine.

The Jehovah's Witness (JW) doctrine does not believe in accepting homologous or autologous blood transfusions, and acute normovolemic hemodilution. The following procedures may also be refused but are at the discretion of each individual's interpretation of the JW doctrine: autologous blood salvage or cell-saver scavenging, closed-circuit acute normovolemic hemodilution, epidural blood patch, heart-lung machine, hemodialysis, labeling or tagging, platelet gel, and plasmapheresis.

HEMORRHAGE CONTROL

When hemorrhage of an extremity is confronted in the ER, elevate the extremity as high as possible above the heart level and compress the area. Apply an elastic compression (ACE) bandage while maintaining the elevation to control the bleeding. Often bleeding cannot be controlled with gauze dressings until the extremity is elevated and an elastic compression dressing is applied.

HEMORRHAGIC SHOCK BLOOD LOSS

	Class I	Class II	Class III	Class IV
Blood loss	Up to 750 cc	750 to 1500 cc	1500 to 2000 cc	> 2000
HR	< 100	> 100	> 120	> 140
BP	Normal	Normal	Decreased	Decreased
RR	14 to 20	20 to 30	30 to 35	> 35
Cap refill	Normal	Slight delay	from 2 to 3 seconds	No filling
Skin	Pink and cool	Pale and cold	Pale, cold, moist	Mottled
Urine	> 30 cc/hr	20 to 30 cc/hr	5 to 15 cc/hr	< 5 cc/hr
Behavior	Slight anxiety	Mild anxiety	Anxious, confused	Lethargic, confused
Fluid	Crystalloid	Crystalloid	Crystalloid and blood	Crystalloid and blood

INSTILLATION OF EYE MEDICATIONS AND APPLICATION OF PATCHES

Review of Eye Medication Instillation and Application of Patches
Pull the lower eyelid downward and ask the patient to look up.

Review of Eye Medication Instillation and Application of Patches
Instill eye drops or a thin line of eye ointment into the cul-de-sac of the lower eyelid. Avoid placing eye drops in the inner canthus as the solution drains immediately into the lacrimal duct and then into the nose. If more than one drug is administered, wait several minutes between drugs.
After administration, ask the patient to blink several times and roll his eyes gently to expose the entire eye surface to the medications.
Ask the patient to apply pressure for a few minutes to the tear duct near the nose to minimize systemic absorption.
Instruct the patient not to tightly squeeze the eyelids together as this will cause the medication to leak out.
To apply a patch, ask the patient to close both eyes and then place a horizontally folded eye patch over the lid. The folded patch fills the indention between the brow and the cheek and when taped will apply a light pressure on the globe. Place a second patch unfolded over the first patch and tape obliquely with paper tape.

INTRAOSSEOUS INFUSIONS

Intraosseous infusion is occasionally the only method of giving fluids when the intravenous route is not available. The sternum can be used on adults and the anterior tibia on children for intraosseous infusion of intravenous solutions and blood products.

IRRIGATION OF THE EYE

Review of Irrigation of the Eye
Wash the entire skin area around the eye.
Gather the following equipment: Warmed irrigating solution of normal saline IV tubing IV cannula (with the needle removed) attached to the tubing or for chemical irrigation, a Morgan Lens may be used. Ophthalmic anesthetic, if ordered by medical provider
Place the patient on the affected side or on the back for bilateral irrigation. Pad well with towels.
Instill ophthalmic anesthetic if ordered.
Run a gentle stream of solution over the eye from the inner canthus to the outer canthus.
Ask the patient to occasionally blink, look up, down, and from side-to-side to assure that the irrigating solution reaches all surfaces of the eye.
Evert (turn inside out) the upper eyelid by placing a cotton swab over the eyelid, pulling the eyelashes down, and then up over the swab to irrigate under the upper lid.

LOCAL ANESTHESIA DURATION

Review of Local Anesthesia Duration	
Lidocaine (Xylocaine)	Lasts for 30 to 60 minutes
Lidocaine with epinephrine	Lasts for 60 to 90 minutes
Marcaine 0.5% (bupivacaine)	Lasts for 3 to 6 hours. Marcaine can be used as a regional block and injection directly into the wound can be avoided. A block is good for the face to avoid distortion that impairs matching of the wound edges.

MUSCULAR PENETRATING INJURIES

Penetrating trauma enters the body through the skin and muscle. The laceration can involve tendons and ligaments. Permanent disability can result if wounds are not thoroughly irrigated at the time of injury. Primary or secondary repair is essential for tendons and ligaments. An x-ray is the first step to rule out the presence of a metal foreign body, such as a nail.

NORMAL CHANGES DURING PREGNANCY

Anatomy and Physiology Changes in the Pregnant Female	
Gastrointestinal	The stomach and intestines are displaced upward. Gastric emptying is delayed.
Hemodynamic	Hemodynamic changes include an increase in cardiac output of approximately 40%, increase in systolic blood pressure of 5 to 15 mmHg, increase in heart rate of 15 to 20 beats per minute, an increased hematocrit of 30% to 35%, and a decreased clotting time.
Renal	Renal blood flow is increased.
Respiratory	The diaphragm is displaced upward by about 1½ to 2 inches. The air passages are engorged because of the increased blood flow. The respiratory rate is increased. Basal metabolism and oxygen consumption are increased. The pCO2 is decreased to about 30 mmHg.
Reproductive	The uterus that is normally the size of a pear increases to contain the fetus and about 1 liter of amniotic fluid. The gravid uterus within a protruding abdomen is prone to penetrating injuries.

O-NEGATIVE BLOOD

O-negative blood can be administered in an emergency until typed and cross-matched blood is available. A person with O-negative blood is considered the universal donor.

OPEN FRACTURES

Review of Open Fractures

Review of Open Fractures	
Definition	An open fracture is a fractured bone with disruption of the skin near the fracture site.
Cause	Either external or internal forces may cause the skin disruption.
Symptoms	Symptoms are disruption of the skin near a fracture site often associated with protrusion of the bone, pain, neurovascular compromise, and bleeding.
Tests	Tests may include x-rays, CT, and MRI.
Management	Management includes collection of a wound culture, cleansing and irrigation of the wound, covering with a sterile dressing, and splinting.
Disposition	Hospital admission may be required for surgery or a transfer to a facility that can provide the necessary care.

ORTHOSTATIC VITAL SIGNS

Review of Orthostatic Vital Signs	
Definition	Orthostatic vital signs are lying, sitting, and standing blood pressure and pulse measurements with less than 1 minute between readings.
Rationale	A patient with a clinically significant circulatory volume loss will have objective findings of a decrease in blood pressure >20 mmHg and an increase in pulse > 20 beats/min. Subjective findings include lightheadedness, nausea, and sweating.
Changes	Drop of systolic blood pressure > 20 mmHg may indicate as much as 15% loss of blood volume.

PENETRATING EYE INJURIES

Penetrating Eye Injuries	
Conjunctival laceration	A fingernail is a common cause of conjunctival laceration. Typically, lacerations < 5 mm are treated with antibiotics and patching. Lacerations > 5 mm may require suturing.
Corneal abrasion	Corneal abrasions occur when a foreign body denudes the epithelium. Diagnosis is made by fluorescein stain. Treatment may include pressure patching for 24 to 48 hours to prevent the eyelid from scraping against the denuded area. Treatment includes antibiotic drops, cycloplegic drops (relieve pain caused by ciliary spasm), and nonsteroidal anti-inflammatory drops (may also help with pain relief).
Corneal laceration	Corneal lacerations are the next step above abrasions. Small lacerations are treated the same as corneal abrasions. Large lacerations require suturing in surgery.

Penetrating Eye Injuries	
Corneal ulcer	A corneal ulceration is often caused by irritation from contact lenses left in the eye too long. The ulcer appears as a white spot on the cornea. Symptoms may include pain, photophobia, vascular congestion, and profuse tearing. Fluorescein stain is used for diagnosis. Treatment may include systemic antibiotics, warm compresses, and an eye patch.
Eyelid wounds	Wounds to the eyelids often mean an injury to the eye. Careful examination of the eye is essential. The eyelids are vascular, and edema develops quickly preventing good approximation of the wound edges. A plastic surgeon is recommended for closure.
Foreign body	Eye foreign bodies consist of anything that will fit into the eye. Symptoms may include pain, hypersensitivity to light, and excessive tearing. Treatment may include local anesthesia to facilitate examination and removal of the foreign object. A needle should never be used to facilitate removal of an object imbedded in the cornea. Special ophthalmic tools are available. Antibiotic ointment is essential, and patching is often necessary to prevent further damage from scraping of the eyelid and for comfort. Organic materials have a high incidence of infection. Metallic objects can cause rust rings if left in the eye for over 12 hours. Ocular burr drills are used to remove rust rings. Topical anesthetics are not for long-term use as the substance retards healing.
Globe rupture	EMERGENT Globe rupture can occur from blunt or penetrating trauma. Symptoms may include altered light perception, a deep anterior chamber, hyphema, and occasionally vitreous hemorrhage. AVOID EYE MANIPULATION DO NOT REMOVE CONTACTS DO NOT USE TOPICAL EYE MEDICATIONS If the penetrating object is still present, stabilize it, and loosely patch both eyes to decrease eye movement. Treatment may include surgery for repair or enucleation.

Penetrating Eye Injuries	
Intraocular foreign bodies	EMERGENT Small projectiles striking the eye at a high rate of speed can penetrate the eye and come to rest in the anterior chamber. A metal fragment from a drill is the most common. Symptoms may be minor discomfort and a good history is essential. X-rays of the eye are used to identify the size and position of the fragment if it is metal. CT is used for non-metal objects. Treatment may include surgical removal of the object, antibiotics, tetanus toxoid, and patching to prevent further damage from scraping of the eyelid and for comfort.

PUPIL EXAMINATION

Review of Pupil Examination	
Shape	The pupil is normally round. An irregular shape can be an acute emergency, an old injury, or secondary to eye surgery. A good history is essential. Tear-shaped pupils are associated with globe ruptures with the tear dropping toward the rupture site.
Size	The size of the pupil changes in response to direct and consensual light (concurrent constriction of one pupil in response to light shined in the other).
Reaction to light	Reaction to light describes a pupil that constricts to light. Documentation for a pupil that constricts from 6 mm to 2 mm in light is 6 → 2.
Accommodation	Accommodation refers to the automatic adjustment in the focal length of the lens of the eye to permit retinal focus of images of objects at varying distances.
OD	Right eye
OS	Left eye
OU	Both eyes
Documentation	PERRLA, pupils are equal, round, regular, and reactive to light and accommodation.

STAB WOUNDS

Many different objects cause stab wounds. A knife is the most common. The tissue damage follows the path of the blade and is dependent of the length of the blade, the velocity of the blow, and the angle of entry. The tissue damage may be adjacent to the presumed path as tissue is often displaced and stretched by the blade.

STATISTICS

According to the United States Department of Justice, it is estimated there are more than 192 million privately owned firearms in the United States of which 65 million are handguns. Firearm-related crime has plummeted since 1993, and then slightly increased in 2005. The average cost of one-gun related crime is $1.79 million, and it is estimated gun violence costs the United States $100 billion a year. In 2005, 71% of all homicides in the United States were committed with a firearm.

SUTURE REMOVAL

Review of Suture Removal Times	
Face	3 to 5 days
Scalp, trunk, hands, and feet	7 to 10 days
Arms and legs	10 to 14 days
Over joints	14 days

VISUAL ACUITY

Visual acuity testing is essential for all eye problems. The test is a measurement of the patient's ability to see. In chemical burns, irrigation takes priority over testing the patient's visual acuity. If the patient normally wears corrective lenses or glasses, the exam is done with the glasses or corrective lens in place. If glasses or lenses are not available, a pinhole can be utilized to measure the visual acuity. Pierce an 18-gauge needle through a card and ask the patient to look through the pinhole. The pinhole can correct an error of up to approximately 20/30.

First, test the affected eye by asking the patient to cover the unaffected eye and read the chart. Second, test the unaffected eye by asking the patient to cover the affected eye and read the chart. Last, test both eyes by asking the patient to read the chart with both eyes open.

The Snellen chart is the most universally used. The patient's distance from the Snellen chart must be 20 feet and is inconvenient in most emergency rooms. The Rosenbaum Pocket Vision Screener that is held 14 inches from the nose is more convenient.

Documentation for Visual Acuity using the Snellen Chart	
20/20	The patient can read what is expected of a person to normally read at 20 feet.
20/20 2	The patient missed two letters, otherwise can read what is expected of a person to normally read at 20 feet. Change the number missed to fit the patient's ability.
20/200	At 20 feet, the patient can only read what the normal person can read at 200 feet. This is the level of legal blindness.
10/200	When the patient must stand at 10 feet from the Snellen chart and can read what the normal person can read at 200 feet. Change the number of feet to describe the patient's ability.
CF/3 ft.	The patient can count fingers at 3 feet. Change the number of feet to describe the patient's ability.
HM/4	The patient can see hand motion at 4 feet.
LP/position	The patient can perceive light and determine the direction it comes from.

Documentation for Visual Acuity using the Snellen Chart	
LP/no position	The patient can perceive the light but is unable to determine the direction.
NLP	The patient is unable to perceive light.

TYPES OF WOUNDS

Types of Wounds	
Open	An abrasion is a superficial wound in which the topmost layers of the skin are scraped off. A gunshot wound is caused by a projectile driving into or through the body. An incision is caused by a sharp-edged object A laceration is a rough, irregular wound caused by blunt-force trauma. A puncture is caused by an object puncturing the skin. A penetrating wound is caused by an object entering the body.
Closed	A contusion (bruise) is caused by blunt force trauma that damages the tissue under the skin. A crush injury is caused by an extreme amount of force applied over a long period of time. A hematoma is caused by damage to a blood vessel that causes blood to collect under the skin.

WOUND MANAGEMENT

Review of Wound Management
Control bleeding with pressure
Ask that local anesthesia be initiated. Clean the wound. Scrub if necessary. If contaminated, irrigate for five to 30 minutes with normal saline. Soak puncture wounds for 15 to 30 minutes.
Set up for débridement of devitalized tissue and approximation of wound edges with sutures, staples, Steri-Strips, or a bonding agent by assembling and arranging instruments, light, sutures, and a kick bucket.
After the wound is débrided and approximated, apply a thin layer of antibiotic ointment and dress with a dry sterile dressing. DO NOT USE PLASTIC BAND-AIDS. Plastic coverings macerate the skin and prevent healing. Facial lacerations are covered with ointment and normally no dressing is applied.
Instruct the patient in proper home wound care. Recommend the time and place for suture or staple removal.

WOUND CLOSURES

Review of Wound Closures	
Tape closures (Steri-Strips)	Used for superficial wounds under minimal tension. An anesthetic is not necessary, and a lower rate of infection is associated with tape closures than with no closure. No follow-up visit is required for tape removal.
Sutures	Sutures approximate wound edges, decrease infections, promote wound healing, and minimize scarring. A local anesthetic is required. A follow-up visit is required for suture removal.
Staples	Staples approximate the wound edges, have a low rate of infection, but do not approximate the wound edges close enough to minimize scarring. A follow-up visit is required to remove the staples.
Tissue Adhesive (Dermabond)	Dermabond is a cyanoacrylate tissue adhesive that forms a strong bond across apposed wound edges providing a flexible water-resistant protective coating and eliminates the need for suture removal. Tissue adhesive should not be used on jagged wounds, animal bites, severely contaminated wounds, ulcers, puncture wounds, mucous membranes (including mucocutaneous junctions) or areas of high moisture content, such as the groin or axillae. The adhesive may be used in place of sutures of 5-0 or smaller to selected wounds on the face, torso and extremities.

PEDIATRIC CONSIDERATIONS

PEDIATRIC PENETRATING INJURIES

The pediatric population has penetrating injuries resulting from violence (guns and knives), play objects (BB guns and sharp pointed toys), equipment used for support (walkers and strollers), and from falls onto sharp objects (glass coffee-tables and sharp pointed toys). Ten percent of children's homicides are by firearms. The relationship of the small pediatric size compared to the size of the common bullet or knife is drastically different than compared to the adult. The penetrating object does more damage to the child.

FUNDAMENTAL CONSIDERATIONS FOR THE INJURED CHILD

Review of Fundamental Considerations for an Injured Child
The child's oropharynx is relatively small and is easily obstructed by the tongue.
Vocal cords are short and concave and collapse easily if the head is hyperflexed or extended.
Lower airway passages are small and easily obstructed by mucus and swelling.
The mediastinum is mobile allowing more damage to the great vessels.
Crying children swallow air and gastric distension can prevent free respiratory movement.

Review of Fundamental Considerations for an Injured Child
Lung sounds can be difficult to auscultate because of crying.
The child's blood volume is less than an adult, but more on a ml/kg basis.
Hypotension is typically not present until the child has lost 20 to 25% of their blood volume.
Low blood pressure is a late sign of hypovolemia in a child and is sign of imminent cardiac arrest.
Bradycardia is a late sign of cardiac decompensation.
The head is large and heavy. The skull offers little protection for the brain as it yields readily to external pressure. The scalp is vascular and bleeds readily.
Brain tissue is easily damaged.
The child is vulnerable to spinal injuries because of the heavy head and underdeveloped bony structure.
The protuberant abdomen of the child is vulnerable to injury. The internal organs are close together and multiple injuries can occur at once.
The pliable rib cage offers little protection for the lungs.
The liver is vulnerable to injury because of its large size.
The large kidneys are not protected well because of little perinephric fat.
The bones are stronger, thicker, and bend more easily than an adult. Even though bones are strong, fractures occur more frequently than sprains. A growth plate fracture can be present and not be seen on x-ray.
The child has a large body surface area with small amounts of subcutaneous fat and is prone to heat loss.

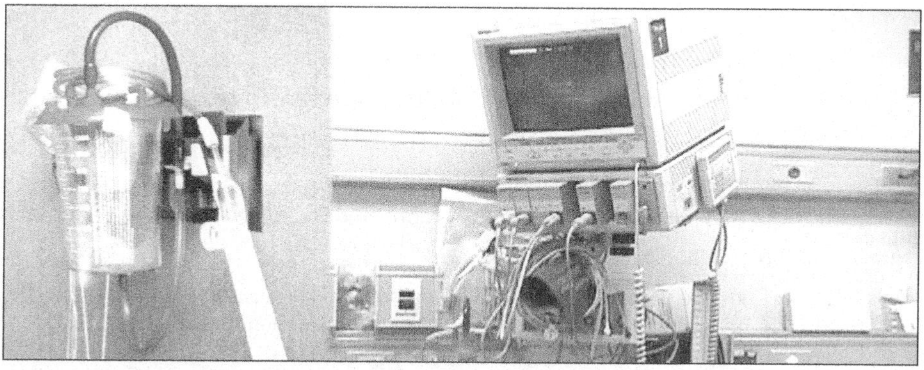

30 STROKE, CVA, AND TIA

For details on triage see Chapter 34, Triage in a Nutshell.

PATIENT'S STORY – INTERVIEW QUESTIONS

1. Have you had a recent injury?
2. When did the symptoms begin?

Time of onset is crucial when considering thrombolytics for a stroke patient. The window of opportunity for thrombolytics is short, usually one to three hours from the onset of symptoms.

   a. If the symptoms are no longer active, how long did they last?
   b. If the symptoms were intermittent, how long did each episode last and how frequent were they?
3. What part of the body is involved?
   a. Are any other symptoms associated with the chief complaint?
   b. Is the patient experiencing any nausea, vomiting, headache, sweating, or slow or irregular heartbeat?
4. How does the problem affect the patient's normal function?
   a. Does the patient have any speech problems?
   b. Does the patient have any weakness in the arms or legs?
   c. Is the patient experiencing any numbness or tingling?
   d. Does the patient have any visual disturbances?
   e. Is the patient able to count fingers, perceive light?
   f. Does the patient have blurred vision or see halos?
5. What was the patient doing when the symptoms began or did anything cause the symptoms, e.g., trauma, strenuous exercise?
6. Has any treatment been initiated, and has it helped?

7. Has the patient had similar problems before?
    a. When was the problem?
    b. What was the diagnosis and treatment?
8. Does the patient have any pertinent past history?
9. Does the patient take any routine medications?
    a. What is the name, dosage, route, and frequency of each medication?
    b. When was the last dose?
10. Does the patient take any complementary or alternative therapies, herbal products, over-the-counter medications or supplements, or natural therapies?
    a. What is the name, dosage, route and frequency of each therapy?
    b. When was the last dose or therapy?
11. Does the patient have allergies to drugs or foods?
    a. What is the name of the allergen?
    b. What was the reaction?
12. If the patient is female and between the ages of 10 to 50 years, when was the first day of her last menstrual period?

NURSING DOMAIN

The nursing domain, nursing diagnosis and plan of care can only be determined after an in-depth interview and consideration of the patient's story.

Domain 12. Comfort. Class 1. Physical comfort.
Domain 4. Activity/Rest. Class 5. Self-care.
Domain 5. Perception/cognition. Class 1. Attention Class 2. Orientation. Class 3. Sensation/perception. Class 4. Cognition. Class 5. Communication.

ANTICIPATED MEDICAL CARE

Review of the Anticipated Medical Care of Stroke, CVA, and TIA	
Exam	Full body
Blood tests	CBC, electrolytes, glucose, renal studies
ECG	ECG for females and males over 35 years of age
X-ray studies	Chest x-ray, CT scan of the brain

Review of the Anticipated Medical Care of Stroke, CVA, and TIA	
Other tests	Arteriogram if actively bleeding, spinal tap post CT if febrile; pregnancy test for women of reproductive age unless they have had a hysterectomy
Diet	NPO
IV	No fluids, intravenous access saline locked to avoid the risk of over-hydration
Medications	Aspirin, Heparin, Nipride, thrombolytics
Other	Ventriculostomy
Disposition	Hospital admission may be required for emergent surgery such as aneurysm clipping or evacuation of a hematoma. Consents are required for both surgery and anesthesia.
Worst-case scenario	The worst-case scenario is an unnoticed decreasing alertness caused by respiratory acidosis resulting in respiratory arrest. Treatment may include endotracheal intubation and mechanical ventilation to correct the acid-base problem.

INITIAL CARE PLAN

> Alcohol-based hand sanitizers are the preferred method for cleaning your hands in most clinical situations. Wash your hands with soap and water whenever they are visibly dirty, before eating, and after using the restroom.

1. Ask the patient to undress, remove all jewelry that might interfere with the examination, and put on an exam gown. Assist as needed.
2. Obtain vital signs including pulse oximetry or test capillary refill. Initiate heart monitoring, non-invasive blood pressure monitor, and pulse oximetry.
3. Place on oxygen if oxygen saturation is < 94%. There is no evidence that the routine use of oxygen is beneficial for an acute stroke. Severe COPD patients may be unable to maintain saturation >88% to 92%.
4. Establish intravenous access and draw laboratory blood specimens.
   a. Draw a variety of tubes that will allow the lab to perform hematology, chemistry, and coagulation studies if the patient is on anticoagulants, has cirrhosis, or if thrombolytic therapy is a possibility.
   b. Perform a point-of-care blood glucose at the bedside. Signs and symptoms of hypoglycemia often mimic the signs and symptoms of a stroke.
   c. Consider drawing other labs, e.g., blood cultures if the patient is febrile; type and screen if thrombolytic therapy is a possibility.
5. Position the patient so as not to increase intracranial pressure.

Bending the patient at the waist, flexing the neck, or flexing the hips can increase intracranial pressure.

6. Keep the patient warm.

Most hospitals have a neurological checklist that makes the initial evaluation easy to document. The form prompts assessment of specific functions and makes comparison of ongoing evaluations easy for multiple users.

7. Perform a focused physical examination.
    a. Evaluate pupil equality and the response to light
    b. Perform a cursory assessment for stroke symptoms
        i. Evaluate for facial droop by asking patient to smile. Normally both sides move equally well. The smile is abnormal when one side of the face does not move as well as the other side.
        ii. Evaluate arm weakness by asking the patient to hold his arms outstretched with his eyes closed. Normally both arms move equally well. The arms are considered abnormal when one arm does not move as well as the other or one arm drifts down compared with the other.
        iii. Evaluate the speech by asking the patient to say, "You can't teach an old dog new tricks." Normally the patient uses correct words with no slurring. The speech is abnormal if the patient slurs words, uses inappropriate words, or is unable to speak.
    c. Evaluate the level of consciousness based on the mnemonic **AVPU** or **ACDU** level of consciousness score.
    AVPU: **A**lert, **V**erbal, **P**ain, **U**nresponsive.
    ACDU: Alert, **C**onfused, **D**rowsy, **U**nresponsive.
    d. Inspect the body surface for injury.
8. Give initial medications covered by hospital protocol, e.g., aspirin.
9. Consider placing drains.
    a. Nasogastric tube for decompression of the stomach to reduce the risk of vomiting and aspiration
    b. Indwelling urinary catheter to monitor urine output hourly.
10. Initiate any diagnostic tests covered by hospital protocol, e.g., STAT laboratory studies and CT scan under a protocol for thrombolytics.
11. Instruct the patient not to eat or drink and teach the patient and family the rationale for the NPO status.
12. Elevate the siderails and place the stretcher in the lowest position.
13. Inform the patient, family, and caregivers of the usual plan of care, and the expected overall time in the ER.

14. Provide the patient with a device to reach someone for assistance and explain how to use it. Ask the patient to call for help before getting off the stretcher.

ONGOING CARE PLAN

Inform the medical provider of adverse changes noted during ongoing evaluation. Document that the medical provider was notified of the adverse change. Document if orders were or were not received.

1. Monitor temperature, heart rate and rhythm, blood pressure, and effectiveness of breathing. Monitor every 15 minutes times four to determine stability.
2. Monitor level of consciousness with the AVPU or ACDU method and compare to the baseline. If the patient appears asleep, wake the patient for evaluation.
3. Monitor motor function and sensation in all extremities and compare to the baseline.
4. Monitor therapy closely for the patient's therapeutic response.
    a. The usual time for a medication effectiveness check is 20 to 30 minutes after giving the drug.
    b. If therapy is not effective, ask the medical provider for a repeat dose or an alternative.
5. Monitor closely for the development of adverse reactions to therapy.
    a. Perform interventions to relieve the adverse reaction.
    b. Ask the medical provider for a remedy.
6. Keep the patient, family, and caregivers well informed of the plan of care and the remaining time anticipated before disposition.
7. Monitor the patient's laboratory and x-ray results and notify the medical provider of critical abnormalities. Remedy abnormalities as ordered.
8. Notify the medical provider when all diagnostic results are available for review. Ask for establishment of a diagnosis and disposition.

DISCHARGE INSTRUCTIONS

1. Provide the patient with the name of the nurse and doctor in the emergency room.
2. Inform the patient of their diagnosis or why a definitive diagnosis couldn't be made. Explain what caused the problem if known.
3. Teach the patient how to take the medication as prescribed and how to manage the common side effects. Instruct the patient not to drive or perform any dangerous tasks while taking narcotic pain medications.
4. For the patient with a transient ischemia attack (TIA), inform the patient that:

a. The medical provider has determined that outpatient therapy is appropriate.

b. Follow-up with the recommended medical provider for evaluation is strongly recommended. A TIA must be thoroughly evaluated to determine, correct, and maybe prevent a stroke.

c. If aspirin therapy is prescribed, take the aspirin regularly once every day with food. The aspirin is used to thin the blood and prevent a recurrence. Enteric-coated aspirin will reduce the risk of gastric irritation.

d. One day of rest is recommended. Avoid strenuous activity or exercise until approved by the follow-up medical provider.

e. If recurrent numbness, visual disturbances, headache, fever, stiff neck, or weakness occur return to the emergency room.

5. Recommend a medical provider for follow-up care. Provide the name, address, and phone number with a recommendation of when to schedule the care.

6. Instruct the patient to call the follow-up medical provider immediately or return to the emergency room if any unusual symptoms develop. Encourage the patient NOT to IGNORE WORSENING OR PERSISTENT SYMPTOMS.

7. Ask for verbal confirmation or demonstration of understanding and reinforce teaching as needed.

COMMONLY ORDERED MEDICATIONS

ATIVAN

Ativan (lorazepam)	
Indications	Extreme agitation
Adult dose	44 mcg/kg IV for agitation 0.25 mg/hr to 2 mg/hr IV infusion
Onset	IV onset 5 to 15 minutes, duration 3 to 6 hours
Compatibility	Compatible with NOTHING, crystallizes easily
Side effects	Over sedation
Note	Expiration for IV mixture is 12 hours. Mix 12 mg/50 ml or 24 mg/100 ml depending on the rate. Do not hang for more than 12 hours. Drug is lost into the bag. Mix Ativan with an equal amount of solution in a syringe before adding to bag. With an IV running, Haldol and opiates can be given.

HEPARIN

Heparin

Heparin	
Indications	Adjunctive therapy in AMI Anticoagulant therapy in prophylaxis and treatment of venous thrombosis, pulmonary embolus, and in atrial fibrillation to reduce the risk of embolus
Adult dose	Generic protocol 80 IU/kg IV initial bolus 18 IU/kg/hr IV (rounded to nearest 50 IU) Adjust to maintain aPTT 1 ½ to 2 times normal
Onset	IV onset 5 min., peak 10 min., duration 2 to 6 hours
Compatibility	Compatible at Y-site with potassium chloride, Aminophylline, Dopamine, Isuprel, Lidocaine, Neo-Synephrine, Levophed
Side effects	Bleeding
Note	Check PTT per hospital protocol.

NIPRIDE

Nipride (nitroprusside)	
Indications	Hypertensive crisis, to reduce afterload in heart failure and pulmonary edema
Adult dose	0.10 mcg/kg/min IV to start and increase every 3 to 5 minutes to desired effect
Onset	IV onset 0.5 to 1 min., peak 1 to 2 min., duration up to 10 min. after the drug is stopped
Compatibility	Compatible at Y-site with Inocor, Dopamine, NTG, dobutamine
Side effects	Hypotension, altered LOC, cyanide toxicity
Note	If blood pressure does not drop after 10 min. of infusion at the maximum dose, the Nipride is considered ineffective. Maximum does is 10 mcg/kg/min. Ask the medical provider for another drug. Nipride is light sensitive and the bag must be covered to protect the drug from the light.

THROMBOLYTICS

TPA	
Indications	Thrombus only utilized if onset of symptoms can be confirmed to have begun within 3 hours of arrival in the ER
Adult dose	0.9 mg/kg IV (maximum 90 mg) with 10% of the dose given as a bolus and the remainder by infusion lasting 60 min.
Streptokinase	
Not recommended for stroke	

VALIUM

Valium (diazepam)	
Indications	Agitation
Adult dose	5 to 10 mg IV every 10 to 15 min., maximum dose 30 mg
Pediatric dose	0.05 mg/kg IV or intraosseous every 10 to 15 min., maximum dose 4.0 mg 0.5 mg/kg rectally maximum dose 20 mg Use a 3 ml syringe without a needle and inject into the rectum.
Onset	IV onset 5 min., peak 15 min.
Compatibility	Valium is not compatible with any medications. Administer into an intravenous line placed in a large vein to reduce the risk of venous damage.
Side effects	Central nervous system depression
Note	Continuous monitoring of the heart, blood pressure, and effectiveness of breathing is essential until the patient has fully returned to their pre-medication responsiveness.

VERSED

Versed (midazolam hydrochloride)	
Indications	For conscious sedation
Adult dose	1 to 2.5 mg IV over 2 min. Wait for 2 minutes to fully evaluate effect before giving another dose. A total dose of over 5 mg IV is not usually necessary. If patients have narcotic medications administered before the Versed, use 30% less Versed.
Pediatric dose	Pediatric patients 12 to 16 years old should be dosed as adults. Pediatric dose is weight-based and usually used only for intubated pediatric patients. Initial loading dose is 0.05 to 0.2 mg/kg IV over 2 to 3 min.
Onset	IV onset 3 to 5 min.
Compatibility	Use normal saline in the IV line before and after the dose.
Side effects	Serious life threatening decreased respiratory tidal volume and respiratory rate
Monitor	Continuous monitoring of heart, blood pressure, breathing effectiveness
Note	Versed is a potent sedative that requires slow administration and individualization of dosage. Versed is 3 to 4 times as potent as Valium. Reversing agent is Romazicon (flumazenil)

RELATED INFORMATION

BABINSKI'S REFLEX

To elicit a Babinski reflex, stroke up on the outer side of sole and across the ball of the foot. Normal is plantar flexion. Abnormal is dorsiflexion of the big toe. A positive Babinski is a sign of a lesion in the pyramidal tract. It may be elicited during unconsciousness after a drug overdose, alcohol intoxication, or seizure.

BELL'S PALSY

Review of Bell's Palsy	
Definition	Bell's palsy is an idiopathic unilateral facial paralysis
Cause	The cause of Bell's palsy is unknown.
Symptoms	Symptoms may include rapid onset of ear and facial pain with maximal paralysis over 2 to 5 days. The patient is unable to move the affected side. The patient may experience difficulty eating.
Tests	No tests are commonly done. Diagnosis is made by history and physical examination, but a brain CT Scan may routinely be performed to confirm the absence of other pathology.
Treatment	Treatment may include steroids, analgesics, and artificial tears. Protection of the eye during sleep is essential to avoid damage to the eye. Moist heat and passive range of motion exercises to improve comfort may be recommended.
Complications	Complications include corneal abrasions, facial muscle atrophy, and residual weakness.
Note	Bell's palsy is the most common of the facial paralyses and found in 23 of 100,000 people annually. It is most common in patients over 40 years old and occurs with equal incidence in both males and females.

CRANIAL NERVES

Review of the Cranial Nerves	
I	Olfactory nerve
II	Optic nerve
III	Oculomotor nerve
IV	Trochlear nerve
V	Trigeminal nerve
VI	Abducens nerve
VII	Facial
VIII	Vestibulocochlear nerve (auditory nerve)
IX	Glossopharyngeal nerve

Review of the Cranial Nerves	
X	Vagus nerve
XI	Accessory nerve (spinal accessory)
XII	Hypoglossal nerve

CT OF THE BRAIN

CT without contrast excludes hemorrhage as the cause of a stroke and can detect surrounding edema and less reliably hemorrhagic infarction. The CT provides an estimate of the extent and location of supratentorial infarction as small as 0.5 to 1 cm. It cannot detect most infarctions for at least 48 hours and often does not detect lesions in the cortical surface or brainstem.

DECEREBRATE POSTURE

The decerebrate posture is characteristic of a patient with decerebrate rigidity resulting from a lesion of the middle lobe of the cerebellum. The extremities are stiff and extended and the head is retracted.

DECORTICATE POSTURE

The decorticate position is characteristic of a patient with a lesion at or above the upper brainstem. The patient is rigidly still with arms flexed, fists clenched, and the legs extended. The words towards the core are a reminder of the arms flexed inward and therefore decorticate posturing.

DIFFERENTIAL DIAGNOSIS OF ACUTE STROKE

Review of Conditions That Cause Acute Neurological Deficits	
Metabolic disturbances	Hyponatremia, hypoglycemia, and nonketotic hyperosmolar hyperglycemia can cause asymmetrical neurological deficits. All patients should have electrolyte and glucose testing.
Intracerebral mass lesions	Brain tumors and abscesses can present with sudden neurological deficits from acute swelling or hemorrhage resulting in compression of an area in the brain. All patients with neurological deficits should have a CT of the brain to rule out intracerebral mass lesions.
Expanding extracerebral masses	Subdural or epidural hemorrhage can present with sudden onset of neurological deficit. These patients usually have a history of trauma. All patients with neurological deficits should have a CT of the brain to rule out extracerebral masses.
Post-seizure paralysis	Todd's paralysis is one-sided paralysis post seizure following a Jacksonian seizure (one-sided seizure). The paralysis is usually on the same side as the seizure. A history of Jacksonian seizures, postictal state, or altered mental status with clearance in a matter of hours often supports the diagnosis.

Review of Conditions That Cause Acute Neurological Deficits	
Acute mono-neuropathies	Bell's palsy, radial nerve palsy, and peroneal nerve palsy can be mistaken for a stroke. A detailed neurological exam will reveal the single peripheral nerve distribution.
Psychogenic causes	Hysteria, malingering, and catatonia can appear suddenly and resemble a stroke. The absence of reflex changes, normal radiographic and laboratory studies, and a known history of psychiatric disorder may point to a psychiatric cause.

STROKE ALGORITHM

Review of Medical Algorithm for Suspected Stroke
Assess ABCs and vital signs.
Provide oxygen by nasal cannula if saturation is < 94%. There is no evidence that the routine use of oxygen is beneficial for an acute stroke. Severe COPD patients may be unable to maintain saturation >88% to 92%.
Establish intravenous access. Draw CBC, electrolytes, and coagulation studies.
Perform bedside blood sugar evaluation.
Perform a brief stroke assessment. Assess for facial drop by asking the patient to smile. Assess extremity weakness by asking the patient to hold both arms out with the eyes closed and look for arm drift. Assess speech by having the patient say you can't teach an old dog new tricks.
Alert the stroke team.
Review the patient's history and establish the onset of symptoms. If less than three hours consider thrombolytics.
Determine stroke severity by use of a stroke scale For a list of various stroke scales utilize this website http://www.strokecenter.org provided by Washington University in St. Louis School of Medicine
Order urgent non-contrast CT of the brain
Review CT results consider the cause of symptoms as hemorrhage or ischemic and consider the use of thrombolytics.

STROKE EVOLUTION

Review of Stroke Classification	
Transient ischemic attack (TIA)	A TIA is an event that temporarily disturbs the blood supply to the brain causing transient neurological deficit.
Reversible ischemic deficit	A reversible ischemic deficit is a neurological deficit that lasts a few days or weeks with no permanent residual.

Review of Stroke Classification	
Stroke in evolution	A stroke in evolution is one that presents with progressive neurological deficits.
Completed stroke	A completed stroke is stable with permanent deficit.

STROKE MANAGEMENT IN THE ER

Review of Medical Stroke Management	
Airway management	Stroke patients may have decreased level of consciousness and be unable to clear their airway. Endotracheal intubation and mechanical ventilation may be necessary to reduce the risk of respiratory compromise.
Blood pressure management	Hypertension > 220 mm Hg systolic or > 120 mm Hg diastolic may be treated with Nipride or another anti-hypertensive agent.
Tests	CT of the brain is used to determine the type of stroke.
Disposition	Surgical intervention may be necessary for a hemorrhage stroke. Heparin therapy may be used for embolic strokes. Thrombolytic agents and neuroprotective agents are used in some centers.

STROKE SYNDROMES

Review of Strokes	
Carotid occlusion	When carotid artery disease produces a fluctuating, stuttering, or progressive defect, early surgical intervention with a carotid endarterectomy may stop further deficit.
Thrombus	An intra-arterial thrombus can produce a deficit that comes and goes or progresses gradually. Management may include treatment with heparin to prevent further thrombus formation. A CT is needed to confirm no evidence of hemorrhage before starting heparin.
Cerebellar hemorrhage	Most hemorrhagic strokes need only supportive treatment. Diagnosis on CT is essential to rule out the need for surgical evacuation.
Subarachnoid hemorrhage	Often subarachnoid hemorrhage is caused by a ruptured or leaking aneurysm. Management may include admission for definitive treatment such as surgical clipping of the aneurysm.
Embolic infarction	Emboli from a cardiac source carry a high risk of recurrence. Predisposing factors are atrial fibrillation, endocarditis, prosthetic heart valve, and mitral valve prolapse. Management is directed towards terminating the arrhythmia, anticoagulation, and correction of the underlying cause.

Review of Strokes	
Thrombotic stroke	Hyper-coagulable states such as pregnancy, cancer, leukemia, sickle cell disease, and other hematologic conditions predispose patients to intravascular thrombosis. Management is directed towards diagnosis and heparin therapy.

SYMPTOMS OF STROKE

Review of Stroke Symptoms	
Onset	Onset is sudden with hemorrhagic stroke and may be stuttering with a thrombolytic arterial occlusion or rupture of an extracerebral artery (subdural or epidural).
Conscious	Loss of consciousness is usually present at the onset of the stroke.
Breathing	Abnormal breathing symptoms may include stertorous breathing due to paralysis of one side of the soft palate and respiratory expiration often puffs out the sides of the cheek and mouth on the affected side.
Pupils	Sometimes the pupils are unequal. The larger pupil is on the side of the hemorrhage. The eyes turn away from the side of paralysis.
Paralysis	Paralysis involves one side of the trunk, face, and extremities. It extends from the midline of the body outward.
Speech	Speech disturbances are common in stroke.

STROKE STATISTICS

According to the American Heart Association, stroke killed 137,119 people in 2006. It's the third largest cause of death, ranking behind heart diseases and all forms of cancer. Stroke is a leading cause of serious, long-term disability in the United States.

GERIATRIC CONSIDERATIONS

TIA AND SUSPECTED STROKE

Ask the older adult about recent unsteadiness or falls. An older adult is less likely to forget or minimize falls and unsteadiness than other symptoms of stroke or transient ischemia attacks (TIA).

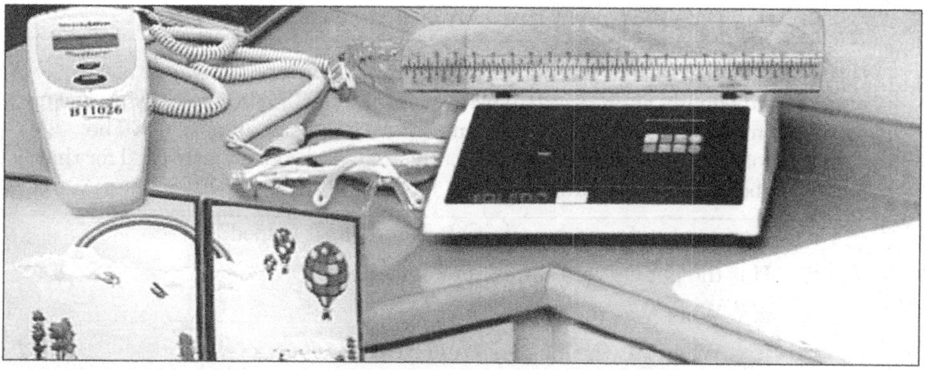

31 SYMPTOMS NOT ASSOCIATED WITH A DEFINED EMERGENCY

For details on triage see Chapter 34, Triage in a Nutshell.

PATIENT'S STORY – INTERVIEW QUESTIONS

1. Have you had a recent injury?
2. When did the symptoms begin?
    a. If the symptoms are no longer active or are intermittent, how long did they last?
    b. If the symptoms were intermittent, how long did each episode last and how frequent were the episodes?
3. Where is the problem?
    a. What region of the body is involved, and does it radiate to any other area of the body?
    b. Are any other symptoms associated with the chief complaint, e.g., nausea, vomiting, headache, sweating, or irregular heartbeat?

Breastfed infants normally have frequent loose, yellow stools.

4. Why is the symptom present?
    a. Did anything cause the symptoms, e.g., trauma, twisting, bending, eating a specific or contaminated food?
    b. What was the patient's activity at the onset of symptoms?
5. How does the problem affect normal body function?
    a. Is pain present?
        i. Does anything make the pain better or worse?
        ii. Is the severity and character of the pain, e.g., pressure, sharp, burning, shooting, dull, or cramping?

b. Does the patient have normal function of the involved area?

> It is appropriate to use the terms mild, moderate, or severe, the words of the patient, and equally appropriate to use a scale of 0 to 10. Zero typically means no pain. The meaning of a 10 is not the same for all nurses or all patients. The definition of 10 must be determined, documented, and consistently used for that patient to be an effective pain evaluation tool.

6. Has any treatment been initiated, and has it helped?
7. Has the patient had similar problems before?
    a. When was the problem?
    b. What was the diagnosis and treatment?
8. Is unlawful activity suspected?
    a. Was law enforcement at the scene?
    b. What agency?

> Medical personnel are obligated to notify law enforcement if unlawful activity is suspected.

9. Does the patient have any pertinent past history?
10. Does the patient take any routine medications?
    a. What is the name, dosage, route, and frequency of each medication?
    b. When was the last dose?
11. Does the patient take any complementary or alternative therapies, herbal products, over-the-counter medications or supplements, or natural therapies?
    a. What is the name, dosage, route and frequency of each therapy?
    b. When was the last dose or therapy?
12. Does the patient have allergies to drugs or foods?
    a. What is the name of the allergen?
    b. What was the reaction?
13. When was the patient's last tetanus immunization?
14. If the patient is female and between the ages of 10 to 50 years, when was the first day of her last menstrual period?

NURSING DOMAIN

The nursing domain, nursing diagnosis and plan of care can only be determined after an in-depth interview and consideration of the patient's story.

> Domain 12. Comfort.
> Class 1. Physical comfort.

Domain 8. Sexuality Class 2. Sexual function

NURSING DOMAIN

The nursing domain, nursing diagnosis and plan of care can only be determined after an in-depth interview and consideration of the patient's story.

Domain 12. Comfort. Class 1. Physical comfort.

ANTICIPATED MEDICAL CARE

Review of the Anticipated Medical Care of Symptoms Not Associated with a Defined Emergency	
Medical provider exam	Local exam for localized symptoms and full body exam if symptoms encompass a body system
Urine tests	Collect a urine specimen; pregnancy test for women of reproductive age unless they have had a hysterectomy
Blood tests	Wait for medical provider's orders
ECG	Wait for medical provider's orders
X-ray	X-rays of suspected bony damage
Diet	NPO
IV	Possible intravenous access for fluid resuscitation with normal saline or Ringer's solution or saline locked access for intravenous medications
Medications	Symptomatic therapy
Disposition	Admission to the hospital may be required depending on the severity of the condition.

INITIAL CARE PLAN

Alcohol-based hand sanitizers are the preferred method for cleaning your hands in most clinical situations. Wash your hands with soap and water whenever they are visibly dirty, before eating, and after using the restroom.

If patient is ambulatory and not bleeding vaginally, ask the patient to collect a clean-catch urine specimen before undressing.

1. Ask the patient to undress to expose the body region involved in the complaint, take off jewelry that might interfere with the examination, and put an exam gown. Assist as needed.

2. If the patient is unstable, initiate continuous heart monitoring, non-invasive blood pressure monitoring, and pulse oximetry.
3. Obtain initial vital signs. Consider obtaining a rectal temperature.

Every patient should have a temperature taken in the ER.

4. Consider the need for intravenous access and drawing of laboratory blood specimens.
    a. Draw a variety of tubes that will allow the lab to perform hematology, chemistry, and coagulation studies. Cirrhotic patients and patients on anticoagulants may need coagulation studies.
    b. Consider drawing other labs, e.g., type and screen, blood cultures.
5. Position the patient to enhance normal body function and comfort.
6. Keep the patient warm.
7. Examine the region of complaint.
8. Evaluate the level of consciousness based on the mnemonic **AVPU** or **ACDU** level of consciousness score.
   AVPU: **A**lert, **V**erbal, **P**ain, **U**nresponsive.
   ACDU: **A**lert, **C**onfused, **D**rowsy, **U**nresponsive.
9. Consider administration of medications covered by hospital protocols, e.g., antipyretics.
10. Consider insertion of drains, e.g., indwelling Foley catheter.
11. Order diagnostic tests covered by hospital protocol.
12. Inform the patient if he can eat or drink.
13. Elevate the siderails and place the stretcher in the lowest position.
14. Inform the patient, family, and caregivers of the usual plan of care and the expected overall time in the ER.
15. If NPO, explain the rationale for the need to abide by the NPO status.
16. Provide the patient with a device to reach someone for assistance and explain how to use it. Ask the patient to call for help before getting off the stretcher.

ONGOING CARE PLAN

1. Inform the medical provider of adverse changes noted during ongoing evaluation. Document that the medical provider was notified of the adverse change. Document if orders were or were not received.
2. Monitor temperature, heart rate and rhythm, blood pressure, and effectiveness of breathing.
3. Monitor therapy closely for the patient's therapeutic response.
    a. The usual time for a medication effectiveness check is 20 to 30 minutes after giving the drug.

   b. If therapy is not effective, ask the medical provider for a repeat dose or an alternative.
4. Monitor closely for the development of adverse reactions to therapy.
   a. Perform interventions to relieve the adverse reaction.
   b. Ask the medical provider for a remedy.
5. Keep the patient, family, and caregivers well informed of the plan of care and the remaining time anticipated before disposition.
6. Monitor the patient's laboratory and x-ray results and notify the medical provider of critical abnormalities. Remedy abnormalities as ordered.
7. Notify the medical provider when all diagnostic results are available for review. Ask for establishment of a diagnosis and disposition.

DISCHARGE INSTRUCTIONS

1. Provide the patient with the name of the nurse and doctor in the emergency room.
2. Inform the patient of their diagnosis or why a definitive diagnosis couldn't be made. Explain what caused the problem if known.
3. Teach the patient how to take the medication as prescribed and how to manage the common side effects. Instruct the patient not to drive or perform any dangerous tasks while taking narcotic pain medications.
4. Recommend a medical provider for follow-up care. Provide the name, address, and phone number with a recommendation of when to schedule the care.
5. Instruct the patient to call the follow-up medical provider immediately or return to the emergency room if the pain or problem worsens in any way or any unusual symptoms develop. Encourage the patient NOT to IGNORE WORSENING OR PERSISTENT SYMPTOMS.
6. Ask for verbal confirmation or demonstration of understanding and reinforce teaching as needed.

RELATED CONDITIONS AND INFORMATION

ALPHA BETA

Alpha-receptors are sites in the autonomic nervous system in which excitatory responses occur when adrenergic hormones, such as, norepinephrine and epinephrine are released. Activation of alpha-receptors causes various physiological reactions, including the stimulation of associated muscles and the constriction of blood vessels. These sites are also called alpha-adrenergic sites. An alpha-blocking agent is a drug that opposes the excitatory effects of norepinephrine released from sympathetic nerve endings at alpha-receptors. These drugs are also called alpha-adrenergic blocking agents. They cause a dilation of peripheral blood vessels and lower peripheral resistance, resulting in a lower blood pressure. They cause a positive chronotropic effect and increase conductivity and contractility. Examples are Regitine (phentolamine) and Dibenzyline (phenoxybenzamine).

Beta-receptors are sites in the autonomic nervous system in which inhibitory responses occur when adrenergic hormones, such as norepinephrine and epinephrine are released. Activation of beta-receptors causes various physiological reactions, such as relaxation of the bronchial muscles, an increase in the heart rate, and increase in the force of cardiac contraction. These sites are also called beta-adrenergic receptors. Beta blocking agents are drugs, such as Lopressor (metoprolol), that oppose the excitatory effects of norepinephrine released from sympathetic nerve endings at beta-receptors. They are used for the treatment of angina, hypertension, arrhythmia, and migraine. These drugs are also called beta-adrenergic blocking agents. The drugs can be selective to beta 1 or to beta 2 receptors. They cause vasoconstriction, increased inotropic effect, and a negative chronotropic affect. They are used for hypertension and ventricular arrhythmias. The generic names of the drugs use the last three letters of lol, e.g., atenolol, metoprolol, propranolol, labetalol.

An agonist is a substance that can combine with a nerve receptor to produce a reaction typical for that substance. An antagonist is a chemical substance that interferes with the physiological action of another, especially by combining with and blocking its nerve receptor.

ARTERIAL BLOOD GAS ANALYSIS

Quickie Arterial Blood Gas Analysis
Draw an arrow next to the pH. Up (↑) for >7.45 down (↓) for <7.35
Draw an arrow next to the PaCO2. Up (↑) for >45 and down (↓) for <35.
If the arrows are in the opposite direction (↑↓) a respiratory problem exists. Acidotic for a pH < 7.35 and alkalotic for a pH > 7.45. In the alphabet, O comes just before P. Arrows in the Opposite direction means a pulmonary problem.
Look at the HCO3 and draw an arrow down (↓) if it is <22 or an arrow up (↑) if it is > 26.
If the arrow is in the same direction as the pH arrow, the problem is a renal or metabolic one. In the alphabet, R comes just before S. **R**enal problem arrows go in the **S**ame direction

BLOOD SUGAR

Point of care blood sugar at the bedside is a priority measure in obtunded children and adults.

FEVER

Fever is a nonspecific symptom of an underlying infectious or inflammatory process.

CHILDHOOD DISEASES

Review of Childhood Diseases

Review of Childhood Diseases	
Chicken pox Varicella	Cause: Virus of the herpes family Symptoms: Blister-like lesions on the face, scalp, or trunk Transmission: Highly contagious, spread by respiratory droplets as in coughing and sneezing Complications: Bacterial infections of the skin, swelling of the brain, and pneumonia. Usually more severe in older children, over 13, and adults Vaccine: Available. Recommended for healthcare workers and all workers that come in contact with young children. Vaccine is not given to pregnant females. Immediate ER Intervention: Isolation
German measles Rubella	Cause: A virus (a virus that normally grows in the lining of the back of the throat and the lungs) Symptoms: Rash and fever for 2 to 3 days. Usually mild in children and young adults. Transmission: Highly contagious, spread by respiratory droplets as in coughing and sneezing Complications: Birth defects in pregnant women, at least a 20% change of damage to the fetus. Vaccine: Available. Recommended for healthcare workers, college and high school students, international travelers, women of childbearing age. Not needed in individuals showing they are immune by blood test. Immediate ER Intervention: Isolation
Measles	Cause: A virus Symptoms: Rash, high fever, cough, nasal drainage, red watery eyes. Symptoms appear 10 to 12 days after exposure. Rash started in about 14 days after exposure and begins at the hairline and spreads to the face and neck. Transmission: Highly contagious, spread by respiratory droplets as in coughing and sneezing Complications: Diarrhea, ear infections, severe infections such as pneumonia and encephalitis, death Vaccine: Available. It is a live, attenuated combination vaccine that protects against measles, mumps, and rubella virus. Recommended for most individuals who are not immune to the disease. Blood tests show immunity. Immediate ER Intervention: Isolation

Review of Childhood Diseases	
Mumps	Cause: A virus Symptoms: Fever, headache, swelling of the salivary glands, most often the parotid gland Transmission: Direct contact with respiratory secretions, saliva, or fomites (inanimate object or substance) Complications: Severe complications are rare Vaccine: Available. Contained in the measles, mumps, and rubella vaccine Immediate ER Intervention: Isolation
Scabies	Cause: Microscopic mite *Sarcoptes scabiei.* Infestation is found worldwide. Symptoms: Pimple-like irritations, rash, especially between the fingers and in skin folds Transmission: Direct, prolonged skin-to-skin contact Complications: Bacterial infections Treatment: Lotions are available to kill the mites. Itching may continue for 2 to 3 weeks after infestation has been cured
Note	The CDC has a resource for diseases, listed alphabetically, on their website at http://www.cdc.gov/az.do.

GUILLAIN BARRÉ SYNDROME

Review of Guillain Barré Syndrome	
Definition	Guillain Barré syndrome is an acute paralytic disease named after Georges Guillain (1876-1961) and Jean Alexandre Barré (1880-1967), French neurologists.
Cause	The syndrome is caused by a decreased myelin at the nerve root and in peripheral nerves. It typically follows a viral febrile illness.
Symptoms	Signs and symptoms may include deceased deep tendon reflexes and a symmetrical ascending paralysis beginning in the lower extremities.
Management	Supportive management of presenting symptoms may include respiratory support with endotracheal intubation and mechanical ventilation.
Disposition	Hospital admission may be required for diagnostic work-up and supportive treatment.

HYPERKALEMIA

Review of Hyperkalemia	
Definition	Hyperkalemia is a serum $K > 5.5$ mmol/L.

Review of Hyperkalemia	
Causes	The causes of hyperkalemia include impaired potassium excretion in acute and chronic renal failure, excessive dietary potassium, and potassium sparing diuretics.
Clinical effects	The clinical effects of hyperkalemia may include cardiac conduction changes, arrhythmias, and may cause ascending muscle weakness.

HYPERKALEMIA EMERGENCY TREATMENT

AZZAAAAAAA Emergency Treatment	
Calcium chloride	5 to 10 ml IV of 10% solution (500 or 1000 mg) Onset 1 to 3 minutes, duration 30 to 60 min.
Sodium bicarbonate	1 mEq/kg IV, onset 5 to 10 min., duration 1 to 2 hours
Insulin and glucose	Insulin 10 unit and 25 grams of glucose IV, onset 30 min., duration 4 to 6 hours
Lasix	40 to 80 mg IV bolus, onset with diuresis
Kayexalate plus sorbitol	15 to 50 grams PO or PR, onset 1 to 2 hours, duration 4 to 6 hours
Hemodialysis or peritoneal dialysis	Onset immediate, duration until completion of dialysis

HYPOCALCEMIA

Review of Hypocalcemia	
Definition	Hypocalcemia is an abnormally low serum calcium level.
Management	Medical management may include 10 to 20 ml of 10% calcium gluconate or 10% calcium chloride at a rate of 1 to 2 ml/min. For severe hypocalcemia, management may include administration of elemental calcium 15 to 20 mg IV per kilogram of body weight every 4 to 6 hours at a rate of 15 to 20 mg/min. or less.

HYPOKALEMIA

Review of hypokalemia	
Definition	Hypokalemia is serum potassium of < 3.5 mmol/L (3.5 mEq/L).

Review of hypokalemia	
Causes	Causes of hypokalemia include: Inadequate intake Excessive losses from the gastrointestinal tract Renal loss from alkalosis of any cause Osmotic diuresis as in hyperglycemia Hyperaldosteronism Renal tubular disorders Drugs Magnesium depletion Treatment with insulin as the cellular ions change
Symptoms	Symptoms may include muscle weakness, ileus, polyuria, and electrocardiogram changes (U-waves, prolonged QT interval, and flat T waves).
Management	If serum K+ > 2.5, administer KCl at a rate 10/mEq/hr to 20 mEq/hr, diluted in 50 to 100 ml of fluid. If serum K+ < 2.5 with ECG changes or evidence of paralysis, may administer KCl at a rate of 40 mEq/hr, dilute in at least 500 ml of fluid.

HYPOMAGNESEMIA

Review of Hypomagnesemia	
Definition	Hypomagnesemia is serum magnesium < 0.7 mmol/L (1.4 mEq/L).
Management	For acute myocardial infarction, loading dose of 1 to 2 grams mixed with 50 to 100 ml of D5W over 5 to 60 min. IV. Follow with 0.5 to 1.0 gm/hr for up to up to 24 hours.

HYPERNATREMIA

Review of Hypernatremia	
Definition	Hypernatremia is serum sodium >150 mmol/L.
Causes	The causes of hypernatremia include loss of water resulting in a water deficit relative to the sodium. Loss of water can result in water loss from the skin or lungs that is not replaced. Renal losses from diabetes insipidus can result from a head injury or neurosurgery. Other causes include conditions that cause water losses that exceed the sodium loss, such as, fever, burns, exposure to high temperature, or from renal losses during osmotic diuresis as in severe hyperglycemia. Hypernatremia may occur in patients who ingest excessive amounts of sodium chloride.

Review of Hypernatremia	
Management	Medical management is correction of the osmolality by replacing the water slowly. Normal saline is used to treat hypovolemic hypernatremia until the volume is restored. Hypervolemic hypernatremia is best treated with hypotonic fluids, loop diuretics, and if necessary, dialysis.

HYPONATREMIA

Review of Hyponatremia	
Definition	Hyponatremia is serum sodium <135 mmol/L or excess body H2O relative to the serum sodium.
Causes	Causes of hyponatremia include conditions when the total water exceeds the increase of sodium; e.g., severe CHF; cirrhosis; nephritic syndrome; sodium loss from the gastrointestinal tract; renal loss such as with diuretics, Addison's disease, diabetes mellitus, SIADH, severe hyperlipidemia, and severe hyper-proteinemic states such as multiple myeloma.
Symptoms	Symptoms may include confusion, anorexia, lethargy, disorientation, and cramps. Sodium <120 may cause seizures, hemiparesis, and coma.
Management	The initial step of medical management is assessment of volume status. Hypovolemic patients receive normal saline. Hypervolemic patients need a fluid restriction. For profound hyponatremia (<120 mmol/L), the sodium must be calculated, and half of the deficit required to correct the sodium is replaced over 24 hours. Hypertonic solutions are always given via central veins.

INTRAVENOUS FLUID CONSIDERATIONS

Solution Osmolarity	Considerations
1/3 NS hypotonic 103 mOsm D¼W hypotonic 126 mOsm ½NS hypotonic 154 mOsm	Hypotonic solutions shift fluid and electrolytes out of the intravascular compartment hydrating intracellular and interstitial compartments. Administer cautiously. Can cause sudden fluid shift from blood vessels to cells. DO NOT GIVE TO HEAD INJURY, STROKE, NEUROSURGICAL, BURN, OR TRAUMA PATIENTS.

Solution Osmolarity	Considerations
D5W 260 mOsm Acts as a hypotonic solution in the body	Isotonic only in the bag. The body burns the dextrose and leaves the water that is a hypotonic solution. DO NOT GIVE TO HEAD INJURY, STROKE, NEUROSURGICAL, BURN, OR TRAUMA PATIENTS.
Ringer's solution isotonic 275 mOsm NS isotonic 308 mOsm	Isotonic solutions are used in the ER. They expand the intravascular compartment contents only. Use isotonic solutions for patients with blood loss or dehydration from fluid loss (vomiting, diarrhea). The body's normal osmolarity is about 290 to 300 mOsm. DO NOT USE FOR PATIENTS WITH HYPERTENSION OR PATIENTS WHO ARE ALREADY OVERLOADED.
D5 ½NS hypertonic 406 mOsm D5NS hypertonic 560 mOsm D5NS hypertonic 560 mOsm D5LR hypertonic 575 mOsm 3% NS 1027 mOsm	Hypertonic solutions draw fluids and electrolytes into the intravascular compartment dehydrating the intracellular and interstitial compartments. DO NOT USE FOR PATIENTS WITH DIABETIC KETOACIDOSIS OR IMPAIRED HEART OR KIDNEY FUNCTION.

MEDICAL RESOURCE PHONE NUMBERS FOR PATIENTS

Medical Resource	Phone Number
Alzheimer's Disease Information	800-272-3900
American Cancer Society	800-227-2345
American Diabetes Association	800-342-2383
American Heart Association	800-242-8721
American Liver Foundation	800-223-0179
American Lung Association	800-586-4872
Arthritis Foundation	800-283-7800
Centers for Disease Control National AIDS Hotline	800-232-4636
Center for Mental Health Services	800-789-2647

Medical Resource	Phone Number
Medicare	800-633-4227
National Child Safety Council	800-222-1464
National Council on Alcoholism and Drug Dependence, Inc.	800-622-2255
National Institute on Aging	800-222-2225
National Kidney Foundation	800-622-9010
National Rehabilitation Information Center	800-346-2742
Office of Minority Health Resource Center	800-444-6472
Sickle Cell Disease Association of America	800-421-8453
Social Security	800-772-1213
Supplemental Security Income	800-772-1213
Women's Health America Group	800-558-7046

MYASTHENIA GRAVIS

Review of Myasthenia Gravis	
Definition	Myasthenia gravis is a neuromuscular disorder resulting in weakness and fatigability of the skeletal muscles.
Cause	The cause of myasthenia gravis is an autoimmune-mediated process.
Symptoms	Symptoms may include muscle weakness provoked by exertion. Characteristic distribution is the eyelids, extraocular muscles, facial weakness with nasal or slurred speech, and limb muscle weakness.
Tests	Diagnosis is not commonly made in the ER. These patients commonly present with acute exacerbation of their symptoms and with associated respiratory compromise (myasthenic crisis).
Management	Management may include symptomatic treatment, protection of the airway, and breathing support with endotracheal intubation and mechanical ventilation, plasmapheresis and/or immunodulatory therapy with high-dose intravenous immunoglobulin and corticosteroids.

PHYSICAL SIGNS AND EPONYMS OF DISEASE

Review of Physical Signs and Eponyms of Diseases

Review of Physical Signs and Eponyms of Diseases	
Babinski's sign	Babinski's sign indicates pyramidal tract disease when stimulation or stroking of the plantar surface of the foot causes extension of the great toe instead of the normal flexion. When the great toe extends the sign is said to be positive. It may be elicited during unconsciousness after a drug overdose, alcohol intoxication, or seizure.
Battle's sign	Battle's sign is present when there is bruising behind the ear indicating basilar skull fracture.
Brudzinski sign	Brudzinski sign is present when flexion of the neck causes flexion of the legs in meningitis.
Cheyne-Stokes respirations	Cheyne-Stokes respirations are repeating cycles of increased breathing depth followed by a decease resulting in apnea. The respirations are seen in central nervous system disorders, uremia, and abnormal sleep patterns.
Chvostek's sign	Chvostek's sign is present when facial spasms (tetany) are caused by tapping over the facial nerve indicating hypocalcemia.
Cullen's sign	Cullen's sign is a bruising around the umbilicus indicating intraperitoneal bleeding.
Gray Turner's sign	Gray Turner's sign is bruising of the flank, occasionally spreading to the groin, indicating retroperitoneal bleeding.
Heberden's nodes	Heberden's nodes are when flicking of the volar surface of the distal phalanx causes the fingers to flex, a sign of pyramidal tract disease.
Hoffmann's sign or reflex	Hoffmann's sign or reflex is when flicking the nail of the second, third for fourth finger causes a reflex that flexes these fingers and sometimes the thumb indicating hyperactive tendon reflexes.
Homans' sign	Homans' sign is when pain is present in the calf when the toe is passively dorsiflexed (moving the toes away from the sole of the foot) indicating early deep vein thrombosis.
Kehr's sign	Kehr's sign is pain referred from the epigastrium to the right shoulder, a phenomenon associated with biliary colic or acute cholecystitis. Kehr's sign can also be from a diaphragm that is irritated by blood in the peritoneum and often seen with a ruptured spleen.
Kernig's sign	Kernig's sign is an inability to extend a flexed leg suggestive of meningeal irritation indicating meningitis.
Kussmaul respiration	Kussmaul respiration is a pattern of deep rapid respirations seen in coma and diabetic ketoacidosis.

Review of Physical Signs and Eponyms of Diseases	
Levine's sign	Levine's sign is a clenched fist held over the chest when describing chest pain and is a sign of angina and acute myocardial infarction.
McBurney's point and sign	McBurney's point is located one-third the distance from the anterior superior iliac spine to the umbilicus. Tenderness at this site is a sign of acute appendicitis.
Murphy's sign	Murphy's sign is severe pain and inspiratory arrest on palpation of the right upper quadrant indicating cholecystitis.
Obturator sign	Obturator sign is when flexion and lateral rotation of the thigh causes hypogastric pain indicating a pelvic abscess or appendicitis.
Psoas sign (Iliopsoas test)	Psoas sign is when extension and elevation of the right leg produces pain. The sign indicates appendicitis.
Quincke's sign	Quincke's sign is an alternating blushing and blanching of the fingernail bed following light compression and is a sign of aortic regurgitation.
Romberg's sign	Romberg's sign is unsteadiness when standing with feet close together and eyes closed indicating an inner ear disorders.
Trousseau's sign	Trousseau's sign is carpal spasm produced by inflating a blood pressure cuff above the systolic pressure indicating hypocalcemia.

REYE'S SYNDROME

Reye's syndrome is a complication that may follow a viral illness in children and includes mitochondria injury to tissues. Fatty infiltration of the liver interferes with the enzymatic conversion of ammonia to urea and is associated with an elevated ammonia level.

ROTAVIRUS

Rotavirus causes severe dehydrating diarrhea in children with vomiting, diarrhea, and low-grade fever. It lasts <24 hours. Diagnosis is made by laboratory results that can be made rapidly with a stool specimen on a culture swab. Treatment includes fluid replacement.

SEPTIC SHOCK

Septic shock in the early stages is characterized by a hyperdynamic state resulting in tachycardia, mild hyperglycemia, and reduced afterload. The goal in treating all forms of shock is restoration of oxygenation and tissue perfusion.

SHOCK

A patient who is tachycardic, pale, cool, clammy, with a thready pulse, and an altered mental state is in shock. The goal in treating all forms of shock is restoration of oxygenation and tissue perfusion.

SICKLE CELL CRISIS

Review of Sickle Cell Crisis

Review of Sickle Cell Crisis	
NOTE	Patients with diagnosed sickle cell disease must receive sickle cell negative red cells. This requirement must be communicated to the blood bank.
Sickle cell crisis	Sickle cell crisis is a vascular occlusive crisis with pain from infarction of the spleen, brain, marrow, kidney, lung, aseptic necrosis of bone, and associated with ankle ulcers. Management includes analgesics (high dose narcotics), intravenous hydration, warmth, and oxygen.
Painful or infarction crisis	Infarction or painful crisis is severe skeletal pain that persists for several days or weeks. Fever is common with changes of hemoglobin concentration. Management includes analgesics (high dose narcotics), intravenous hydration, warmth, and oxygen.
Sequestration crisis	Usually in infants and children, sequestration crisis is a sudden pooling of red cells in the spleen with a fall in hemoglobin. Uncommonly fatal. Management includes analgesics (high dose narcotics), intravenous hydration, warmth, and oxygen.
Hemolytic crisis	Hemolytic crisis is uncommon and associated with a fall in hemoglobin and a marked increase in jaundice. Management includes analgesics (high dose narcotics), intravenous hydration, warmth, and oxygen.

THROMBOPHLEBITIS

Review of Thrombophlebitis	
Definition	Thrombophlebitis is an inflammation of a vein associated with a formation of a thrombus.
Symptoms	Symptoms may include tenderness, aching, positive Homans' sign (pain in the calf when the toe is passively moved away from the sole of the foot [dorsiflexed]), and differences in calf circumference.
Tests	Tests may include venous Doppler study.
Management	Management may include elevation, rest, anticoagulants to reduce the risk of further thrombus formation, and monitoring for signs of pulmonary embolus (dyspnea, tachycardia, chest pain). The goal is to present a thrombus from becoming an embolus that reaches the lung.
Disposition	Hospitalization may be required to monitor heparin therapy. Ligation proximal to the thrombus may be necessary.

THYROID STORM

Thyroid storm or thyroid crisis is a potentially life-threatening condition for people with hyperthyroidism. The thyroid released large amounts of thyroid hormone is a short period of time. It can be trigged by serious infection, surgery, or by using iodine for a scan. Emergency medical treatment is required. Intravenous propranolol (Inderal) can be ordered for a patient with a thyroid storm. The drug is used to keep the heart rate under 100 beats/min in order to maintain adequate cardiac output and avoid heart failure.

URINE SPECIFIC GRAVITY

Urine specific gravity is a measure of urine concentration or density. Normal values range from 1.003 to 1.030. Specific gravity reflects the state of hydration and the kidneys ability to reabsorb water. The specific gravity on a point of care dip test can be used as a quick measure of dehydration.

VARICELLA-ZOSTER SHINGLES

Review of shingles	
Causes	Shingles are caused by the virus varicella-zoster, the same virus that causes chicken pox. The chicken pox virus becomes dormant in the sensory ganglia and reactivates to produce shingles. The virus is held in check by cell-mediated immunity. If the immunity declines such as in advanced age, disease states, or AIDS, the virus reverts to its infectious state and shingles results.
Symptoms	Skin eruptions follow the tract of a cranial or spinal nerve. Symptoms may include severe pain or mild itching along the tract followed within 5 days by swelling, redness, and clusters of clear vesicles that develop into blisters. The symptoms do not cross the midline. The symptoms are most commonly in areas supplied by the trigeminal nerve and thoracic ganglia. Approximately 10 to 20% of Americans will develop shingles. They are more commonly seen in immunocompromised persons and those beyond the age of 80.
Management	Diagnosis is made by clinical appearance. Laboratory tests are necessary to accurately differentiate between herpes zoster and herpes simplex. Management may include analgesics and topical and oral antiviral agents. The most common complication is the debilitating complication of post herpetic neuralgia. Prompt treatment of the acute zoster with antiviral agents may decrease the incident of post herpetic neuralgia.

Review of shingles	
Contagion	New lesions appear for 2 to 3 days and within 14 days, the lesions become pustular and crusty. At this point, the lesions no longer contain the virus. Varicella-zoster immune globulin prevents or modifies the clinical illness in susceptible immunocompromised persons who are exposed to the virus. It is most effective immediately post exposure but may be effective up to 96 hours after exposure. Types of exposure for the use of immune globulin are (1) direct exposure of 1 hour or more, (2) sharing the same hospital room with an infectious patient, (3) prolonged direct face-to-face contact with an infectious patient (health-care worker), and (4) continuous exposure to household members. The immune globulin is recommended for exposed hospital personnel who never had chicken pox. The most frequent adverse reaction of the globulin is discomfort at the injection site.

CHICKEN POX

Review of Chicken Pox	
Causes	The Varicella zoster virus causes chicken pox.
Symptoms	Symptoms may include an itchy rash that forms blisters (average 300 to 400 lesions on the body) and then dry and scab in 4 to 5 days. The rash is sometimes associated with fever and malaise.

Review of Chicken Pox	
Contagion	Highly contagious, by adulthood more than 90% of Americans have had chicken pox. Contagious 1 to 2 days before the rash appears and until all the blisters have formed scabs. Disease develops 10 to 21 days after contact. Spreads by direct contact and through the air. Varicella vaccine is available since March of 1995, for use in healthy children 12 months of age or older. A blood test is available to test for immunity. New lesions appear for 2 to 3 days and within 14 days the lesions become pustular and crusty. At this point, the lesions no longer contain the virus. Varicella-zoster immune globulin prevents or modifies the clinical illness in susceptible immunocompromised persons who are exposed to the virus. The globulin is most effective immediately post exposure but may be effective up to 96 hours after exposure. Types of exposure for the use of immune globulin are (1) direct exposure of 1 hour or more, (2) sharing the same hospital room with an infectious patient, (3) prolonged direct face-to-face contact with an infectious patient (health-care worker), and (4) continuous exposure to household members. The immune globulin is recommended for exposed hospital personnel who never had chicken pox. The most frequent adverse reaction of the globulin is discomfort at the injection site.

VARICELLA ZOSTER COMPLICATIONS

Review of Varicella Zoster Complications	
Complications	Varicella zoster may cause various complications including bacterial infections of the skin and soft tissues in children and pneumonia in adults. Infections may be severe and include septicemia, toxic shock syndrome, necrotizing fasciitis, osteomyelitis, bacterial pneumonia, and septic arthritis. Other complications may include cerebellar ataxia, encephalitis, and hemorrhagic complications leading to bleeding disorders including disseminated intravascular coagulation.

PEDIATRIC CONSIDERATIONS

CIAMPEDS

Review of CIAMPEDS History Technique Emergency Nurses Association 1998	
(C) Chief Complaint	What is the chief complaint? What is the duration of the complaint?
(I) Immunizations	Are they up to date?

Review of CIAMPEDS History Technique Emergency Nurses Association 1998	
Isolation	Has the child been exposed to any communicable disease?
(A) Allergies	Are there any known allergies? What was the reaction?
(M) Medications	Is the child taking any medications including over the counter medications or herbal preparations? When was the dose given and how much? Is the child on any immunosuppressive medications?
(P) Past Medical History	Is there a significant history of illness, surgery, or hospitalization? Is there a known chronic illness?
(P) Parents Impression	What is different about the child's condition that concerns the parent?
(E) Events Surrounding the Illness or Injury	How long has the child been ill? Was the onset rapid or slow? Has anyone else been ill? If an injury, when did the injury occur? Was it witnessed? What happened?
(D) Diet	How much has the child been eating and drinking? When was the last time the child ate or drank?
(D) Diapers	When was the child's last void? How much was it? When was the child's last bowel movement? What did it look like and how large?
(S) Symptoms	What symptoms are present? When did the symptoms begin? Have they gotten better or worse?

IMMUNIZATION

Immunization recommendations by the American Academy of Pediatrics and American Academy of Family Medical providers	
Immunization	Age
Hepatitis B	1 to 2 months, 6 to 18 months
Rotavirus	2 to 6 months
Diphtheria, Tetanus, Pertussis	15 to 18 months 4 to 6 years

Immunization recommendations by the American Academy of Pediatrics and American Academy of Family Medical providers	
Haemophilus influenzae type b	12 to 15 months
Pneumococcal	15 to 15 months
Inactivated poliovirus	6 to 18 months, 4 to 6 years
Influenza	6 months and yearly thereafter
Measles, mumps, rubella	12 to 15 months
Varicella	12 to 15 months
Hepatitis A	12 to 15 months

Pediatric Urine Output

Urine output in a child is 1 to 2 ml/kg per hour. Most cases of shock in children are from hypovolemia. The goal in treating all forms of shock is restoration of oxygenation and tissue perfusion.

Pediatric Fever

A rectal temperature of 100.4° F (38° C) is consistent with a fever in pediatric patients.

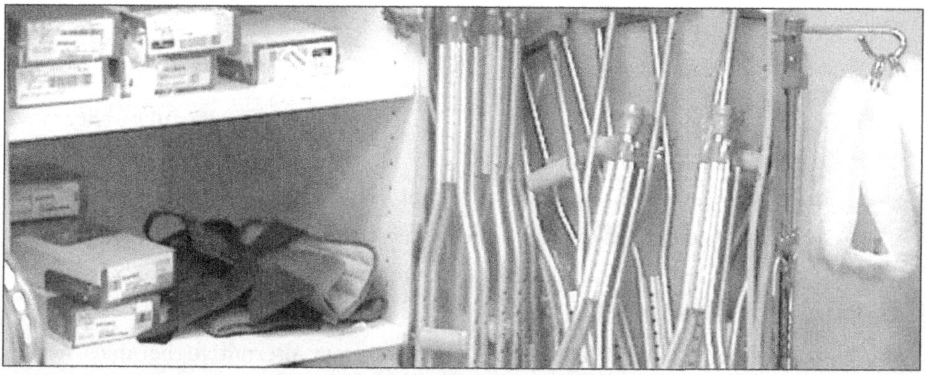

32 TRAUMATIC INJURY AND HEAD INJURY

For details on triage see Chapter 34, Triage in a Nutshell.

PATIENT'S STORY – INTERVIEW QUESTIONS

1. Consider the nature of the emergency.
   a. For a fall > six feet, consider #17 Falls and Spinal Injury.
   b. For a MVC, consider #24 Motor Vehicle Crash
   c. For laceration, consider #23 Laceration.
   d. For a penetrating wound, consider #29 Stabbing, Gunshot, and Penetrating Injury.
   e. For serious bleeding, consider #21 Hemorrhage.
2. When did the injury occur?
3. Where is the injury located and are any associated symptoms present?
4. What caused the injury; e.g., a trip and fall or slip and fall, a falling object, a direct blow from a fist or an object?
5. How does the problem affect normal function?
   a. Is the patient's level of consciousness altered?
   b. What is the appearance of the injured site?
   c. Were any body parts amputated and were the body parts found?
   d. Is any deformity present?
   e. Is neurovascular function and use normal?
6. Has any treatment been initiated, and has it helped?
7. Has the patient had injury to that area before?
   a. What type of injury?
   b. What was the treatment?
8. Is unlawful activity suspected?

a. Was law enforcement at the scene?

b. What agency?

Medical personnel are obligated to notify law enforcement if unlawful activity is suspected.

9. Does the patient have any pertinent past history?
10. Does the patient take any routine medications?
    a. What is the name, dosage, route, and frequency of each medication?
    b. When was the last dose?
11. Does the patient take any complementary or alternative therapies, herbal products, over-the-counter medications or supplements, or natural therapies?
    a. What is the name, dosage, route and frequency of each therapy?
    b. When was the last dose or therapy?
12. Does the patient have allergies to drugs or foods?
    a. What is the name of the allergen?
    b. What was the reaction?
13. When was the patient's last tetanus immunization?
14. If the patient is female and between the ages of 10 to 50 years, when was the first day of her last menstrual period?

NURSING DOMAIN

The nursing domain, nursing diagnosis and plan of care can only be determined after an in-depth interview and consideration of the patient's story.

Domain 12. Comfort. Class 1. Physical comfort.
Domain 5. Perception/Cognition. Class 1. Attention Class 2. Orientation. Class 3. Sensation/perception. Class 5. Communication
Class 4. Activity/Rest Class 2. Activity/exercise Class 5. Self-care.

ANTICIPATED MEDICAL CARE

Review of the Anticipated Medical Care of Traumatic Injuries and Head Injury	
Medical provider Exam	Local exam for localized symptoms and full body exam if symptoms involve a body system, such as a head injury

Review of the Anticipated Medical Care of Traumatic Injuries and Head Injury	
Urine test	Urine dip for blood if an injury of the abdominal cavity is present. Otherwise, urine tests are not usually ordered for traumatic injuries or head injury. A pregnancy test for women of reproductive age unless they have had a hysterectomy would be reasonable.
Blood tests	Labs are not usually ordered unless blood loss is significant, the patient has a history of anemia, or surgery is anticipated.
ECG	Not usually ordered unless injury is suspected to involve the chest
X-ray	X-ray of any areas of suspected bony damage, CT, MRI
Diet	NPO
IV	Normal saline or Ringer's solution for fluid resuscitation
Medications	Antiemetics, antipyretics, analgesics
Disposition	Hospital admission may be required for serious injury.
Worst-case scenario	The worst-case scenario is neurovascular compromise of a dislocated joint that goes unnoticed. Management is to relocate the dislocation before x-rays if necessary, to save the limb.

INITIAL CARE PLAN

NEUROVASCULAR COMPROMISE IS EMERGENT. Notify the medical provider immediately.

Alcohol-based hand sanitizers are the preferred method for cleaning your hands in most clinical situations. Wash your hands with soap and water whenever they are visibly dirty, before eating, and after using the restroom.

TRAUMATIC INJURIES

1. Ask the patient to undress the area of injury and take off jewelry that might compromise circulation if the area swells. Assist as needed.

Rings on the fingers must be removed for injuries of the arm or hand. Rings on the toes must be removed for injuries of the leg or foot.

2. Inspect for swelling, deformity, and disruption of the skin.
3. Palpate the region for crepitus and point tenderness.

4. Perform a neurovascular assessment. Use the mnemonic five P's plus two and assess:
    a. **P**ain
    b. **P**ulses
    c. **P**aralysis
    d. **P**aresthesia
    e. **P**allor
    f. ca**P**illary refill
    g. tem**P**erature
5. Splint for deformity, pain, bony crepitus, edema, ecchymosis, vascular compromise, open wounds, and paralysis or paresthesia.
    a. Use a splint that will immobilize the joints below and above the injury.
    b. Avoid manipulation of the bone.
    c. Rigid splints such as plastic devices and metal splints are used for lower extremity fractures.
    d. Soft splints such as pillows and slings are used for upper extremity fractures.
    e. Traction splints are used for femur and proximal tibial fractures.
6. Practice the mnemonic **PRICE**.
   Protect the injured area and keep out of harm's way; do not leave an injured foot in the way of a passerby. Cover skin that is not intact with a sterile dressing.
   Rest the area. Do not allow the patient to use or bear weight on an injured extremity.
   Ice the area with an ice pack saddled around the injured area.
   Compress the area with light pressure from the ice pack or a compression bandage to reduce the risk of swelling.
   Elevate the injured area above the level of the heart. Ice and elevation are essential ER procedures.
7. Instruct the patient not to eat or drink and teach the patient and family the rationale for the NPO status.
8. Elevate the siderails and place the stretcher in the lowest position.
9. Inform the patient, family, and caregivers of the usual plan of care and the expected overall time in the ER.
10. Provide the patient with a device to reach someone for assistance and explain how to use it. Ask the patient to call for help before getting off the stretcher.

HEAD INJURIES

1. Ask the patient to undress, remove jewelry that might interfere with the exam, and put on an exam gown. Assist as needed.

2. Obtain vital signs.
3. Place on heart, blood pressure, and continuous pulse oximetry, if available.
4. Perform a head-to-toe physical examination.

> If two nurses are at the bedside, one can ask the following questions and document the answers of the other who performs the exam. Document positive and negative findings.

a. What is the size and reaction of the pupils?

b. Does the patient have any head pain or injuries to the head?
Is the tongue or mouth injured?
Is any drainage present from the nose or ears?

c. Is the trachea midline?
Is jugular venous distention present (unable to detect under fluorescent light)?

d. Does the chest expand equally?
Is subcutaneous emphysema present?
Are the heart tones within normal limits?
Are the heart tones diminished?
Are any murmurs present?
Does the patient complain of chest pain?
Is the chest tender to palpation?

e. Are the lung sounds clear on the right and left?
Are wheezes or crackles present?
Are the lung sounds decreased or absent in any area of the lungs?

f. Is the abdomen soft, flat, rigid, or distended?
Are bowel sounds normal, hypoactive, hyperactive, or absent?
Does the patient complain of abdominal pain?
Is the patient's abdomen tender to palpation?

g. Is the patient incontinent?
Examination of the genitalia may be deferred if trauma is not suspected.
Do the genitalia appear normal?
Does the patient have bleeding from the urethral meatus or vagina?
Is priapism present?
Does the patient complain of genital pain?
Is the perineal area or genitalia tender to palpation?

h. Does the patient complain of pain when light pressure is applied to the iliac crests?
Is the pelvis stable or unstable?

i. Does the patient have normal motion and sensation in the upper and lower extremities?
Are distal pulses present in the upper and lower extremities?

j. Does the patient have normal movement of his back?
Does the patient complain of back pain?
While keeping the back immobilized, turn the patient.
Inspect the posterior surfaces.
Does the patient have obvious back injuries?
Is the back tender to palpation?

k. Does skin inspection reveal any damage to the skin; e.g., abrasions, lacerations, bruises, needle tracks, or petechiae?

5. Give initial medications covered by hospital protocol, e.g., tetanus toxoid.
6. Consider collecting wound cultures. Clean and dress wounds.
7. Consider placing drains; e.g., nasogastric tube to reduce the risk of vomiting and aspiration, indwelling urinary catheter for monitoring hourly urinary output.
8. Order diagnostic tests covered by hospital protocol, e.g., x-rays of areas with suspected bony damage.
9. Instruct the patient not to have any food or drink and teach the patient and family the rationale for the NPO status.
10. Place and maintain the bed siderails up.
11. Inform the patient, family, and caregivers of the usual plan of care, the expected overall time in the ER.
12. Provide the patient with a device to reach someone for assistance and explain how to use it. Ask the patient to call for help before getting off the stretcher.

ONGOING CARE PLAN

Inform the medical provider of adverse changes noted during ongoing evaluation. Document that the medical provider was notified of the adverse change. Document if orders were or were not received.

TRAUMATIC INJURY

1. Monitor vital signs.
2. Monitor the neurovascular status distal to the injury. Use the mnemonic five P's plus two.
   a. **P**ain
   b. **P**ulses
   c. **P**aralysis
   d. **P**aresthesia
   e. **P**allor
   f. ca**P**illary refill
   g. tem**P**erature
3. Monitor therapy closely for the patient's therapeutic response.

   a. The usual time for a medication effectiveness check is 20 to 30 minutes after giving the drug.

   b. If therapy is not effective, ask the medical provider for a repeat dose or an alternative.

4. Monitor closely for the development of adverse reactions to therapy.

   a. Perform interventions to relieve the adverse reaction.

   b. Ask the medical provider for a remedy.

5. Keep the patient, family, and caregivers well informed of the plan of care and the remaining time anticipated before disposition.

6. Monitor the patient's laboratory and x-ray results and notify the medical provider of critical abnormalities. Remedy abnormalities as ordered.

7. Notify the medical provider when all diagnostic results are available for review. Ask for establishment of a diagnosis and disposition.

HEAD INJURY

1. Monitor temperature, heart rate and rhythm, blood pressure, and effectiveness of breathing.

2. Monitor the level of consciousness using the Glasgow Coma Scale and notify the medical provider of adverse changes.

3. Monitor therapy closely for the patient's therapeutic response.

   a. The usual time for a medication effectiveness check is 20 to 30 minutes after giving the drug.

   b. If therapy is not effective, ask the medical provider for a repeat dose or an alternative.

4. Monitor closely for the development of adverse reactions to therapy.

   a. Perform interventions to relieve the adverse reaction.

   b. Ask the medical provider for a remedy.

5. Keep the patient, family, and caregivers well informed of the plan of care and the remaining time anticipated before disposition.

6. Monitor the patient's laboratory and x-ray results and notify the medical provider of critical abnormalities. Remedy abnormalities as ordered.

7. Notify the medical provider when all diagnostic results are available for review. Ask for establishment of a diagnosis and disposition.

DISCHARGE INSTRUCTIONS

1. Provide the patient with the name of the nurse and doctor in the emergency room.

2. Inform the patient of their diagnosis or why a definitive diagnosis couldn't be made. Explain what caused the problem if known.

3. Teach the patient how to take the medication as prescribed and how to manage the common side effects. Instruct the patient not to drive or perform any dangerous tasks while taking narcotic pain medications.

4. For the patient with a soft tissue injury teach the mnemonic **PRICE**. When the injured area is not managed properly, the patient pays the **PRICE** of increased pain and disability.
   Protect the injured area and keep out of harm's way; do not leave an injured foot in the way of a passerby. Cover skin that is not intact with a sterile dressing when in a dirty environment.
   Rest the area. Do not use the injured extremity. Use crutches or a wheelchair to rest an injured lower extremity.
   Ice the area.
   Compress the area with light pressure from a compression bandage or ice pack to reduce the risk of swelling.
   Elevate the injured area above the level of the heart.
5. Inform the patient with a fracture that splints can become too tight if swelling develops.
   a. Watch carefully for loss of the normal color in the fingers or toes and increased pain.
   b. Call the follow-up medical provider or return to the ER if a problem develops.
6. Teach crutch-walking to the patient unable to bear weight.
   a. Inform the patient not to bear weight on the injured leg and not to bear the body's weight on the crutches up against the armpit. This can cause serious and permanent nerve damage.
   b. Keep the arms straight and support the body's weight on the crutch handles. The two crutches serve as a support for the injured leg and swing with that leg. Move the crutches and the injured leg forward at the same time, then pick up the crutches and step forward on the uninjured leg.
   c. Take care to keep the rubber tips clean and tightly affixed to the crutch. Do not use on wet surfaces or on ice. Depend on a wheelchair if your arms cannot support your weight on crutches.
   d. Notify the follow-up medical provider if any problems develop regarding the use of the crutches.
7. Instruct the patient with a sutured laceration that:
   a. The laceration must be kept clean and dry.
   b. The dressing applied in the ER should be removed after one to two days and the wound left open to the air. Some lacerations of the face and scalp are not covered with a dressing in the ER. The wound may be covered with a dry sterile dressing if needed to protect the area.
   c. Elevate the area when possible to reduce the risk of swelling.
   d. The laceration should be cleaned with mild soap and water and an antibiotic over-the-counter ointment applied two times a day for the first three days.
   e. Ask the patient to follow-up as recommended for suture removal.

8. Some lacerations contaminated with dirt or bacteria are not sutured. These are considered dirty wounds and further care is necessary at home.
   a. Soak the area in warm water and prescribed solution for twenty minutes three times a day for the first three days.
   b. Keep the wound covered with a dry sterile dressing between soaks. If the wound is dry and clean after three days of soaks, stop the soaking, and keep it clean, dry, and covered.
   c. Not all dirty wounds need antibiotics. If antibiotics are prescribed, take them until the pills are gone. Do not stop when the wound looks better.
   d. Redness, swelling, red streaks, and pus are signs of infection. Notify the follow-up medical provider if any of these symptoms develop.
9. Recommend a medical provider for follow-up care. Provide the name, address, and phone number with a recommendation of when to schedule the care.
10. Instruct the patient to call the follow-up medical provider immediately or return to the emergency room if the pain or problem worsens in any way or any unusual symptoms develop. Encourage the patient NOT to IGNORE WORSENING OR PERSISTENT SYMPTOMS.
11. Ask for verbal confirmation or demonstration of understanding and reinforce teaching as needed.

COMMONLY ORDERED MEDICATIONS

DILAUDID

Dilaudid (hydromorphone)	
Indications	Moderate to severe pain
Dose	Typical dose 1 to 5 mg IV. Titrate to response. No maximum dose.
Onset	IV onset rapid, peak 15 to 30 minutes, duration 3 to 4 hours
Side effects	Drowsiness, dizziness, confusion, sedation, increased intracranial pressure, nausea, vomiting, urinary retention, respiratory depression
Monitor	CNS changes, respiratory effectiveness, allergic rash
Note	Dilaudid 5 mg equivalent to Morphine 10 mg IM. Dilute to 4 or 5 ml with NS or sterile water for injection and administer slowly over at least 2 to 3 min. Antidote is naloxone.

SOLUTION OSMOLARITY

Solution Osmolarity	Considerations
1/3 NS Hypotonic 103 mOsm D¼W Hypotonic 126 mOsm ½NS Hypotonic 154 mOsm	Hypotonic solutions shift fluid and electrolytes out of the intravascular compartment, hydrating intracellular and interstitial compartments. Administer cautiously. Can cause sudden fluid shift from blood vessels to cells. DO NOT GIVE TO HEAD INJURED, STROKE, NEUROSURGICAL, BURNED, OR TRAUMA PATIENTS.
D5W 260 mOsm Acts as a hypotonic solution in the body	Isotonic only in the bag, the body burns the dextrose and leaves water, a hypotonic solution. DO NOT GIVE TO HEAD INJURED, STROKE, NEUROSURGICAL, BURNED, OR TRAUMA PATIENTS.
Ringer's solution Isotonic 275 mOsm NS Isotonic 308 mOsm	Isotonic solutions are used in the ER. They expand the intravascular compartment only. Use isotonic solutions for patients with blood loss, dehydration from fluid loss (vomiting, diarrhea). The body's osmolarity is about 290 to 300 mOsm. DO NOT USE FOR HYPERTENSIVE OR CHF PATIENTS WHO ARE ALREADY OVERLOADED.
D5 ½NS Hypertonic 406 mOsm D5NS Hypertonic 560 mOsm D5NS Hypertonic 560 mOsm D5LR Hypertonic 575 mOsm	Hypertonic solutions draw fluids and electrolytes into the intravascular compartment, dehydrating the intracellular and interstitial compartments. DO NOT USE FOR DIABETIC KETOACIDOSIS, IMPAIRED HEART OR KIDNEY FUNCTION.

MANNITOL

Mannitol	
Indications	Increased intracranial pressure, edema
Effect	Increased osmolarity of glomerular filtrate, raising the osmotic pressure of fluid in the renal tubules, increasing urinary output and decreasing intracranial pressure

Mannitol	
Adult dose	0.5 to 1 gram/kg IV over 5 to 10 min., additional doses can be given 0.25 to 2 grams/kg IV every 4 to 6 hours
Onset	IV onset ½ to 1 hour, peak 1 hour, duration 6 to 8 hours
Side effects	Seizures, rebound intracranial pressure
Note	For head injury, use in conjunction with hyperventilation. Use with caution in renal failure.
Monitor	Intake and output, monitor fluid status, osmolarity (not to exceed 310 mOsm/kg)

NIPRIDE

Nipride (nitroprusside)	
Indications	Hypertensive crisis, to reduce afterload in heart failure and pulmonary edema
Adult dose	0.10 mcg/kg/min. IV, increase every 3 to 5 min. to desired effect
Onset	IV onset 0.5 to 1 min., peak 1 to 2 min., duration up to 10 min. after the drug is stopped
Compatibility	Compatible at Y-site with Inocor, dopamine, NTG, dobutamine
Side effects	Hypotension, altered consciousness, cyanide toxicity
Note	Light sensitive, cover drug bag

TETANUS AND DIPHTHERIA TOXOID, ADSORBED FOR ADULTS

Tetanus and Diphtheria Toxoid, Adsorbed for Adults	
Indications	Immunization against tetanus and diphtheria
Dose	0.5 ml IM for adults and children 7 years and older
Side effects	Local reactions such as erythema, induration, and tenderness are common. Systemic reactions include fever, chills, myalgias, and headache. Local reactions are usually self-limiting. Sterile abscess and subcutaneous atrophy may occur at the injection site.
Monitor	Injection site
Note	The goal is to keep tetanus immunization current not specifically to prevent tetanus infection from the current wound. Persons in the United States have a right not to be immunized. Children can receive a religious exception and be in public school without the recommended immunizations.

VERSED

Versed (midazolam hydrochloride)

Versed (midazolam hydrochloride)	
Indications	Conscious sedation
Adult dose	1 to 2.5 mg IV over 2 min., every 2 min., over 5 mg IV is seldom necessary. If patients have narcotic medications before the Versed, use approximately 30% less Versed.
Pediatric dose	0.05 to 0.2 mg/kg IV loading dose, over 2 to 3 min. Versed is seldom used in pediatric patients who are not intubated. Pediatric patients 12 to 16 years old should be dosed as adults.
Onset	IV onset 3 to 5 minutes
Compatibility	Use normal saline in the IV line before and after the dose.
Side effects	Serious life threatening decreased respiratory tidal volume and respiratory rate
Monitor	Heart, blood pressure, respiratory effectiveness
Note	Versed is a potent sedative that requires slow administration and individualization of dosage. Versed is 3 to 4 times as potent as Valium. Reversing agent is Romazicon (flumazenil).

RELATED CONDITIONS AND INFORMATION

AMPUTATION

Review of Amputations	
Definition	An amputation is a traumatic separation of a digit or limb from the body.
Symptoms	Symptoms include loss of part or tissue, and may include bleeding, hypovolemic shock, and pain.
Tests	Tests may include x-rays to determine bony damage.
ER Management	Management includes control of bleeding with pressure dressings, elevation, cleansing of the wound, splinting and dressing with sterile dressings.
Disposition	Hospital admission may be required for surgical intervention or a transfer to a facility with a reclamation team.
Note	Keep the amputated part covered with saline moistened gauze in a watertight plastic bag or container. Place the bag or container in ice and water.

ASSESSMENT

Review of Assessment and Interventions for Bone and Tissue Injury
Inspect for swelling, deformity, and disruption of the skin.
Palpate the region for crepitus and point tenderness.

Review of Assessment and Interventions for Bone and Tissue Injury
Neurovascular assessment. Use the mnemonic five P's plus two. **P**ain **P**ulses **P**aralysis **P**aresthesia **P**allor ca**P**illary refill tem**P**erature
Splint for deformity, pain, bony crepitus, edema, ecchymosis, vascular compromise, open wounds, and paralysis or paresthesia.
Ice the area. Place a large ice pack like a saddle over the area. Use the ice pack to apply light compression to the area to reduce the risk of swelling.
Elevate the area. Sit the patient up for facial, head and chest injuries and elevate extremities as high as possible to reduce the risk of swelling.

CLAVICLE FRACTURE

Clavicle fractures are usually best treated without surgery with good outcomes. Management includes either the use of a shoulder sling or a figure-of-eight support. Most fractures heal with limited deformity. Incorrect application of a figure-of-eight support has the potential of injury to the radial nerve.

COMMON HEAD INJURIES

Review of Common Head Injuries	
Anatomical location	The brain is covered with three fibrous membranes. The pia mater is the thick membrane covering nearest the brain; the arachnoid mater is a thinner membrane between the pia and dura; and the dura is the outermost covering. A mnemonic is PAD starting from the brain the pia, arachnoid, and dura membranes form a pad to protect and hold the brain. To define the location of a hematoma or bleed, use the prefix epi (above) or the prefix sub (below) with the name of the membrane.
Cerebral concussion	A cerebral concussion is a mild closed-head injury with a history of loss of consciousness. Amnesia and headache are common.
Cerebral contusion	Cerebral contusion is a closed-head injury with bruising of the brain.
Epidural hematoma	An epidural hematoma is located above (epi) the dura and is usually from an arterial source.
Intracerebral hemorrhage	An intracerebral hemorrhage is a hemorrhage inside the brain.
Penetrating head injury	A penetrating head injury is a wound from a missile that has penetrated the skull.

Review of Common Head Injuries	
Scalp Laceration	A scalp laceration bleeds profusely but is seldom life threatening.
Skull fracture	Skull fractures may have obvious deformity or be visible only on x-ray or CT. If the skull is indented, it may need to be repaired. The skull fracture is not a threat to life. The potential damage to the brain caused by pressure from the fracture or the associated bleeding or swelling may be a threat to life.
Subarachnoid hematoma	A subarachnoid hematoma is a hematoma located below (sub) the arachnoid membrane and is usually an arterial bleed.
Subdural hematoma	A subdural hematoma is a hematoma located below (sub) the dura usually from a venous source. A subdural hematoma can develop days or weeks after an injury.

COMPARTMENTAL SYNDROME

Review of Compartmental Syndrome	
Definition	A compartmental syndrome is a condition in which tissue is severely constricted in its space causing damage to the tissue. The syndrome occurs several hours post injury. It is not commonly seen at the time of injury.
Cause	Trauma causes inflammation and swelling of tissue. At times, more swelling than can be contained within the compartment without constriction damage to the tissue. This condition is called compartmental syndrome.
Symptoms	Symptoms may include progressive pain, sensory deficits, muscle weakness, and a tense swollen area. It usually occurs in the forearm and lower leg.
Tests	Tests may include measurement of muscle compartment pressure. A reading of greater than 35 to 45 mmHg is indicative of the need for fasciotomy.
Management	Management includes elevation TO the level of the heart to assure venous outflow. Elevation above the heart decreases perfusion. Ongoing monitoring of size and tenseness of the injured area is essential.
Disposition	Hospital admission may be required for potential surgical fasciotomy or repair of neurovascular damage.

CRUSH INJURIES

Review of Crush Injuries	
Definition	A crush injury is destruction caused by extreme pressure against the tissue resulting in damage to skin, muscle, nerves, and bone.

Review of Crush Injuries	
Cause	The cause of crush injuries is an external force.
Symptoms	Symptoms may include pain, loss of neurovascular function distal to the injury, hemorrhage, hypovolemic shock, swelling, and ecchymosis.
Tests	Tests may include x-rays and CT.
Management	Management may include: Control of bleeding. Fluid resuscitation with normal saline to increase urinary output and facilitate excretion of myoglobin. Elevation, cleansing and irrigation of wounds. Monitoring of urinary output volume and urinary myoglobin. Monitoring of neurovascular function.
Disposition	Hospital admission may be required for surgical débridement, fasciotomy, or amputation.

DISLOCATED SHOULDER

Review of Dislocated Shoulder	
Definition	A dislocated shoulder is a displacement of the humerus from its normal position in the shoulder joint.
Causes	An anterior dislocation of the shoulder usually occurs when the patient falls on an extended arm. Posterior dislocation is rare but can occur with seizure activity.
Symptoms	Symptoms may include severe pain in the shoulder, inability to move the arm, and deformity at the shoulder. Approximately 60% of shoulder dislocations are recurrent.
Management	Management includes placement of the extremity in the position of maximum comfort, support with a pillow or a sling, and monitoring of distal pulses, movement, and sensation. Medical management may include radiographic plane films prior to relocation unless neurovascular compromise is present, conscious sedation for relocation in the ER, and immobilize in a sling and swathe post relocation.
Discharge Instructions	Discharge Instructions include an ice pack (30 minutes out of every two hours) and elevation for the first 24 to 48 hours to minimize inflammation and swelling. The first shoulder dislocation is immobilized with a sling and swathe for six weeks. Failure to immobilize the joint for six weeks will predispose the shoulder to recurrent dislocations. Ask the patient to call the recommended follow-up medical provider if signs of decreased circulation or numbness occur.

FACIAL FRACTURES

Review of Facial Fractures	
Definition	A facial fracture is any fracture of a facial bone.
Symptoms	Symptoms may include pain, swelling, ecchymosis, and deformity of the face.
Ongoing monitoring	Ongoing monitoring includes looking for increasing edema, compromised airway, bleeding, and changes of level of consciousness, pupil size, eye movement, and vital signs.
Management	Management includes placing the patient in a high sitting position to maintain a clear airway, managing secretions, and decreasing edema with an ice pack to cool the area. Ice and elevation are essential ER procedures. Medical management may include prophylactic antibiotics and hospital admission for treatment and airway support.
Types	Maxillary fractures account for approximately 25% of all facial fractures. Le Fort I (horizontal fracture of the body of the maxilla), Le Fort II (called a pyramidal fracture that incorporates the central maxilla, nasal area and ethmoid bones), and Le Fort III are facial fractures of increasing severity originated from the work of René Le Fort in 1901. A tripod fracture is the extensive fracture of the zygomatic process. Orbit fracture is a fracture of the orbit of the eye.

FACIAL INJURIES

Review of Facial Injuries	
Definition	Facial injury is any facial bony or soft tissue injury.
Symptoms	Symptoms may include pain, swelling, ecchymosis, and deformity of the face.
Ongoing monitoring	Ongoing monitoring includes looking for increasing edema, compromised airway, bleeding, and changes of level of consciousness, pupil size, eye movement, and vital signs.
Management	Management includes placing the patient in a high sitting position to maintain a clear airway, managing secretions, and decreasing edema with an ice pack to cool the area. Ice and elevation are essential ER procedures. Medical management may include prophylactic antibiotics and hospital admission for treatment and airway support.

FRACTURE MANAGEMENT IN THE ER

Review of ER Management of Fractures

Review of ER Management of Fractures	
Expose	Remove all clothing and jewelry near the suspected fracture site.
Perform a physical assessment	Inspect the injured area for color, position, and obvious differences as compared to the uninjured side. Look for a break in the skin and assess for bleeding and deformity. Palpate the extremity for pain, pallor, pulses, paresthesia, and paralysis (five Ps).
Need to splint	Splint for deformity, pain, bony crepitus, edema, ecchymosis, vascular compromise, open wounds, and paralysis or paresthesia.
Immobilize	Select a splint that will immobilize the joints below and above the injury. Avoid manipulations of the bone. Rigid splints, such as plastic devices and metal splints are used for lower extremity fractures. Soft splints such as pillows and slings, are used for upper extremity fractures. Traction splints are used for femur and proximal tibial fractures.
PRICE	Protect, rest, ice, compress, and elevate the site. Ice and elevation are essential ER procedures.
Medications	Administer analgesics.
Diagnostic Testing	X-rays views should include the joints above and below the injury.
On-going monitors	Frequently reassess the five Ps (pain, pallor, pulses, paresthesia, and paralysis).
Disposition	Hospitalization may be required for definitive stabilization, traction, external fixation, and closed or open reduction.

FRACTURE TYPES

Review of Fractures Types	
Closed	Closed means the skin over the site is intact.
Comminuted	Comminuted means the bone is splintered into fragments.
Complete	Complete means the bony continuity is interrupted.
Displaced	Displaced means the proximal and distal segments of bone are not aligned.
Greenstick	Greenstick means the bone is bent.
Impacted	Impacted means the distal and proximal fracture sites are wedged together.
Open	Open means the skin over the fracture site is not intact.

FEMUR FRACTURES

Review of Femur Fractures

Review of Femur Fractures	
Definition	Definition of a femur fracture is a disruption of the continuity of the femur. A hip fracture is a fracture of the proximal femur ordinarily at the neck or ball.
Cause	The causes of femur fractures are commonly major trauma, falls, motor vehicle crashes, and slip and falls in the elderly.
Symptoms	Symptoms may include pain, inability to bear weight, shortening and rotation of the leg, and hypovolemic shock. The goal in treating all forms of shock is restoration of oxygenation and tissue perfusion.
Radiographic studies	Studies may include x-ray of the hip or area of suspected bony damage to the femur and chest x-ray.
Splint	Splinting may include immobilization of the leg with a traction splint or a traction pin.
Diagnostic laboratory studies	Pre-operative laboratory studies may include type and screen and coagulation studies if the patient is on anticoagulants or is cirrhotic.
Diet	NPO
IV	Normal saline
Ongoing evaluations	Ongoing evaluation consists of monitoring sensation, movement, and circulation distal to the fracture.
Disposition	Hospital admission may be required for open surgical reduction, internal fixation, or continued traction.

HEAD INJURY

Review of Head Injury	
Definition	A head injury is damage to the brain or craniofacial area.
Causes	Causes include a blunt acceleration and deceleration forces, a penetrating missile, or a secondary injury from hypoxemia, cerebral edema, hypercapnia, hypotension, and increased intracranial pressure.
Symptoms	Early signs may include headache, nausea, vomiting, amnesia (both of past and current events), a change in the patient's normal level of consciousness, and a change in speech or mentation. Late signs may include a dilated and nonreactive pupil, unresponsiveness, posturing, increased systolic blood pressure, bradycardia, and changes in respiratory rate and rhythm.

Review of Head Injury	
Ongoing monitoring	Use the Glasgow Coma Scale as a baseline and for ongoing monitoring. Monitor pupil size, shape, equality, reaction to light, and external movement. Inspect for contusions and development of ecchymosis and drainage from the ears or nose. Perform ongoing evaluation of sensation and motor ability and compare to the baseline. Monitor vital signs including core temperature.
Tests	Tests may include a CT scan of the brain, skull x-rays, MRI, and ABG.
Management	Medical management may include intubation if the Glasgow Coma Scale is less than 8. If the patient's level on consciousness is acutely decreased, the patient may be unable to clear his airway. Hyperventilation may be used to maintain PaCO2 between 30 and 35 mmHg with 100% oxygen. A bag-valve mask with an attached reservoir may be used if the patient is not intubated. Fluid support is necessary to maintain stability but use caution not to over hydrate. Orogastric or nasogastric tube may be used for decompression of the stomach to reduce the risk of vomiting and aspiration. The head should be kept positioned midline. Rotation of the head or flexion of the neck can increase intracranial pressure. Mannitol, a diuretic, may be used to decrease intracranial pressure. Hourly urine output is essential when using Mannitol. A normal core temperature must be maintained with heating or cooling blankets. Antipyretic and sedatives may be ordered if indicated. Hospital admission may be required for surgery, further diagnostic workup, treatment, and support. Transfer to another facility may be indicated.

JOINT DISLOCATIONS

Review of Joint Dislocations	
Definition	A joint dislocation is a displacement of a bone from its normal position in the joint.
Cause	The cause is commonly traumatic movement beyond the normal range of motion.
Symptoms	Symptoms include pain, deformity, swelling, inability to move the joint, and neurovascular compromise.
Tests	Tests may include x-ray of the joint.
Management	Medical management may include temporary immobilization of the joint, conscious sedation, and immediate reduction. Hospital admission may be required for observation and supportive treatment.

Review of Joint Dislocations	
Comments	DISLOCATION OF THE KNEE OR ELBOW IS EMERGENT In the knee, the peroneal nerve and vein may be permanently damaged. An angiogram may be necessary to evaluate vascular compromise.

KNEE INJURY

Review of Knee Injuries	
Definition	A knee injury is caused when the joint is stressed beyond the normal range of motion. Injuries are commonly strains and tears to the medial meniscus, collateral ligament, and cruciate ligament.
Symptoms	Symptoms may include swelling, pain, tenderness, loss of range of motion, inability to bear weight, and bruising.
Management	Management may include x-ray to rule out fracture, a knee immobilizer or ace wrap, and referral to outpatient follow-up.
Discharge Instructions	Instructions include resting the leg (non-weight bearing) by using crutches, cooling the area with ice 30 minutes out of every two hours for the first 24 to 48 hours, compressing the area with a knee immobilizer or Ace wrap, and elevating whenever possible. For a ligament tear, referral to an orthopedic surgery for repair within 48 hours is often recommended.

NURSEMAID ELBOW (RADIAL HEAD SUBLUXATION)

Review of Nursemaid Elbow	
Definition	Nursemaid elbow is dislocation of part of the elbow in children altering the normal alignment of the joint without fracture. This typically occurs in children under 6 years of age. As the child grows older the elbow structures fit tighter and there is less room for subluxation.
Symptoms	Symptoms may include pain and limited motion of the elbow.
Management	Management may include x-ray of the elbow to rule out fracture and reduction of the dislocation. If pain continues after reduction, a sling can be used.
Discharge Instructions	Instructions include an ice pack on the elbow 30 minutes out of every 2 hours for the first 24 to 48 hours and acetaminophen for pain. If neurovascular dysfunction develops call the doctor immediately or return to the emergency room.

OPEN FRACTURES

Review of Open Fractures

Review of Open Fractures	
Definition	The definition of an open fracture is a fracture of the bone with disruption of the skin near the fracture site either from external or internal forces.
Cause	The cause of an open fracture is commonly trauma.
Symptoms	Symptoms include disrupted skin near the fracture site, and may include protrusion of the bone, pain, neurovascular compromise, and bleeding.
Tests	Tests include x-rays, CT, and MRI.
Management	Management includes a wound culture, cleansing and irrigation of the wound, a sterile dressing, and a splint.
Disposition	Hospital admission may be required for surgery or transfer to a facility that can provide the necessary care.

PELVIC FRACTURES

Review of Pelvic Fractures	
Definition	A pelvic fracture is a fracture of the pelvis.
Cause	The cause is usually trauma.
Symptoms	Symptoms may include deformity and swelling at the site of fracture, shortening or abnormal rotation of the leg, and pain. Pelvic fracture in males is the most common cause of injury to the posterior urethra.
Tests	X-ray, CT, cystogram
Management	Management may include splinting with a simple sheet and towel clamp method by wrapping the pelvis tightly with a sheet and securing with towel clamps if the patient is hemodynamically unstable, resuscitation with normal saline. A large amount of blood loss can accompany an unstable pelvic fracture.
Disposition	Stable fractures are treated with bed rest. Unstable fractures may require hospital admission for surgery or transfer to a facility that can surgically repair the pelvis.
Associated injury	Associated injuries include injury of the perineum, genitalia, and rectum.
Note	The ischial ramus is often the cause of a fracture sustained when someone pulls a chair out from another causing them to fall and land on a hard floor. This type of fracture is normally stable, and the patient is able to ambulate.

PREGNANCY AND TRAUMA

Review of Anatomy and Physiology Changes in the Pregnant Female

Review of Anatomy and Physiology Changes in the Pregnant Female	
Gastrointestinal	The stomach and intestines are displaced upward. Gastric emptying is delayed
Hemodynamic	Hemodynamic changes include cardiac output increase of approximately 40%, systolic blood pressure increase of 5 to 15 mmHg, heart rate increases 15 to 20 beats per minute, hematocrit increases (30% to 35%), and a decreased clotting time.
Renal	Renal blood flow is increased.
Respiratory	The diaphragm is displaced upward by about 1½ to 2 inches. The air passages are engorged because of the increased blood flow. The respiratory rate is increased. Basal metabolism and oxygen consumption are increased. The pCO2 is decreased to 30 mmHg.
Uterus	The uterus that is normally the size of a pear increases to contain the fetus and about 1 liter of amniotic fluid.

SPRAINED ANKLE

Review of Ankle Sprain	
Causes	An ankle sprain is an injury that tears ligaments or tendons around the ankle joint.
Symptoms	Symptoms include post injury pain, swelling, limited use, and bruising.
Management	Practice the mnemonic **PRICE.** **P**rotect the injured area and keep out of harm's way; do not leave an injured foot in the way of a passerby. Cover damaged skin with a sterile dressing. **R**est the area. Do not allow the patient to use or bear weight on an injured extremity. **I**ce the area with an ice pack saddled around the injured area. **C**ompress the area. Either with light pressure from the ice pack or a compression bandage to reduce the risk of swelling. **E**levate the injured area above the level of the heart. When the injured area is not managed properly, the patient pays the PRICE of increased pain and disability. Medical management may include radiographic plane films to rule out fracture; pain medications; and a splint, wrap, or boot to immobilize the area.

Review of Ankle Sprain	
Discharge Instructions	Teach the mnemonic PRICE. Use ice 30 minutes out of every two hours for the first 24 to 48 hours. Inform the patient that healing takes 4 to 6 weeks and pain, swelling, bruising, and stiffness are common. Instruct the patient to watch for decreased sensation and circulation if the ankle is splinted. Inform the patient that minor fractures may not be evident at the ER visit and if symptoms worsen, repeat x-rays could show a fracture. Recommend a follow-up medical provider with a recommendation of when to schedule follow-up care.

GERIATRIC CONSIDERATIONS

HEAD INJURIES

Due to the cerebral atrophy seen in older adults, they can tolerate a large subdural hematoma for a longer period of time without any obvious symptoms.

PEDIATRIC CONSIDERATIONS

HEAD INJURIES

If a child begins to play or run immediately after getting a bump on the head, serious injury is unlikely. Children often vomit ONCE after a head injury.

INJURED CHILD CONSIDERATIONS

Review of Cardinal Considerations for an Injured Child
The child's oropharynx is relatively small and is easily obstructed by the tongue.
Vocal cords are short and concave and collapse easily if the head is hyperflexed or extended.
Lower airway passages are smaller and easily obstructed by mucus and swelling.
The mediastinum is more mobile allowing more damage to the great vessels.
Crying children swallow air and gastric distension can prevent free respiratory movement.
Lung sounds can be difficult to auscultate because of crying.
The child's blood volume is less than adult, but more on a ml/kg basis.
Hypotension is usually not present until the child has lost 20% to 25% of their blood volume
Low blood pressure is a LATE sign of hypovolemia in a child and is sign of imminent cardiac arrest.
Bradycardia is a LATE sign of cardiac decompensation.
The head is larger and heavier. The skull offers less protection for the brain as it yields readily to external pressure. The scalp is vascular and bleeds more readily.

Review of Cardinal Considerations for an Injured Child
Brain tissue is more easily damaged.
The child is more vulnerable to spinal injuries because of the heavy head and less developed bony structure.
The protuberant abdomen of the child makes it vulnerable to injury. The internal organs are close together and multiple injuries occur at once.
The pliable rib cage offers little protection for the lungs.
The liver is vulnerable to injury because of its large size.
The large kidneys are not protected well because of less perinephric fat.
Bones are stronger, thicker, and bend more easily. Even though bones are strong, fractures occur more frequently than sprains. A growth plate fracture can be present and not be seen on x-ray.
The child has a larger ratio of body surface area and less subcutaneous fat; therefore, is more prone to heat loss.

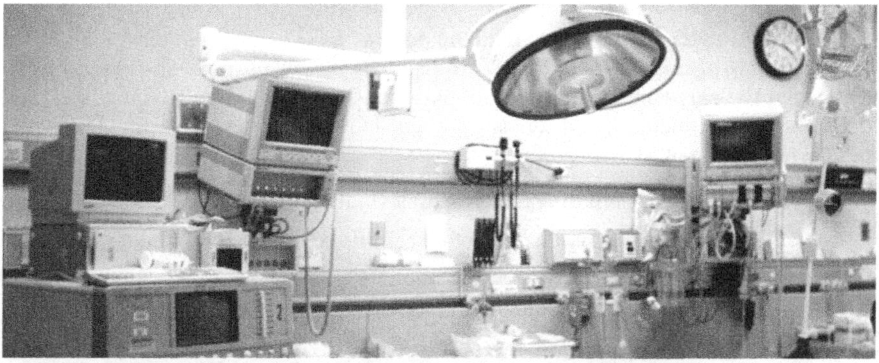

33 WEAKNESS, UNCONSCIOUS OR ALTERED CONSCIOUSNESS, SYNCOPE AND NEAR SYNCOPE

For details on triage see Chapter 34, Triage in a Nutshell.

PATIENT'S STORY – INTERVIEW QUESTIONS

1. Have you had a recent injury?
2. When did the symptoms begin?
    a. If the symptoms are no longer active, how long did they last?
    b. If the symptoms were intermittent, how long did each episode last and how frequent were the episodes?
3. Does the problem affect the whole body?
    a. Is the problem localized to a specific area of the body?
    b. Are other symptoms associated with the chief complaint; e.g., nausea, vomiting, headache, sweating, a slow heart rate or an irregular heartbeat?
4. Is the cause known?
5. How does the problem affect normal function?
    a. Is pain present?
        i. Where is the pain located and is radiation present?
        ii. What is the character of the pain; e.g., pressure, sharp, burning, shooting, dull, or cramping?
        iii. What is the severity of the pain?

> It is appropriate to use the terms mild, moderate, or severe and equally appropriate to use a scale of 0 to 10. Zero typically means no pain. The meaning of a 10 is not the same for all nurses or all patients. The definition of 10 must be determined, documented, and consistently used for that patient to be an effective pain evaluation tool.

   b. Is the patient able to perform normal daily activities?

6. Was any treatment started before coming to the hospital and if so, has it helped?
7. Has the patient had similar problems before?
   a. When was the problem?
   b. What was the diagnosis and treatment?
8. Is unlawful activity suspected?
   a. Was law enforcement at the scene?
   b. What agency?

> Medical personnel are obligated to notify law enforcement if unlawful activity is suspected.

9. Does the patient have any pertinent past history?
10. Does the patient take any routine medications?
    a. What is the name, dosage, route, and frequency of each medication?
    b. When was the last dose?
11. Does the patient take any complementary or alternative therapies, herbal products, over-the-counter medications or supplements, or natural therapies?
    a. What is the name, dosage, route and frequency of each therapy?
    b. When was the last dose or therapy?
12. Does the patient have allergies to drugs or foods?
    a. What is the name of the allergen?
    b. What was the reaction?
13. When was the patient's last tetanus immunization?
14. If the patient is female and between the ages of 10 to 50 years, when was the first day of her last menstrual period?

NURSING DOMAIN

The nursing domain, nursing diagnosis and plan of care can only be determined after an in-depth interview and consideration of the patient's story.

> Domain 12. Comfort.
> Class 1. Physical comfort.

Domain 5. Perception/Cognition Class 1. Attention. Class 2. Orientation, Class 3. Sensation/perception. Class 4. Cognition. Class 5. Communication.

ANTICIPATED MEDICAL CARE

Review of the Anticipated Medical Care of Weakness, Unconsciousness, Altered Consciousness, Syncope, and Near Syncope.	
Exam	Full body
Urine tests	Urine test for toxicology screening; pregnancy test for women of reproductive age unless they have had a hysterectomy
Blood tests	CBC with platelet count, electrolytes, glucose, BUN, creatinine, liver function studies, chemistries, magnesium, calcium, coagulation studies, drug serum levels of regular medications and known recreational drugs including alcohol, ammonia levels for patients with a history of cirrhosis, blood cultures if febrile
ECG	ECG for all ages
Radiographic studies	C-spine, chest x-ray, x-ray of suspected bony damage, CT of the brain without contrast
Other tests	Lumbar puncture (after CT) for cell count, glucose, gram stain, culture and sensitivity of spinal fluid
Diet	NPO
IV	Normal saline or Ringer's solution
Management	Protection of the airway including endotracheal intubation and mechanical ventilations, arterial blood gases, hyperventilation with 100% oxygen, a nasogastric tube to decompress stomach and reduce the risk of vomiting and aspiration, an indwelling urinary catheter for hourly urine output monitoring
Medications	Narcan for suspected narcotic overdose, Dextrose 50% 50 ml for hypoglycemia; thiamine 50 to 100 mg IV for alcohol abuse; flumazenil for suspected benzodiazepine abuse, antiemetics for nausea, antipyretics for fever
Disposition	Hospital admission may be required if the diagnosis is unknown or inpatient treatment is needed.

INITIAL CARE PLAN

> Alcohol-based hand sanitizers are the preferred method for cleaning your hands in most clinical situations. Wash your hands with soap and water whenever they are visibly dirty, before eating, and after using the restroom.

1. Ask the patient to undress, remove jewelry that might interfere with the exam and put on an exam gown. Assist as needed.
2. Obtain vital signs including pulse oximetry or test capillary refill.
3. Place on oxygen if saturation is < 94%. Severe COPD patients may be unable to maintain saturation >88% to 92%.
4. Consider performing orthostatic blood pressure and pulse.
5. Consider obtaining a rectal temperature if the patient is obtunded.
6. Establish intravenous access and draw laboratory blood specimens.
    a. Draw specimen tubes for a variety of tests to include hematology, chemistries, and coagulation studies. The tests commonly ordered include CBC, with platelet count, electrolytes, glucose, BUN, creatinine, liver function studies, calcium, and coagulation studies.
    b. Draw tubes for drug serum levels of regular medications and recreational drugs, including alcohol. Establish ammonia levels for patients with a history of cirrhosis and blood cultures if the patient is febrile.
7. Obtain arterial blood gas.
8. Assess for the following signs:
    a. Babinski's sign. Stimulation or stroking of the plantar surface of the foot causes extension of the great toe instead of the normal flexion. A sign of pyramidal tract disease. It may be elicited during unconsciousness after a drug overdose, alcohol intoxication, or seizure.
    b. Battle's sign. Bruising behind the ear. A sign of basilar skull fracture.
    c. Brudzinski. Flexion of the neck causes flexion of the legs in meningitis.
    d. Kernig's sign. The inability to extend a flexed leg, indicating meningeal irritation. A sign of meningitis.
9. Collect a urine specimen for possible toxicology screen.
10. Position the patient to protect the airway. Use the high Fowler's position if conscious; or if unresponsive, position in the recovery position on their right side with the head dependent and the left leg bent at the knee to stabilize them.
11. Keep the patient warm.
12. Consider administration of medications covered by hospital protocols.

a. Consider Narcan to rule out narcotic overdose
0.4 to 2 mg IV, every 2 to 3 min., give up to 10 mg over 30 min. A maximum dose has not been established. However, if the patient does not respond after 10 mg of Narcan, the diagnosis of an opioid overdose must be questioned.

b. Consider Romazicon for possible benzodiazepine overdose
1st dose 0.2 mg IV over 15 sec,
2nd dose 0.3 mg IV over 15 seconds,
3rd dose 0.5 mg IV over 30 seconds.
If no response, may repeat every minute until response is adequate or the maximum of 3 mg are given.

c. If hypoglycemia is determined by bedside testing, consider Dextrose 50% 50 ml IV to protect the brain from hypoglycemia.

d. Consider thiamine IV, if alcohol abuse is suspected.
100 mg IV over 5 min. to metabolize the alcohol.

13. Consider inserting drains.
    a. Indwelling urinary catheter to monitor output hourly.
    b. Nasogastric tube to decompress stomach and prevent vomiting and aspiration.
14. Order diagnostic tests covered by hospital protocol.
    a. X-ray of the chest
    b. CT scan of the brain without contrast
15. Instruct the patient not to eat or drink and teach the patient and family the rationale for the NPO status.
16. Elevate the siderails and place the stretcher in the lowest position.
17. Inform the patient, family, and caregivers of the usual plan of care and the expected overall time in the ER.
18. Provide the patient or family with a device to reach someone for assistance and explain how to use it. Ask the patient to call for help before getting off the stretcher.

ONGOING CARE PLAN

Inform the medical provider of adverse changes noted during ongoing evaluation. Document that the medical provider was notified of the adverse change. Document if orders were or were not received.

1. Evaluate the level of consciousness based on the mnemonic **AVPU** or **ACDU** level of consciousness score and compare to the baseline.
   AVPU: **A**lert, **V**erbal, **P**ain, **U**nresponsive.
   ACDU: **A**lert, **C**onfused, **D**rowsy, **U**nresponsive.
2. Monitor temperature, heart rate and rhythm, blood pressure, and effectiveness of breathing.

3. Monitor neurological status and document on a flow sheet if available.
4. Monitor therapy closely for the patient's therapeutic response.
   a. The usual time for a medication effectiveness check is 20 to 30 minutes after giving the drug.
   b. If therapy is not effective, ask the medical provider for a repeat dose or an alternative.
5. Monitor closely for the development of adverse reactions to therapy.
   a. Perform interventions to relieve the adverse reaction.
   b. Ask the medical provider for a remedy.
6. Keep the patient, family, and caregivers well informed of the plan of care and the remaining time anticipated before disposition.
7. Monitor the patient's laboratory and x-ray results and notify the medical provider of critical abnormalities. Remedy abnormalities as ordered.
8. Notify the medical provider when all diagnostic results are available for review. Ask for establishment of a diagnosis and disposition.

DISCHARGE INSTRUCTIONS

1. Provide the patient with the name of the nurse and doctor in the emergency room.
2. Inform the patient of their diagnosis or why a definitive diagnosis couldn't be made. Explain what caused the problem if known.
3. Teach the patient how to take the medication as prescribed and how to manage the common side effects. Instruct the patient not to drive or perform any dangerous tasks while taking narcotic pain medications.
4. Recommend a medical provider for follow-up care. Provide the name, address, and phone number with a recommendation of when to schedule the care.

COMMONLY ORDERED MEDICATIONS

DEXTROSE

Dextrose	
Indications	Hypoglycemia
Adult dose	50 ml of D50W
Pediatric dose	2 ml/kg of D25W IV or IO for children D12.5W for neonates
Onset	IV onset immediate, PO onset rapid
Compatibility	May be mixed with normal saline or Ringer's solution
Side effects	Hyperglycemia, peripheral vein irritation with high concentration solutions

Dextrose	
Note	The solution is hypertonic and may damage peripheral veins. A D50W filled syringe of 50 ml can be diluted with 50 ml NS to make D25W or with 150 ml to make D12.5W. A maximum concentration of 25% dextrose in water should be infused in a peripheral vein. The concentration for neonates is 12.5%.
Monitor	Blood sugar levels

NARCAN

Narcan (naloxone)	
Indications	Respiratory and neurological depression due to opioid overdose
Dose	0.4 to 2 mg IV every 2 to 3 min. A maximum dose has not been established. However, if the patient does not respond after 10 mg of Narcan, the diagnosis of an opioid overdose must be questioned.
Pediatric dose	< 5 years or < 20 kg 0.1 mg/kg > 5 years or > 20 kg 2.0 mg
Onset	IV onset 1 min., duration 45 min.
Side effects	Nervousness, ventricular tachycardia, increased systolic blood pressure in high doses
Monitor	Monitor for the return of pre-narcotic status

ROMAZICON

Romazicon (flumazenil)	
Indications	Valium, Versed, benzodiazepine overdose
Adult dose	First dose 0.2 mg IV over 15 sec, Second dose 0.3 mg IV over 15 seconds, Third dose 0.5 mg IV over 30 seconds. If no response, may repeat every minute until response is adequate or the maximum of 3 mg is given.
Onset	IV onset 1 minute, peak 10 min., duration unknown
Side effects	Nausea, vomiting, seizures, dizziness, agitation, pain at the injection site
Note	Effects of flumazenil may wear off before the benzodiazepine. Repeat dose to the maximum levels.
Monitor	Monitor respiratory effectiveness.

SODIUM BICARBONATE

Sodium Bicarbonate

Sodium Bicarbonate	
Indications	Metabolic acidosis
Adult	8.4% solution, 1 mEq/kg IV, then 0.5 mEq/kg IV every 10 min., then base dose on ABG analysis.
Pediatric dose	4.2% solution, 1 mEq/kg IV per dose or 0.3 x kg IV x base deficit
Onset	IV onset rapid, peak rapid
Side effects	Circulatory collapse
Note	A 50 ml syringe of 8.4% solution provides 50 mEq of sodium bicarbonate.

THIAMINE

Thiamine (vitamin B1)	
Indications	Chronic alcoholism, malnourished and cachectic patients
Adult dose	100 mg IV undiluted over 5 min. or diluted with IV solution and given at 100 mg or less over 5 min.
Onset	IV onset unknown
Compatibility	Compatible with alkaline solutions
Note	Give IV push early in the ER course to detoxify the patient. Hanging in a liter of fluid (banana bag) delays the therapeutic effect of the thiamine until late in the ER course.

RELATED INFORMATION

CAUSES FOR LOSS OF CONSCIOUSNESS MNEMONIC

Mnemonic AEIOU TIPS HAT for Causes of Loss of Consciousness	
A	<u>Alcohol</u> Suspected by history from friends, family members, and the alcoholic smell of the patient. Confirmed by blood alcohol level. Alcoholic cirrhosis can cause increased ammonia and urea toxins leading to an encephalopathy altering the level of consciousness. Supportive therapy, fluid resuscitation, thiamine, and the passage of time are the treatment.
E	<u>Epilepsy</u> Not all seizures are convulsive in nature and may appear as a cessation of activity. Postictal states include unresponsiveness. Confirmed by witnessed seizure activity, history, or decreased serum levels of anticonvulsant medication. Management includes medications to stop seizure activity, e.g., Valium or Ativan and intravenous anti-convulsant medications in loading doses.

Mnemonic AEIOU TIPS HAT for Causes of Loss of Consciousness	
I	Insulin (hypo or hyperglycemia) Blood glucose levels and metabolic acidosis on arterial blood gases confirm diabetic coma. Management may include reversal of elevated glucose levels with insulin, reversal of decreased glucose levels with glucose, and temporary near reversal of metabolic acidosis (increase of the pH > 7.25) with sodium bicarbonate (decrease of hyperglycemia also increases the pH over time to normal limits).
O	Overdose Confirmed by blood toxin levels. Management may include toxin removal by alkalinization, antidotes, decontamination, elimination, forced diuresis, or hemodialysis and supportive care.
U	Uremia (toxic condition associated with renal insufficiency) Confirmed by elevated BUN and creatinine, associated with hyperkalemia, metabolic acidosis, and anemia. Management may include fluid restriction, diuresis, and hemodialysis.
T	Trauma or Tumors Trauma is suspected from signs of cranial trauma. Confirmed by CT scan of the brain showing a space-occupying lesion. Management may include admission for surgical intervention or supportive care.
I	Infections or Ischemia Infection is confirmed by evidence of diagnostic findings of sepsis (elevated WBC, shock state). Ischemia to the brain can be caused by hypoxia, anemia, hypoventilation, hypoglycemia, and TIA or stroke. Management may include rapid administration of intravenous antibiotics for infections, corrective measures to reverse electrolyte disturbances, transfusion for anemia, and supportive measures for TIA or stroke. The goal in treating all forms of shock is restoration of oxygenation and tissue perfusion.
P	Psychiatric (less than 5% of cases) All psychiatric patients die from organic causes. The history of a mental health disorder is not an indicator of a psychiatric coma. True psychiatric coma is not commonly seen in the ER.

Mnemonic AEIOU TIPS HAT for Causes of Loss of Consciousness	
S	Stroke Stroke patients may have a decreased level of consciousness and be unable to clear their airway. Endotracheal intubation and mechanical ventilation are necessary to reduce the risk of respiratory compromise. Hypertension > 220 mm Hg systolic or > 120 mm Hg diastolic is treated with Nipride or other anti-hypertensive agent. CT scan of the brain is used to determine the type of stroke. Surgical intervention may be necessary for a hemorrhage stroke. Heparin therapy may be used for embolic strokes. Thrombolytic agents and neuroprotective agents are used in some centers.
H	Hypoxemia Insufficient oxygenation of the brain is usually caused by inadequate ventilation or inadequate gas exchange at the alveolar capillary membrane level. Hypoxia is confirmed by ABG analysis revealing a respiratory acidosis (a $PaCO_2 > 45$, an acidotic $pH < 7.35$), and a $PaO_2 <$ normal). Management may include maneuvers to ensure airway patency and adequate ventilation, correcting the acid-base imbalance with hyperventilation, finding the cause of the hypoxemia, and correction. Endotracheal intubations and mechanical ventilation may be necessary.
A	Acidosis Acid-base imbalance is either metabolic or respiratory and confirmed by ABG analysis. Management may include treatment of the cause and reversal of the acid-base imbalance with hyperventilation or buffering solutions.

Mnemonic AEIOU TIPS HAT for Causes of Loss of Consciousness	
T	Thermoregulation The core temperature confirms a thermoregulation problem. Management may include techniques to warm or cool the body to a normal temperature. Severe Hypothermia Less than 30° C (86° F) Death usually occurs below 25.6° C (78° F) Active internal rewarming may include warm intravenous fluids at 43° C (109.4° F), warm humid oxygen 42° to 46° (107.6° to 114.8° F), peritoneal lavage, extra corporeal rewarming, hemodialysis, and esophageal rewarming tubes. Discontinue when core temperate is > 35° C (95° F) to reduce the risk of hyperthermia. Severe Hyperthermia Cardinal signs and symptoms may include hot and dry skin with no sweating, a core temperature of > 40.6° C (> 105° F), prostration, rapid pulse, rapid respirations, and a low blood pressure. Diagnostic findings may include an elevated WBC and BUN, protein in the urine, respiratory alkalosis or metabolic acidosis, abnormal ECG, and abnormal clotting studies that may culminate to DIC. Treatment includes placing in a cool environment, removing all clothing, putting into a cool shower on a gurney, and directing fans on the patient. Chilled normal saline may be used for intravenous fluids; however, these patients are not volume depleted and 1 to 2 liters over the first 4 hours is usually adequate. Lactated Ringer's (Hartmann's solution) is not recommended because the liver may not be able to metabolize lactate. Chlorpromazine (Thorazine) is used to reduce shivering. Continue cooling until the core temperature reaches 39° C (102° F).

MENINGITIS

Review of Acute Bacterial Meningitis	
Definition	Acute bacterial meningitis is a bacterial infection of the cerebral spinal fluid.
Cause	The causes include acute otitis media, pneumonia, a head injury with a cerebral spinal fluid leak, sickle cell anemia, Hodgkin's disease, and alcoholism.

Review of Acute Bacterial Meningitis	
Symptoms	Classic symptoms are fever, headache, and neck stiffness. Other symptoms may include vomiting, altered consciousness, sleepiness, sensitivity to light, stiff neck and back, and seizures. 50% of the patients with meningitis have onset over 24 hours following respiratory symptoms and 50% over 1 to 2 days following respiratory symptoms. Infants have irritability, lethargy, and anorexia. Positive Kernig's sign and Brudzinski sign are a signs of meningitis but may be absent in the very young or the very old.
Laboratory findings	Laboratory findings may include an elevated WBC, cerebral spinal fluid with leukocytosis, and a positive gram stain.
Management	Management may include symptomatic treatment of fever, headache, vomiting, and fluid resuscitation. Diagnostic workup may include CBC, electrolyte and renal study function studies, chest x-ray, CT of the brain, and spinal tap post CT (CT first to rule out masses and situations where the LP would risk herniation of the brain), INTRAVENOUS ANTIBIOTICS STARTED IN THE ER, and hospital admission.
Mortality	THE RISK OF DYING FROM MENINGITIS CAN BE REDUCED TO 15% BY STARTING ANTIBIOTICS EARLY.
Contagion	Bacterial meningitis is spread from the exchange of respiratory and throat secretions. It is not spread by causal contact. People in the same household are considered to be at increased risk. Vaccines are available for some strains and Hib vaccine was added to the childhood immunization in the mid-nineties. The vaccine for meningitis is used to control outbreaks of some types of meningitis in the United States.

VIRAL MENINGITIS

Review of Viral Meningitis	
Definition	Viral meningitis is a viral infection of the cerebral spinal fluid.
Cause	One or more viruses cause viral meningitis.
Symptoms	Symptoms may include fever, headache, stiff neck, sensitivity to light, drowsiness, confusion, and altered consciousness. Fever, irritability, sleepiness, and anorexia may be seen in the infant. The symptoms last 7 to 10 days and the person usually recovers completely.
Tests	Diagnostic workup may include CBC, electrolyte and renal study function studies, chest x-ray, CT of the brain, and spinal tap post CT (CT first to rule out masses and situations where the LP would risk herniation of the brain).

Review of Viral Meningitis	
Management	Management may include supportive treatment for relief of symptoms, resting in bed, fluid resuscitation, antipyretics, and analgesics. No definitive treatment exists.
Contagion	The viruses are contagious. Entero viruses are common in the summer and fall. Many people are exposed to them. Less than 1 in every 1000 persons infected develop meningitis. The enterovirus is spread through direct contact with respiratory secretions; e.g., saliva, sputum, or nasal sections. Shaking hands with an infected person or touching something handled by an infected person and then touching your own nose, mouth, or eyes can introduce the virus. The virus is also present in the stool, and handling stool in diapers can lead to introduction of the virus. The incubation period is 3 to 7 days. The virus can be spread beginning about 3 days after infection until about 10 days after the symptoms develop. Hand washing and disinfection of objects and surfaces contaminated with the virus are effective ways to inactivate the virus.

RECURRENT DISTURBANCES IN CONSCIOUSNESS

Causes of Recurrent Weakness, Faintness, and Disturbances of Consciousness	
Arrhythmias	Bradyarrhythmias, e.g., 2nd and 3rd degree AV blocks, Stokes-Adams attacks; ventricular asystole, sinus bradycardia, carotid sinus syncope Tachyarrhythmias, e.g., ventricular tachycardia
Decreased blood to the brain	Hypoxia Anemia Hypoventilation Hypoglycemia TIA
Hypovolemia	Blood loss or fluid loss
Inadequate vasoconstrictors	Vasovagal Postural hypotension
Mechanical reduction of venous return	Valsalva (Expiratory effort against a closed glottis that increases pressure within the thoracic cavity and thereby impedes venous return of blood to the heart. Named after Antonio Maria Valsalva [1666-1723], an Italian anatomist.) Cough Micturition
Reduced cardiac output	Obstruction of left ventricular outflow or pulmonary flow, pump failure, cardiac tamponade

SEIZURES VERSUS SYNCOPE

Seizures	Syncope
Occurs day or night, regardless of the patient's posture.	Rarely occurs when recumbent.
Cyanosis or plethora may occur in seizure.	Pallor is invariable.
Often heralded by an aura of localizing significance.	No advance knowledge of impending attack.
Injury from falling is common.	Injury is rare.
Return to alertness is usually slow.	Return to alertness is prompt.
Urinary and bowel incontinence are common.	Urinary and bowel incontinence is rare.
Repeated spells of unconsciousness of several per day or per month are indicative of seizures. Not all seizures are convulsive with intense, paroxysmal, and involuntary muscular contraction.	

PEDIATRIC CONSIDERATIONS

SIGNS AND SYMPTOMS OF HYDROCEPHALUS

Review of Hydrocephalus Signs and Symptoms	
Infant	Child
Increased head circumference	Nausea
Setting sun eyes	Headache
Widening sutures	Altered LOC
Dilated scalp veins	Papilledema
Irritability	Diplopia
High pitched cry	Seizures
Seizures	

MENINGITIS SIGNS AND SYMPTOMS BY AGE

Review of Meningitis Signs and Symptoms by Age		
< 2 months old	3 months to 2 years old	> 2 years old

Review of Meningitis Signs and Symptoms by Age		
< 2 months old	3 months to 2 years old	> 2 years old
Altered LOC	Altered LOC	Altered LOC
Apnea	Ataxia	Fever
Bulging fontanel	Bulging fontanel	Headache
Cyanosis	Fever	Irritability
Fever	High-pitched cry	Petechiae/purpura
Irritability	Irritability	Positive Brudzinski sign
Petechiae/purpura	Petechiae/purpura	Positive Kernig's sign
Poor feeding	Seizures	Seizures
Seizures	Stiff neck	Stiff neck

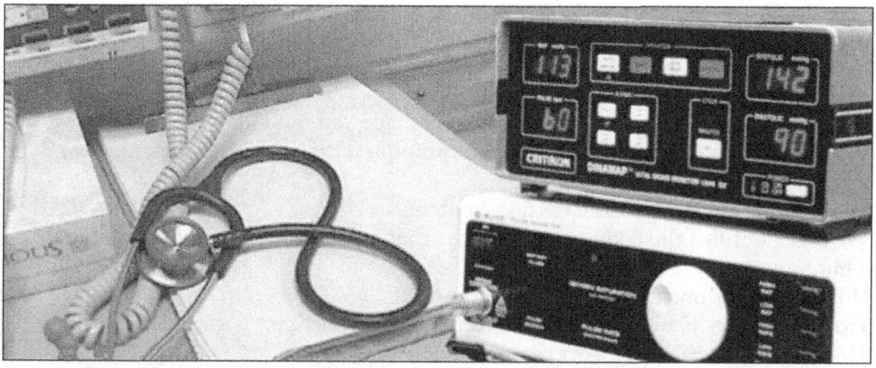

34 TRIAGE IN A NUTSHELL

RAPID ABC ASSESSMENT

1. Is the patient's airway patent?
    a. The airway is patent when speech is clear, and no noise is associated with breathing.
    b. If the airway is not patent, consider clearing the mouth and placing an adjunctive airway.
2. Is the patient's breathing effective?
    a. Breathing is effective when the skin color is within normal limits and the capillary refill is 2 to 3 seconds.
    b. If breathing is not effective, consider administering oxygen and placing an assistive device.
3. Is the patient's circulation effective?
    a. Circulation is effective when the radial pulse is present, and the skin is warm and dry.
    b. If circulation is not effective, consider placing the patient in the recumbent position, establishing intravenous access, and giving a 200 ml fluid bolus (medical provider order required).

Abdominal problems can be minor or life threatening. Triage plays an important role in management. Patients often feel it is necessary to exaggerate their pain because of the fear of not being treated promptly. Look for symptoms of tachycardia, sweating, pallor, toxic appearance, and guarding to accurately determine the urgency for treatment.

The patient's identity, chief complaint, and history of present illness are developed by interview. The standard questions are **who, what, when, where, why, how, and how much.**
Who identifies the patient by demographics, age, sex, and lifestyle.
What develops the chief complaint that prompted the patient to seek medical advice.
When determines the onset of the symptom.
Where identifies the body system or part that is involved and any associated symptoms.
Why identifies precipitating factors or events.
How describes how the symptom affects normal function.
How much describes the severity of the affect.

PATIENT IDENTIFICATION

1. What is the patient's name?
2. What is the patient's age and sex?
3. What is the name of the patient's current medical provider?
4. Does the patient live alone or with others?

CHIEF COMPLAINT

The chief complaint is a direct quote stating the main symptom that prompted the patient to seek medical attention. A symptom is a change from normal body function, sensation, or appearance. A chief complaint is usually three words or less and not necessarily the first words of the patient. Some investigation may be needed to determine the symptom that prompted the patient to come to the ER. When the patient, or other, gives a lengthy monologue, a part of the whole is quoted.

1. In one to three words, what is the main symptom that prompted the patient to seek medical attention?
   a. Use direct quotes to document the chief complaint. Acknowledge the source of the quote; e.g., the patient states, John Grimes the paramedic states, Mary Jones the granddaughter states.
   b. Always consider if the person speaking on behalf of the patient is interested in what is best for the patient.
   c. Never change the chief complaint stated by the patient even if the patient's perception of the problem is not valid, such as the patient states chest pain but the patient points to the umbilicus as the area of pain. Quote chest pain and document that the patient points to the umbilicus as the area for pain.
2. Patients with limited English proficiency must be offered an interpreter by federal law. When using an interpreter, always document the name of the person who is doing the interpreting and their relationship to the patient.

PATIENT'S STORY – INTERVIEW QUESTIONS

1. **When** was the onset of symptoms?
2. **Where** is the problem located and are any associated symptoms present?
3. **Why** are the symptoms present?
    a. Was an injury sustained?
    b. Did any event or circumstance bring on the symptoms?
4. **How** does the symptom affect normal function?
5. **How much** is normal function affected and when was normal function last present?
    a. What are the current vital signs?
    b. What objective symptoms are present?
6. **What** is the nature of the emergency?
7. Based on the nature of the emergency, determine if the patient's medical problem presents a threat to life, limb, or vision; project a timetable for the anticipated threat; and determine when care is needed. Many emergency rooms have used three level triage systems over the years. However, evidence shows that the five-level system provides for more accuracy in sorting patients. The system/process your facility implements, will determine the triage level the scenario falls into. Some systems are based on resources needed by the patient and others are time based. An example of presentations that fit into one type of five level system include;

- Level 1 Resuscitation: Medical care is required immediately. Condition is or may be a threat to life, limb, or vision if immediate care is not received. Reassess on an ongoing basis until conditions warrants otherwise.
- Level 2 Emergent: Care is required within 15 minutes. This is considered a high-risk patient requiring rapid interventions in less than 15 minutes.
- Level 3 Urgent: Conditions that could potentially progress to a serious problem requiring emergency intervention. May be associated with significant discomfort. Care is required within 30 minutes. Reassess in 30 minutes
-
- Level 4 Less Urgent: Conditions where the patient would benefit from being seen within 60 minutes. These may be age related or have a potential for complication. Reassess within 60 minutes.
- Level 5 Non-Urgent: Conditions that may be acute or part of a chronic problem with or without evidence of deterioration. The investigation or interventions for some of these illnesses or injuries could be delayed or even referred to other areas of health care delivery. Reassess every 2 hours.
- Airway, breathing, or circulation compromise are emergent.

- Chest pain and stroke are Level 2 patients in a 5-level system unless they present unconscious or with airway potential. Atypical chest pain scenarios are always considered and the evidence from the American Heart Association should be incorporated into chest pain and stroke triage guidelines.
- Dislocated elbows and knees with perfusion problems are emergent.
- Extremity injuries with neurovascular compromise are a level 2 triage until seen by a medical provider.
- Eye problems threaten vision and are second only to emergencies that threaten life, placing them as a Level 2 category. Among the true emergent problems are angle-closure glaucoma, retinal artery occlusion, ruptured globe, intraocular foreign bodies, and ocular chemical burns.
- Penetrating wounds of the trunk that are not obviously superficial are considered to enter the body cavity until proven otherwise. The patient is a Level 2 emergent until a medical provider determines the depth of the wound.
- Poisoning and overdoses are Level 2 emergent until proven otherwise by the medical provider, unless they are unconscious; they then become a Level 1.
- Postpartum DIC and hemorrhage are Level 2 emergent.
- Pregnancy and delivery problems such as abruptio placenta, amniotic fluid embolism, and breech and cord presentations are Level 2 emergent.
- Snakebite is Level 2 emergent until the snake is deemed nonpoisonous by the medical provider.
- Spinal tenderness associated with an injury are considered a potential spinal cord injury until proven otherwise
- Teeth that are avulsed are a dental emergency, however this does not necessarily make them a Level 1 patient. The time the tooth has been out of the socket plays a key role in whether or not the tooth has a chance to survive reimplantation. Determine the physical area of the emergency room that will best meet the needs of the patient. Primary (baby) teeth are seldom reimplanted.
- Develop a rapport with the patient and family.

TRIAGE SYSTEMS

STANDARDIZED ER TRIAGE SCALE AND ACUITY CATEGORIZATION: JOINT ENA/ACEP STATEMENT

The ENA Board of Directors approved the following statement from the Emergency Nurses Association (ENA) and American College of Emergency Medical providers (ACEP) Joint Five-Level Triage Task Force: ACEP and ENA believe that quality of patient care would benefit from implementing a standardized ER triage scale and acuity categorization process. Based on expert consensus of currently available evidence, ACEP and ENA support the adoption of a reliable, valid 5-level triage scale.

Electronic resource: Emergency Nursing Association. Retrieved August 29, 2010, from http://www.ena.org/about/position/jointstatements/Pages/Default.aspx .

EMERGENCY SEVERITY INDEX (ESI)

1. Immediate (airway obstruction, the patient is dying)
2. High risk scenarios (severe distress / pain)
3. Patient will need two or more resources
4. Patient will need only one resource
5. Patient will not require any resources

The Emergency Severity Index system is a simple five-level triage tool that categories emergency room patients by first determining the potential for a threat to life (Is the patient dying?), limb, or organ and then estimates the recourses needed based on previous experience with similar patients.

Examples of Resources for the ESI Triage System
Consultation from a specialty provider
Diagnostic laboratory tests, e.g. blood, urine, body fluids
Electrocardiography, e.g., ECG
Intravenous fluids
Medicine given by the intravenous, intramuscular, or nebulized route
Procedures, e.g., repair of a laceration, insertion of a catheter, or conscious sedation,
Radiographic studies, e.g., x-rays, CT, MRI, ultrasound, angiography

Examples of What are Not Resources for the ESI Triage System
Diagnostic point-of-care testing such as blood glucose
History, physical, pelvic exam not done by a specialty provider
Intravenous saline or heparin lock without intravenous fluid infusion
Medicines given by mouth, tetanus toxoid immunization, and prescription refills
Simple procedures such as wound check, dressings, crutches, splints, slings

FIVE LEVEL SYSTEMS

Each of the five level systems below has additional modifiers and details that help the triage nurse in selection of the appropriate level for each patient.

Australian Level	Time to Treatment
1 Immediately life threatening	Immediate
2. Imminently life threatening	10 minutes
3. Potentially life threatening	30 minutes
4. Potentially serious	60 minutes

Australian Level	Time to Treatment
5. Less Urgent	120 minutes

Canadian Level	Time to Treatment
1 Resuscitation	Immediate
2 Emergent	<15 minutes
3. Urgent	<30 minutes
4. Less urgent	<60 minutes
5 Non-urgent	<120 minutes

ONGOING EVALUATIONS AND INTERVENTIONS

Inform the medical provider of adverse changes noted during ongoing evaluation. Document that the medical provider was notified of the adverse change. Document if orders were or were not received.

1. Initiate any appropriate standing orders for patients.
2. Ongoing evaluations are required for waiting patients. The frequency and extent of evaluation are based on your protocols, which determine what is normal and customary for an emergency patient with similar problems in a hospital setting.

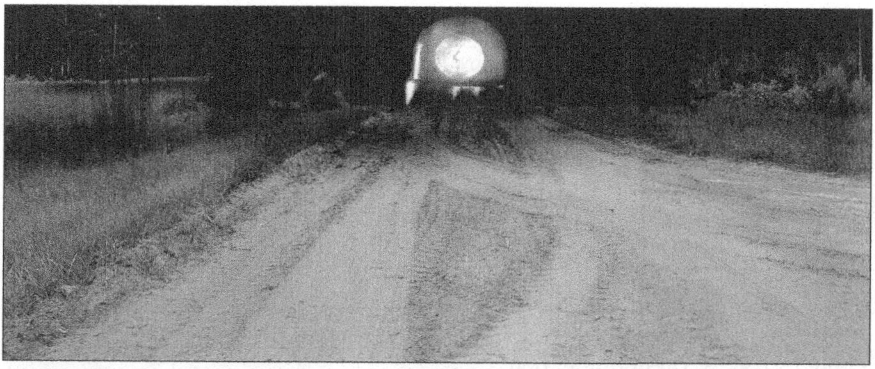

35 DISASTER EVENTS AND HOMELAND SECURITY ISSUES, NATURAL DISASTERS, BIOLOGICAL, NUCLEAR, INCENDIARY, CHEMICAL AND EXPLOSIVE (B-NICE) INCIDENTS

INTRODUCTION

This chapter provides basic information that should be familiar to all healthcare workers, such as the types of disasters, indications of an intentional release of a biological agent, the triage steps, protective equipment and when to use it, disaster zones, and decontamination principles and practices.

First, be sure to obtain as much information from first responders regarding the incident in an effort to utilize the correct hospital response.

If the incident is a suspected terrorist event, be aware, terrorists have been known to use secondary devices to injure, maim, or kill law enforcement and medical personnel. Also, an incident can involve more than one B-NICE component. Next, alert security and follow established hospital protocols to detect suspicious persons close to the decontamination area, treatment area, or entrances to the facility. Victims of the attack are sent to the decontamination area of the hospital, usually in the emergency room, through a separate decontamination area entrance, not the emergency triage and waiting areas. Find where the decontamination area is in your hospital and practice giving verbal directions to reach that area.

Be proactive, learn the basics of disaster management and be prepared for a disaster. This chapter is a beginning.

Useful websites for disaster situations are http://www.fema.gov/hazard/types.shtm and http://www.bt.cdc.gov/

DEFINITIONS OF ABBREVIATIONS:

- START: Simple Triage and Rapid Treatment
- MCI: Mass Casualty Incident
- CDC: Centers for Disease Control and Prevention
- B-NICE: Biological, Nuclear, Incendiary, Chemical, and Explosive
- PPE: Personal Protective Equipment

ANTICIPATED MEDICAL CARE

Review of the Anticipated Medical Care during a Mass Casualty Incident	
Exam	Full body exam is waived if decontamination is required.
Urine tests	If decontamination is necessary, waived until more appropriate time
Blood tests	If decontamination is necessary, waived until more appropriate time
ECG	As appropriate for complaints
X-rays	As appropriate for complaints
Other	Decontamination
Diet	NPO
IV	If necessary, normal saline or Ringer's solution
Disposition	If an urgent or emergent complaint, hospitalization may be required for observation and treatment.
Worst-case scenario	The worse-case scenario is when the emergency room is inadequately prepared and becomes overwhelmed, resulting in loss of life of patients and staff.

PATIENT'S STORY – INTERVIEW QUESTIONS

1. When was the onset of symptoms?
2. Where is the problem located and are any associated symptoms present?
3. Why are the symptoms present?
4. Was an injury sustained?
5. Did any event or circumstance bring on the symptoms?
6. How does the symptom affect normal function?
7. How much is normal function affected and when was normal function last present?
8. What are the current vital signs?
9. What objective symptoms are present?
10. What is the nature of the emergency?
11. Based on the nature of the emergency, determine if the patient's medical problem presents a threat to life, limb, or vision; project a timetable for the anticipated threat; and determine when care is needed.
    a. EMERGENT: Medical care is required immediately. Condition is or may be a threat to life, limb, or vision if immediate care is not received.
    b. URGENT: Care is required within 20 minutes to 2 hours. Condition does or could present a threat to life, limb, or vision if not treated. Reassess in 30 minutes.

c. NON-URGENT: Care can be delayed more than 2 hours. Condition does not present a threat to life, limb, or vision if delayed more than 2 hours. Reassess in 1 to 2 hours.

d. Develop a rapport with the patient and family.

STANDARD CLIENT'S INTERVIEW IN SUSPECTED TERRORISM SITUATIONS

The standard questions are who, what, when, where, why, how, and how much. In a terrorism incident, the identity and a complete history can be delayed if decontamination is required. Much of this information would be obtained after any necessary decontamination.

Who identifies the patient by demographics, age, sex, and lifestyle. This may also give vital information in the investigation following a terrorism event.

What determines the chief complaint that prompted the patient to seek medical advice or the incident or exposure that occurred resulting in their transportation for treatment. What are the symptoms exhibited? How are the patient's normal functions affected?

When determines the onset of symptoms or the time the incident or exposure occurred. When did the incident or exposure occur?

Where identifies the body system or part involved and any associated symptoms. Obtaining the location of the incident is also of importance since it may give vital information in an investigation process if several similar incidents have occurred.

Why identifies precipitating factors, events or information provided to the patient prior to the incident including notes, letters, phone calls, etc. What were the circumstances of the exposure? Has the patient traveled outside the country within the last 10 days?

How describes how the symptoms affect normal function and how an agent may have been disseminated (e.g., gas, dirty bomb, contaminated object, etc.). Was there an incendiary device used in the exposure?

How Much/How Long describes the severity of the affect, duration of the affect, and duration of the exposure.

NURSING DOMAIN

The nursing domain, nursing diagnosis and plan of care can only be determined after an in-depth interview and consideration of the patient's story.

Domain 12. Comfort. Class 1. Physical comfort.
Domain 11. Safety/Protection Class 1. Infection. Class 2. Physical Injury. Class 4. Environmental Hazards.

NATURAL DISASTERS

CYCLONES

A cyclone is a storm or system of winds that rotates about a center of low atmospheric pressure clockwise in the southern hemisphere and counterclockwise in the northern hemisphere. It advances at a speed of 20 to 30 miles an hour. It often brings abundant rain and usually has a diameter of 50 to 900 miles. It is usually violent in the tropics and moderate elsewhere.

EARTHQUAKES

Earthquake is a term used to describe both the incident and the resulting ground shaking and radiated seismic energy caused by the sudden slip on a fault, by volcanic or magmatic activity, or by other sudden stress changes in the earth.

In the United States, Alaska is the most earthquake prone state. After a significant earthquake, the policies for mass casualty incidents need to be initiated for patient care.

EXTREME HEAT

Temperatures that hover 10 degrees or more above the average high temperature and last several weeks are defined as extreme heat. Humid or muggy conditions add to the discomfort of high temperatures and occur when a dome of high atmospheric pressure traps hazy, damp air near the ground. Excessively dry and hot conditions can provoke dust storms and low visibility. Droughts occur when a long period passes without substantial rainfall. Heat combined with a drought is a dangerous condition.

Individuals at high risk from extreme heat
Adults 65 years old and older
Children under 4 years of age
Individuals who overexert themselves during work or exercise
Overweight individuals
Persons with physical conditions including heart disease, hypertension, and those taking medications for depression, insomnia, or poor circulation

FLOOD

A flood is dangerous due to the unpredictability of flood waters. The danger continues after the rain stops and the flood water recedes. Hazards that could be encountered include carbon monoxide, confined spaces, electrical hazards, falls, fire, hazardous materials, heat stress, motor vehicles, and musculoskeletal hazards.

FLOOD FACTS

- Many automobiles will float in 2 feet of water.
- 12 inches of moving water may sweep an automobile off the road.
- An average person may be swept off their feet in 6 inches of moving water.

HURRICANES

A hurricane is a severe tropical cyclone with wind speeds in excess of 74 mph. As a hurricane moves ashore, it brings high winds, tornadoes, torrential rains, storm surge, and subsequent flooding.

LANDSLIDES AND MUDSLIDES

Landslides occur when masses of rock, earth, or debris move down a slope. Debris flows, also known as mudslides, are a common type of fast-moving landslide that tends to flow in channels, such as valleys and roadways.

HAZARDS FROM LANDSLIDES AND MUDSLIDES:

- Rapidly moving water and debris that can lead to trauma
- Broken electrical, water, gas, and sewage lines that can result in injury or illness
- Disrupted roadways and railways that can endanger motorists and disrupt transport and access to health care

TORNADOES

A tornado is a rotating funnel of air that extends from a cloud to the ground. They can travel for many miles at speeds of 250 miles per hour or more. These storms change direction without warning, randomly destroying homes and utility lines, uprooting trees, and hurling large objects over long distances. Tornadoes usually accompany severe thunderstorms.

TSUNAMIS

Tsunamis are a series of enormous waves created by an underwater disturbance such as an earthquake, landslide, meteorite, or volcanic eruption.

VOLCANIC ERUPTIONS

Volcanoes spew hot, dangerous gases, ash, lava, and rock that are powerfully destructive. The most common cause of death from a volcano is suffocation. Volcanic eruptions can result in additional threats to health, such as floods, mudslides, power outages, drinking water contamination, and wildfires. Health concerns after a volcanic eruption include infectious disease, respiratory illness, burns, injuries from falls, and vehicle accidents related to the slippery, hazy conditions caused by ash. Electronic resource: CDC. Retrieved March 7, 2007, from http://www.bt.cdc.gov/disasters/volcanoes/facts.asp.

WILDFIRES

A wildfire is a fire that is out of control and generally viewed as undesirable by land managers. It needs to be put out or suppressed. Wildfires can result in electrical hazards, carbon monoxide poisoning, musculoskeletal injuries, heat exposure, structural instability, confined spaces, fire injuries, respiratory hazards, fatigue.

WINTER WEATHER

Winter storms can result in downed utility lines, flooding, highways closures, hypothermia, roads closures, and storm surges.

DISASTER TRIAGE

Disaster triage involves prioritizing patients using the **START** (**S**imple **T**riage **A**nd **R**apid **T**reatment) system. A 30 to 60 second period is allowed for the initial triage.

TRIAGE TAG COLOR CODES

Black: Unlikely to survive. No spontaneous effective respiration present after repositioning to open the airway.
Red: Cannot wait for treatment. Are unlikely to survive with immediate treatment.
Yellow: Need monitoring by trained professionals and frequent evaluation. Will need hospital care.
Green: Can wait a number of hours or until the next day. Displaying injuries that can be controlled or treated for a limited time in the field.
White: Ambulatory with or without minor injuries. No medical or significant treatment needed.

1. Respiratory
   a. Every patient will be assessed for respiratory rate and adequacy.
   b. If a patient is not breathing, check for foreign objects causing obstruction in the mouth. Remove loose dentures.
   c. Reposition the head, using cervical spine precautions if this does not delay assessment.
   d. If the above procedures do not initiate respiratory efforts, TAG THE PATIENT BLACK.
   e. If the victim's respiratory rate is >30 per minute, TAG THE PATIENT RED.
   f. Victims who have respirations <30 per minute are NOT TO BE TAGGED AT THIS TIME. ASSESS THESE PATIENTS FOR PERFUSION.
2. Perfusion
   a. The best method to assess perfusion is capillary nail bed refill.
   b. Press nail beds or lips and release. Color should return to these areas within two seconds.
   c. If it takes more than two seconds, the patient is showing signs of inadequate perfusion AND MUST BE TAGGED RED.
   d. If the color returns within two seconds, the patient is NOT TAGGED UNTIL THE MENTAL STATUS IS ASSESSED.
   e. If capillary refill cannot be assessed, palpate the radial pulse. In most cases, if the radial pulse cannot be felt, the systolic blood pressure will be below 80 mmHg.
   f. Hemorrhage control techniques are part of the perfusion section. Control significant bleeding by direct pressure and elevate the lower extremities.
   g. Utilize the walking wounded to assist with hemorrhage control on themselves or another patient.
3. Mental Status

a. The mental status evaluation is used for patients whose respirations and perfusion are adequate. To test mental status, the rescuer should ask the victim to follow a simple command, e.g., open and close your eyes or squeeze my hands. Make sure you are speaking his language.

b. If the patient cannot follow these commands, then TAG RED.

c. If the patient can follow these commands, then TAG YELLOW.

d. Only after all patients have been triaged can patients be treated.

DECONTAMINATION PRINCIPLES

Decontamination is of first priority for any contaminated patient. The patient and all staff are in danger when contamination is present. Initial decontamination is usually performed at the scene by emergency crews, but in an emergency situation it CANNOT be assumed all patients have been decontaminated. Some persons may have exited the scene prior to the arrival of first responders. Since the events on September 11, 2001, most facilities have developed plans for the decontamination of persons involved in B-NICE events. Most decontamination involves at least triage and three-stage decontamination for patients to remove clothing, wash themselves, and be prioritized. Articles removed, including jewelry and accessories, must be bagged and tagged for proper disposal.

UP, UP, AND AWAY

All areas of decontamination, triage, and treatment must be established:

- Uphill
- Upwind
- Upstream from the incident area

ZONES IN DISASTER AREAS

The disaster area is divided into three zones: hot (red), warm (yellow), and cold (green).

- **Hot zones** are also known as red zones or exclusion and restricted zones. They are the areas where the actual incident occurred, or contaminated persons arrive from for treatment. This area must be isolated and only persons with appropriate personal protective equipment (PPE) should be allowed in the area to extract contaminated individuals.
- **Warm zones** are also known as yellow zones and decontamination or contamination reduction zones. They are the area where decontamination is performed. Only staff with the appropriate PPE should enter this area and perform decontamination of affected persons. This area must have a water supply and the ability to contain contaminated water. The hospital will have a specific written disaster plan for this type of situation and has specific training for personnel involved in the decontamination procedures.
- **Cold zones** are also known as the green zone and the support zone. They are the area where patients are directed after complete decontamination and for continued treatment.

HOT (RED) ZONE DECONTAMINATION

- Immediate area surrounding the incident.

- Only personnel in appropriate PPE should enter this area.
- Contaminated supplies and equipment should be left in this area until the immediate need is over, and it can be decontaminated properly.
- Decontamination procedures should not normally be performed in this area.

WARM (YELLOW) ZONE DECONTAMINATION

- The area in which decontamination should be performed.
- At a minimum, three-stage decontamination should be performed.
- All clothing and jewelry on contaminated persons should be removed and packaged for later disposal.
- In general, soap and copious amounts of water are the best and safest products to use during skin decontamination.
- When performing skin decontamination, be sure to wash all areas including wounds and all orifices. Pay special attention to skin folds, the nares, the ears, and the genitalia. Wash these areas carefully but totally. Rinse the eyes with copious amounts of water or saline solution.

COLD (GREEN) ZONE DECONTAMINATION

- The area where extended care can be provided.
- Staging and the command post are in this area or located outside the zoned areas and uphill, upwind, and upstream of the hot zone.
- This staging area is where individuals don their PPE and await entry into the warm and/or hot zones.
- The rehabilitation area is also located in the cold zone.

PERSONAL PROTECTIVE EQUIPMENT (PPE)

Donning is dressing out in the personal protective equipment. Doffing is the removal of the personal protective equipment. The equipment is designed to protect the respiratory tract, and the skin including hands and feet.

RESPIRATORY PPE

- Level A: Supplied air and self-contained breathing apparatus (SCBA) protects against gases, vapors, aerosols, and oxygen-deficient environments.
- Level B: SCBC or positive pressure air respiratory (SAR) with SCBA protects against gases, vapors, aerosols but not necessarily oxygen-deficient environments with the use of a positive pressure air respirator. There must also be an air monitoring meter in use.
- Level C: Air purification respiratory (APR) protects against some vapors and aerosols.
- Level D: No breathing apparatus. No protection

SKIN PROTECTIVE CLOTHING PPE

- Level A: Vapor protection. A fully encapsulated, chemical resistant suit protects against gases, vapors, liquids, and solids.
- Level B: Splash protection. A chemical resistant suit protects against liquids and solids.

- Level C: Hooded. A splash protection, chemical resistant suit protects against liquids and solids.
- Level D: No protective clothing. No protection.

GLOVES AND BOOTS PPE

- Level A: Chemical resistant
- Level B: Chemical resistant
- Level C: Chemical resistant
- Level D: No boots or gloves. No protection

DONNING (DRESSING IN) PPE (LEVEL A, B, OR C)

1. Identify the type of exposure and if the PPE provided is appropriate protection.
2. Undergo brief medical evaluation by assigned medical officer. The items identified by the evaluation are blood pressure, hydration status, and adequate rest.
3. Examine PPE, including the respirator and mask for tears, holes, cracks, or rips.
4. An assistant should help with dressing in PPE.
5. Change into minimal clothing, shoe covers, and gloves. This will be the last layer removed.
6. Don the second layer of PPE, e.g., splash protective suit or a pair of scrubs, with shoe covers and gloves. Tape these to the second layer of PPE with duct tape. Fold and leave tab on the duct tape for easy removal.
7. Don the outer protective cover, which will also include shoe covers.
8. Don chemical resistant boots. Tape these to the outer protective suit with duct tape. Fold and leave tab on the duct tape for easy removal.
9. Zip the suit and tape closed with duct tape. Fold and leave tab on the duct tape for easy removal.
10. Don chemical resistant gloves and tape to the outer suit with duct tape. Fold and leave tab on the duct tape for easy removal.
11. Have the assistant write your name in large, easy to read letters on the back of the outer suit.
12. Prior to entering the decontamination area, don your mask and respiratory equipment. The hood should be pulled over the mask and then taped to the mask with duct tape. Fold and leave tab on the duct tape for easy removal.
13. Turn on respiratory device.

DOFFING (REMOVING) PERSONAL PROTECTIVE EQUIPMENT (PEELING AN ONION)

1. If you've been in the hot zone leave contaminated equipment in the hot zone before entering the warm zone for decontamination.

2. Step into the first pool closest to the hot zone. The decontamination personnel will wash and rinse the outer suit and provide assistance with removal of the suit, gloves, and boots. LEAVE THE RESPIRATOR MASK IN PLACE.
3. Step into the second pool. The decontamination personnel will wash and rinse the minimal layer of clothing and provide assistance with the removal of the clothing, gloves, and shoe covers. REMOVE THE RESPIRATOR AT THIS TIME.
4. A final shower may be provided prior to you dressing in clean dry clothing and entering the rehabilitation area for a medical evaluation, rehabilitation, and debriefing.

CATEGORIES OF BIOLOGICAL DISEASES AND AGENTS

The Centers for Disease Control and Prevention defines three categories of biologic agents with potential to be used as weapons, based on ease of dissemination or transmission, potential for major public health impact, e.g., high mortality, potential for public panic and social disruption, and requirements for public health preparedness. Chemical agents are categorized differently and are listed after the following biological diseases and agents.

ANTHRAX INFECTIONS

Cutaneous: 95% of the infections occur when the bacterium enters the body through a disruption in the integrity of the skin. Symptoms started as a raised lesion on the skin and progress to an ulcer with a characteristic black center. Deaths are rare with the appropriate antimicrobial therapy.

Inhalation: Respiratory symptoms progressing to severe and death over several days. Case fatality rates are upwards of 90% to 100%

Gastrointestinal: Initial symptoms of intestinal tract inflammation progress to severe. Case fatality rates are in the range of 25% to 75%.

Treatment includes ciprofloxacin or doxycycline for adults and children, or levofloxacin for adults.

CATEGORY A

Category A diseases and agents are high priority. U.S. public health system and primary healthcare providers must be prepared to address various biological agents, including pathogens that are rarely seen in the United States. High-priority agents include organisms that pose a risk to national security because they can be easily disseminated or transmitted from person to person, result in high mortality rates and have the potential for major public health impact, might cause public panic and social disruption, and require special action for public health preparedness. The following tables are examples of category diseases and agents.

EXAMPLES OF CATEGORY A DISEASES AND AGENTS

Anthrax Inhalation	
Category	A
Quarantine	No quarantine
Decontamination	Decontamination is necessary

Anthrax Inhalation	
Incubation	1 to 43 days
Signs and Symptoms	Initial: 2 to 4 days of fever, cough, malaise, myalgia Terminal: 1 to 2 days of high fever, dyspnea, cyanosis, hemorrhagic mediastinitis and pleural effusion, rapid progress to shock and death
Vaccine	Yes
Treatment	Ciprofloxacin or doxycycline is recommended for adults and children, or levofloxacin for adults
Post Exposure Treatment	Ciprofloxacin: Adults 500 mg PO BID for 8 weeks or doxycycline 100 mg PO BID for 8 weeks
Differential Diagnosis	Tularemia, plague, and community acquired pneumonia if infiltrate is present Hantavirus pulmonary syndrome Bacterial, fungal, or tubercular mediastinitis Fulminate mediastinal tumor Dissecting aortic aneurysm if the mediastinum is widened without fever

Smallpox	
Category	A
Quarantine	Yes. Strict respiratory and contact isolation
Incubation	7 to 17 days
Signs and Symptoms	Sudden onset of fever, malaise, headache, backache, vomiting, transient erythematous rash, exanthema. Lesions begin on the face, hands, forearms and spread to the lower extremities and trunk. Lesions are on the palms and soles of the feet. Synchronous progress with maculas, vesicles, pustules, and scabs
Vaccine	Yes
Treatment	Supportive care
Post Exposure Treatment	Vaccination within 2 to 4 days of exposure

Smallpox	
Differential Diagnosis	**Smallpox** Incubation: 7 to 17 days Prodrome: 2 to 4 days Distribution: centrifugal (proceeding in a direction away from a center or axis) Progression: synchronous Scab formation: 10 to 14 days Scab separation: 14 to 28 days after the rash **Chickenpox** Incubation: 14 to 21 days Prodrome: minimal to none Distribution: centripetal (proceeding in a direction towards a center or axis) Progression: asynchronous Scab formation: 4 to 7 days Scab separation: <14 days after the rash

Pneumonic Plague	
Category	A
Quarantine	Strict respiratory droplet isolation
Incubation	1 to 3 days
Signs and Symptoms	Fever, cough, chest pain, weakness, hemoptysis, rapidly developing pneumonia with shortness of breath, respiratory failure, and shock
Vaccine	Not protective against pneumonic plague. No longer made in the United States of America
Treatment	Streptomycin, gentamicin, tetracyclines, and chloramphenicol are effective against pneumonic plague.
Post Exposure Treatment	Doxycycline 100 mg PO BID for 7 days after exposure

Pneumonic Plague	
Differential Diagnosis	Other bioterrorism threats, e.g., inhalation anthrax, tularemia, melioidosis Other pneumonias, e.g., community acquired pneumonias, influenza, hantavirus pulmonary syndrome Hemorrhagic leptospirosis
Note	Other forms of plague including bubonic and septicemia can be transmitted through bites from vector (rodent fleas) or exposure to infected body substances. Bubonic plague is the most common form of plague and presents with a painful swollen lymph gland called a bubo.

Pneumonic Tularemia	
Category	A
Quarantine	No person to person transmission
Decontamination	Decontamination is necessary if aerosol exposure is suspected
Incubation	Typically, 3 to 5 days. Range 1 to 21 days
Signs and Symptoms	Sudden onset of fever, chills, myalgia, headache, nonproductive cough, segmental lobar infiltrates, hilar adenopathy, and effusions
Vaccine	Currently under review by the FDA
Treatment	Ciprofloxacin, doxycycline, streptomycin, or gentamicin and supportive care
Post Exposure Treatment	Ciprofloxacin 500 mg PO BID for 14 days or doxycycline 100 mg PO BID for 14 days
Differential Diagnosis	Community acquired pneumonia Atypical: Legionella, mycoplasma, streptococcal pneumonia, influenza Brucellosis Q fever Pneumonic plague Inhalation anthrax Hantavirus pulmonary syndrome Histoplasmosis

Viral Hemorrhagic Fevers (VHF)	
Viral hemorrhagic fevers	Filoviridae family (Ebola, Marburg) Arenaviruses (Junin, Lassa, Guanarito, Sabia, Machupo)
Category	A
Quarantine	Strict respiratory and contact isolation
Incubation	Typically, 5 to 10 days with a range of 2 to 16 days
Signs and Symptoms	Fever, headache, malaise, dizziness, myalgia, nausea, vomiting, flushing, periorbital edema, positive tourniquet test hypotension, mucous membrane bleeding, ecchymosis, and shock. Description of tourniquet test: Operator applies a blood-pressure cuff to the upper arm and inflates it to a point midway between diastolic and systolic pressure. For example, if your blood pressure is 120/80, the cuff is inflated to 100 mmHg. The cuff pressure is maintained for 5 minutes then released. The test is positive if 10 or more petechiae per square inch.
Vaccine	Investigational only
Treatment	Supportive care, no anti-platelet drugs or intramuscular injections are to be given. Use caution with sedation and analgesia. Correct coagulopathy, ribavirin may be effective
Post Exposure Treatment	The use of ribavirin may be considered for a significant exposure
Differential Diagnosis	Bacterial: typhoid fever, rickettsioses, leptospirosis, meningococcemia Falciparum malaria Vasculitis Thrombotic uremic syndrome Heat stroke Hemolytic uremic syndrome.
Note	When a viral hemorrhagic fever is suspected, obtain recent travel information

CATEGORY B

Category B diseases and agents are the second highest priority. These agents include those that are moderately easy to disseminate, result in moderate morbidity rates and low mortality rates, and require specific enhancements of the Centers for Disease Control and Prevention's diagnostic capacity and enhanced disease surveillance. The following tables are examples of category B diseases and agents.

EXAMPLES OF CATEGORY B DISEASES AND AGENTS

Ricin	
A stable toxin easily made from the mash that remains after processing castor beans	
Category	B
Quarantine	No quarantine
Decontamination	Required
Incubation	Onset of symptoms can be within hours of exposure. Death can occur within 36 to 48 hours.
Signs and Symptoms	Inhalation: cough, chest tightness, difficulty breathing, nausea, muscle aches, airway inflammation, pulmonary edema, cyanosis Ingestion: internal bleeding, vomiting blood, bloody diarrhea, renal and hepatic and splenic system collapse Injection: renal, hepatic, and splenic system collapse; gastrointestinal hemorrhage and multi-organ failure
Vaccine	No
Treatment	Supportive care, no antidote available
Post Exposure Treatment	No antidote available
Differential Diagnosis	Diagnosis of ricin exposure is difficult and may not be determined until after postmortem examination

Botulism Inhalation	
Category	B
Quarantine	No quarantine
Incubation	24 to 72 hours
Signs and Symptoms	Early nausea, vomiting, diarrhea, cranial neuropathy, ptosis, blurred or double vision, difficulty swallowing or talking, decreased salivation, progressive bilateral descending flaccid paralysis leading to respiratory paralysis and death
Vaccine	No
Treatment	Ventilatory assistance, supportive care, botulinum antitoxin
Post Exposure Treatment	Monitor for symptoms

Botulism Inhalation	
Differential Diagnosis	Cerebral vascular accident Myasthenia gravis Guillain-Barré Syndrome Tick paralysis Atropine poisoning Paralytic shellfish or puffer fish poisoning
Note	Botulism is the most lethal substance known to man

CATEGORY C

Category C diseases and agents are the third highest priority agents. These agents include emerging pathogens that could be engineered for mass dissemination in the future because of availability, ease of production and dissemination, potential for high morbidity and mortality rates, and major health impact. Examples are emerging infectious diseases, such as Nipah virus and hantavirus.

INDICATIONS OF AN INTENTIONAL RELEASE OF A BIOLOGICAL AGENT

Indications of an intentional release of a biological agent include an unusual temporal or geographic clustering of illness (e.g., persons who attended the same public event or gathering) or patients presenting with clinical signs and symptoms that suggest an infectious disease outbreak, especially if occurring in otherwise healthy persons; an unusual age distribution for common diseases, e.g., an increase in what appears to be a chickenpox-like illness among adult patients, but which might be smallpox; and a large number of cases of acute flaccid paralysis with prominent bulbar palsies, suggestive of a release of botulinum toxin. Resource: CDC MMWR Weekly October 19, 2001

Biological agent characteristics presenting the greatest concern for intentional release are those that:

- can cause disease by an aerosol route;
- are relatively stable in an aerosol form;
- have access to a large civilian population which is easily accessible and susceptible;
- are recognized for their individual high morbidity and mortality rate;
- are identified for the high probability of person-to-person transmission;
- are difficult to diagnose, making it difficult to provide adequate treatment or post-exposure prevention;
- have been developed previously for use as a biological agent.

In a mass casualty incident (MCI) in which resources are scarce or very limited, it may become necessary to perform a negative triage which would allow for the care and treatment of those with the greatest likelihood of survival and would result in withholding treatment from those with severe exposure and symptoms or prognosis of imminent death.

Patients contaminated in B-NICE events should only have airway and C-spine precautions addressed prior to decontamination to avoid unnecessary contamination and allow for rapid decontamination.

CHEMICAL AGENTS

Chemical agents are categorized as biotoxins, blister agents/vesicants, blood agents, caustics (acids), choking/lung/pulmonary agents, incapacitating agents, long-acting anticoagulants, metals, nerve agents, organic solvents, riot control agents/tear gas, toxic alcohols, and vomiting agents. Examples are listed in the table below.

Chemical Agents	
Biotoxins	Abrin, ricin, and strychnine
Blister agents/vesicants	Mustards, lewisite chlor arsine agents, phosgene oxime
Blood agents	Arsine and cyanide
Caustics (acids)	Hydrofluoric acid, hydrogen fluoride acid
Choking/lung/pulmonary agents	Ammonia, bromine, chlorine, hydrogen chloride, osmium tetroxide, phosgene, phosphine, phosphorus (elemental, white or yellow)
Incapacitating agents	BX, fentanyl and other opioids
Long-acting anticoagulants	Super warfarin
Metals	Arsenics, mercury, thallium
Nerve Agents	G Agents (sarin, soman, tabun) V agents (VX)
Organic solvents	Benzene
Riot control agents/tear gas	Various agents and combinations of agents (bromobenzyl cyanide, chloroacetophenone, chloropicrin, dibenzoxazepine)
Toxic alcohols	Ethylene glycol
Vomiting agents	Adamsite

The following tables present more detailed information regarding quarantine, decontamination, onset of symptoms, the signs and symptoms, and treatment of nerve agents.

Chemical Nerve Gas	
Types	Sarin (also known as GB) is a clear liquid. Tabun (also known as GA) is a clear liquid. Soman (also known as GD) is a clear liquid. VX is an amber liquid.

Chemical Nerve Gas	
Quarantine	No
Decontamination	Yes
Onset	Can occur within seconds of exposure
Signs and Symptoms	Chemically similar to organophosphate poisoning. Regardless of the exposure route, the signs and symptoms are the same: rhinorrhea, chest tightness, pinpoint pupils, shortness of breath, excessive salivation, sweating, nausea, vomiting, abdominal cramps, involuntary defecation and urination, muscle twitching, seizures, confusion, flaccid paralysis, respiratory failure, and death
Treatment	Mark 1 kit or 600 mg 2-PAM and 2 mg atropine and rapid decontamination. Keep adequate doses for all staff in the area readily available

Nerve Agent Effects and Disposition	
Immediate	Effects: unconscious, talking but not walking, or moderate to severe effects to two or more body systems (gastrointestinal, central nervous system, respiratory failure, death) Clinical signs: seizing, postictal, cardiac arrest, respiratory distress and failure, apnea
Delayed	Effects: recovering from exposure or antidote Clinical signs: diminished secretions, improving respirations
Minimal	Effect: walking and talking Clinical signs: constricted pupils, rhinorrhea, mild to moderate dyspnea
Expectant	Effect: unconscious Clinical signs: cardiac respiratory arrest
Disposition	Monitor patients exposed to nerve agents for at least 16 to 18 hours post exposure to evaluate for delayed symptoms.

Blister Agents/ Vesicants: Mustard Gas, Sulfur Mustard	
Type	Blister Agent
Quarantine	No
Decontamination	Yes

Blister Agents/ Vesicants: Mustard Gas, Sulfur Mustard	
Onset	On contact
Signs and Symptoms	Hyper excitability seizures, erythema, insomnia, nausea, vomiting pruritic rash, blistering, photophobia, lacrimation, conjunctival and scleral edema, nasal burning pain, epistaxis, cough, wheezing, dyspnea, and airway obstruction
Treatment	Sodium thiosulfate IV and rapid decontamination
Eyes	Mild: tearing, itching, burning, gritty feeling. Onset 4 to 12 hours Moderate: all of the above with reddening, lid edema and pain. Onset 3 to 6 hours Severe: all of the above with severe swelling and pain, corneal damage. Onset 1 to 2 hours
Airway	Mild: rhinorrhea, sneezing, epistaxis, hoarseness, hacking cough. Onset 2 to 24 hours Severe: all of the above, productive cough, dyspnea. Onset 2 to 6 hours
Skin	Mild: erythema. Onset 2 to 24 hours Severe: erythema, vesication. Onset 2 to 24 hours

Blister Agent and Vesicant Triage and Disposition	
Immediate	Less than 4 hours up to 12 hours after exposure Clinical signs of dyspnea
Delayed	More than 4 hours for eyes and skin or 12 hours for respiratory after exposure Clinical Signs include eye lesions, impaired vision, skin lesions over 2 to 50% of the body surface area, cough, sputum production, dyspnea
Minimal	More than 4 hours after exposure Clinical signs include minor eye lesions with no vision impairment, skin lesions <2% of the body surface area in non-critical areas, cough, sore throat
Expectant	Less than 4 hours after exposure Clinical signs include dyspnea and skin lesions covering 50% or more body surface area

Blister Agent and Vesicant Triage and Disposition	
Disposition	Monitor patients for 6 hours who have a minor exposure and 48 hours for those with significant exposure for delayed reaction. Those that survive significant exposure for 24 to 48 hours have a higher likelihood of survival.

In a terrorist attack, many of the explosive devises combine conventional explosives and radioactive materials. The table below defines a dirty bomb and outlines decontamination, priorities, and treatment.

Dirty Bomb Radiological Agent	
Definition	A dirty bomb, or radiological dispersion device, is a bomb that combines conventional explosives, such as dynamite, with radioactive materials in the form of powder or pellets. The idea behind a dirty bomb is to blast radioactive material into the area around the explosion. This could possibly cause buildings and people to be exposed to radioactive material. The main purpose of a dirty bomb is to frighten people and make buildings or land unusable for a long period of time.
Decontamination	Victims will have radioactive dust on their clothing. If many people are covered with dust, it will not be feasible to conduct a careful survey of each person. Assume all of the dust is radioactive. Set up a facility where each person can remove and discard their outer clothing, wash as thoroughly as possible, and don coveralls or wrap in blankets. This facility should be upwind and far enough from ground zero to prevent radiation levels from interfering with monitoring of patients.
Priorities	Physical injuries are more serious than radioactive contamination. Deal with life-threatening conventional injuries first. When the patients are stable, turn your attention to the radioactive contamination. Patients who were treated and are now stable should be evacuated from radiation areas.

Dirty Bomb Radiological Agent	
Treatment	Follow the established hospital policy for handling radiation incidents. Personnel should not eat, drink, smoke, etc., at the accident site, in the ambulance, or at the hospital until they have been released by the radiation safety officer. Continue the decontamination process until the dosimetry readings come within normal limits. All vomit, feces, urine and metal should be saved to be preserved for possible assessment of dose received.
Note	In any suspicious event which involves incendiary or explosive devices, evaluate and monitor for possible use of a biological, chemical or radiological agent as well.

Planning, education, drills, and evaluation make up the emergency operations preparation cycle. The Centers for Disease Control and Prevention (CDC) has preparedness and bioterrorism readiness plans and templates for healthcare facilities. Tabletop, functional and full-scale drills meet regulatory agency requirements. The website for the CDC is http://www.cdc.gov.

All nurses need a basic understanding of disaster terms, decontamination, zones, and general procedure. The information is available. Are you ready?

REFERENCES

Ackley, Betty; Ladwig, Gail; Makic, Mary Beth; Melody Zanotti. Nursing Diagnosis Handbook: An Evidence-based Guide to Planning Care. 12th Ed. Elsevier. 2017.

American Academy of Pediatrics and American Heart Association. Pediatric Advanced Life Support. American Heart Association, 2015.

American College of Surgeons, Advanced Trauma Life Support for Doctors. 8th Ed. First Impression, 2008.

American Heart Association. Advanced Cardiac Life Support. American Heart Association, 2015.

Duffy, Virginia. Behavioral First Aid. 1st Ed. Blue Note Books, 2006

Emergency Nurses Association. Sheehy's Emergency Nursing Principles and Practice. 8th Ed. Mosby, 2020.

Emergency Nurses Association. TNCC Trauma Nursing Core Course Provider Manual. ENA, 2020.

Emergency Nurses Association. Sheehy's Manual of Emergency Care. Mosby, 2013.

Harrison's Principles of Internal Medicine. 20th Ed. New York: McGraw-Hill, Inc., 2019.

Herdman, T.H. & Kamitsum, S. Nursing Diagnosis Definitions and Classification 2018-2020. Oxford: Wiley Blackwell.

Lynch, Virginia A. Forensic Nursing Science. 2nd Ed. Elsevier Mosby, 2011.

Nursing 2020 Drug Handbook. Lippincott Williams & Wilkins, 2020.

Potter, Patricia A. Pocket Guide to Physical Assessment. 2nd Ed. St. Louis: The C.V. Mosby Company, 1990.

Rosen's Emergency Medicine, 9th Ed. Mosby, An Imprint of Elsevier. 2018

Taber's Cyclopedic Medical Dictionary. 23rd Ed. F.A. Davis Company, 2017.

INDEX

Made in the USA
Monee, IL
09 July 2026

56825485R00325